Clinical Forensic Medicine

FORENSIC
SCIENCE AND MEDICINE

Steven B. Karch, MD, SERIES EDITOR

CLINICAL FORENSIC MEDICINE

A Physician's Guide

SECOND EDITION

Edited by

Margaret M. Stark, LLM, MB, BS, DGM, DMJ, DAB

The Forensic Medicine Unit, St. George's Hospital Medical School, London, UK

Foreword by

Sir John Stevens

Commissioner of the Metropolitan Police Service, London, UK

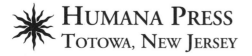

HUMANA PRESS
TOTOWA, NEW JERSEY

© 2005 Humana Press Inc.
999 Riverview Drive, Suite 208
Totowa, New Jersey 07512
www.humanapress.com

This publication is printed on acid-free paper. ∞

ANSI Z39.48-1984 (American Standards Institute) Permanence of Paper for Printed Library Materials.

Production Editor: Amy Thau
Cover design by Patricia F. Cleary

Printed in the United States of America. 10 9 8 7 6 5 4 3 2 1
eISBN: 1-59259-913-3
Library of Congress Cataloging-in-Publication Data

Clinical forensic medicine : a physician's guide / edited by Margaret M.Stark.-- 2nd ed.
   p. ; cm. -- (Forensic science and medicine)
 Rev. ed. of: A physician's guide to clinical forensic medicine. c2000.
 Includes bibliographical references and index.
 ISBN 1-58829-368-8 (alk. paper)
 1. Medical jurisprudence.
 [DNLM: 1. Forensic Medicine--methods. W 700 C641 2005] I. Stark,
Margaret. II. Physician's guide to clinical forensic medicine. III. Series.
 RA1051.P52 2005
 614'.1--dc22

                       2004024006

Dedication

In memory of Smokey and to Amelia and Feline Friends once again!

Foreword

The Metropolitan Police Service (MPS), now in its 175th year, has a long tradition of working with doctors. In fact, the origin of the forensic physician (police surgeon) as we know him or her today, dates from the passing by Parliament of The Metropolitan Act, which received Royal Assent in June of 1829. Since then, there are records of doctors being "appointed" to the police to provide medical care to detainees and examine police officers while on duty.

The MPS has been involved in the training of doctors for more than 20 years, and has been at the forefront of setting the highest standards of working practices in the area of clinical forensic medicine. Only through an awareness of the complex issues regarding the medical care of detainees in custody and the management of complainants of assault can justice be achieved. The MPS, therefore, has worked in partnership with the medical profession to ensure that this can be achieved.

The field of clinical forensic medicine has developed in recent years into a specialty in its own right. The importance of properly trained doctors working with the police in this area cannot be overemphasized. It is essential for the protection of detainees in police custody and for the benefit of the criminal justice system as a whole. A book that assists doctors in the field is to be applauded.

Sir John Stevens

Preface to the Second Edition

The field of clinical forensic medicine has continued to flourish and progress, so it is now timely to publish *Clinical Forensic Medicine: A Physician's Guide, Second Edition*, in which chapters on the medical aspects of restraint and infectious diseases have been added.

Police officers are often extremely concerned about potential exposure to infections, and this area is now comprehensively covered. The results of the use of restraint by police is discussed in more detail, including areas such as injuries that may occur with handcuffs and truncheons (Chapters 7, 8, and 11), as well as the use of crowd-control agents (Chapter 6). The chapter on general injuries (Chapter 4) has been expanded to include the management of bites, head injuries, and self-inflicted wounds.

Substance misuse continues to be a significant and increasing part of the workload of a forensic physician, and the assessment of substance misuse problems in custody, with particular emphasis on mental health problems ("dual diagnosis"), has been expanded. Substance misuse is too often a cause of death in custody (Chapter 10).

Traffic medicine is another area where concerns are increasing over the apparent alcohol/drugs and driving problem. There has been relevant research conducted in this area, which is outlined Chapter 12.

Forensic sampling has undergone enormous technological change, which is reflected in the chapter on sexual assault examination (Chapter 3).

The chapter on the history and development of clinical forensic medicine worldwide has been updated (Chapter 1). Chapters on fundamental principles (Chapter 2), nonaccidental injury in children (Chapter 5), and care of detainees (Chapter 8) are all fully revised, as are the appendices (now containing a list of useful websites). Although the subject is constantly evolving, some fundamental principles remain.

I was very pleased with the response to the first book, and there appears to be a genuine need for this second edition. I hope the good practice outlined in this book will assist forensic physicians in this "Cinderella speciality."

Margaret M. Stark

Preface to the First Edition

"Clinical forensic medicine"—a term now commonly used to refer to that branch of medicine involving an interaction among the law, the judiciary, and the police, and usually concerning living persons—is emerging as a specialty in its own right. There have been enormous developments in the subject in the last decade, with an increasing amount of published research that needs to be brought together in a handbook, such as *A Physician's Guide to Clinical Forensic Medicine*. The role of the health care professional in this field must be independent, professional, courteous, and nonjudgemental, as well as well-trained and informed. This is essential for the care of victims and suspects, for the criminal justice system, and for society as a whole.

As we enter the 21st century it is important that health care professionals are "forensically aware." Inadequate or incorrect diagnosis of a wound, for example, may have an effect on the clinical management of an individual, as well as a significant influence on any subsequent criminal investigation and court proceedings. A death in police custody resulting from failure to identify a vulnerable individual is an avoidable tragedy. Although training in clinical forensic medicine at the undergraduate level is variable, once qualified, every doctor will have contact with legal matters to a varying degree.

A Physician's Guide to Clinical Forensic Medicine concentrates on the clinical aspects of forensic medicine, as opposed to the pathological, by endeavoring to look at issues from fundamental principles, including recent research developments where appropriate. This volume is written primarily for physicians and nurses working in the field of clinical forensic medicine—forensic medical examiners, police surgeons, accident and emergency room physicians, pediatricians, gynecologists, and forensic and psychiatric nurses—but such other health care professionals as social workers and the police will also find the contents of use.

The history and development of clinical forensic medicine worldwide is outlined, with special focus being accorded the variable standards of care for detainees and victims. Because there are currently no international standards of training or practice, we have discussed fundamental principles of consent, confidentiality, note-keeping, and attendance at court.

The primary clinical forensic assessment of complainants and those suspected of sexual assault should only be conducted by those doctors and nurses who have acquired specialist knowledge, skills, and attitudes during both theoretical and practical training. All doctors should be able to accurately describe and record injuries, although the correct interpretation requires considerable skill and expertise, especially in the field of nonaccidental injury in children, where a multidisciplinary approach is required.

Avoidance of a death in police custody is a priority, as is the assessment of fitness-to-be-detained, which must include information on a detainee's general medical problems, as well as the identification of high-risk individuals, i.e., mental health and substance misuse problems. Deaths in custody include rapid unexplained death occurring during restraint and/or during excited delirium. The recent introduction of chemical crowd-control agents means that health professionals also need to be aware of the effects of the common agents, as well as the appropriate treatments.

Custodial interrogation is an essential part of criminal investigations. However, in recent years there have been a number of well-publicized miscarriages of justice in which the conviction depended on admissions made during interviews that were subsequently shown to be untrue. Recently, a working medical definition of fitness-to-be-interviewed has been developed, and it is now essential that detainees be assessed to determine whether they are at risk to provide unreliable information.

The increase in substance abuse means that detainees in police custody are often now seen exhibiting the complications of drug intoxication and withdrawal, medical conditions that need to be managed appropriately in the custodial environment. Furthermore, in the chapter on traffic medicine, not only are medical aspects of fitness-to-drive covered, but also provided is detailed information on the effects of alcohol and drugs on driving, as well as an assessment of impairment to drive.

In the appendices of *A Physician's Guide to Clinical Forensic Medicine*, the relevant ethical documents relating to police, nurses, and doctors are brought together, along with alcohol assessment questionnaires, the mini-mental state examination, and the role of appropriate adults; the management of head-injured detainees, including advice for the police; the Glasgow Coma Scale, and an example of a head injury warning card; guidance notes on US and UK statutory provisions governing access to health records; an alcohol/drugs impairment assessment form, along with a table outlining the peak effect, half-life, duration of action, and times for detection of common drugs.

Margaret M. Stark

Contents

Contributors

KARI BLAHO-OWENS, PhD • Research Administration, University of Tennessee Health Science Center, Memphis, TN

JACK CRANE, MB BCH, FRCPath, DMJ (Clin & Path), FFPath, RCPI • The Queen's University of Belfast and Northern Ireland Office, State Pathologist's Department, Institute of Forensic Medicine, Belfast, Northern Ireland, UK

JUDITH A. HINCHLIFFE, BDS, DipFOd • School of Clinical Dentistry, University of Sheffield, Forensic Odontologist, General Dental Practitioner, and Honorary Clinical Lecturer, Sheffield, UK

STEVEN B. KARCH, MD • Assistant Medical Examiner, City and County of San Francisco, CA

MARY NEWTON, HNC • Forensic Sexual Assault Advisor, Forensic Science Service London Laboratory, London, UK

FELICITY NICHOLSON, MB BS, FRCPath • Consultant in Infectious Diseases and Forensic Physician, London, UK

GUY NORFOLK, MB ChB, LLM, MRCGP, DMJ • Consultant Forensic Physician and General Practitioner, Stockwood Medical Centre, Bristol, UK

NICHOLAS PAGE, MB BS, DCH, DRCOG, DMJ, MRCGP • General Practitioner and Forensic Physician, Ludlow Hill Surgery, Nottingham, UK

ROY N. PALMER, LLB, MB BS, LRCP, MRCS, DRCOG • Barrister-at-Law, H. M. Coroner, Greater London (Southern District), Croydon, UK

JASON PAYNE-JAMES, LLM, MB, FRCS, DFM, RNutr • Consultant Forensic Physician, London, UK

DEBORAH ROGERS, MB BS, DCH, DRCOG, MRCGP, DFFP, MMJ • Honorary Senior Lecturer, The Forensic Medicine Unit, St. George's Hospital Medical School, London, UK

RICHARD SHEPHERD, MB BS, FRCPath, DMJ • Senior Lecturer, The Forensic Medicine Unit, St. George's Hospital Medical School, London, UK

MARGARET M. STARK, LLM, MB BS, DGM, DMJ, DAB • Honorary Senior Lecturer, The Forensic Medicine Unit, St. George's Hospital Medical School, London, UK

SIR JOHN STEVENS • Commissioner of the Metropolitan Police Service, London, UK

AMANDA THOMAS, MB BS, DCH, MmedSc, MA, FRCPCH • Consultant Community Paediatrician, Department of Community Paediatrics, St. James' University Hospital, Leeds, UK

IAN F. WALL, MB ChB(Hons), FRCGP, DMJ, DOccMed • Consultant Forensic Physician and General Practitioner, Kettering, UK

Value-Added eBook/PDA

This book is accompanied by a value-added CD-ROM that contains an eBook version of the volume you have just purchased. This eBook can be viewed on your computer, and you can synchronize it to your PDA for viewing on your handheld device. The eBook enables you to view this volume on only one computer and PDA. Once the eBook is installed on your computer, you cannot download, install, or e-mail it to another computer; it resides solely with the computer to which it is installed. The license provided is for only one computer. The eBook can only be read using Adobe® Reader® 6.0 software, which is available free from Adobe Systems Incorporated at www.Adobe.com. You may also view the eBook on your PDA using the Adobe® PDA Reader® software that is also available free from www.adobe.com.

You must follow a simple procedure when you install the eBook/PDA that will require you to connect to the Humana Press website in order to receive your license. Please read and follow the instructions below:

1. Download and install Adobe® Reader® 6.0 software

You can obtain a free copy of the Adobe® Reader® 6.0 software at www.adobe.com

Note: If you already have the Adobe® Reader® 6.0 software installed, you do not need to reinstall it.

2. Launch Adobe® Reader® 6.0 software

3. Install eBook: Insert your eBook CD into your CD-ROM drive

PC: Click on the "Start" button, then click on "Run"

At the prompt, type "d:\ebookinstall.pdf" and click "OK"

Note: If your CD-ROM drive letter is something other than d: change the above command accordingly.

MAC: Double click on the "eBook CD" that you will see mounted on your desktop. Double click "ebookinstall.pdf"

4. Adobe® Reader® 6.0 software will open and you will receive the message "This document is protected by Adobe DRM" Click "OK"

Note: If you have not already activated the Adobe® Reader® 6.0 software, you will be prompted to do so. Simply follow the directions to activate and continue installation.

Your web browser will open and you will be taken to the Humana Press eBook registration page. Follow the instructions on that page to complete installation. You will need the serial number located on the sticker sealing the envelope containing the CD-ROM.

If you require assistance during the installation, or you would like more information regarding your eBook and PDA installation, please refer to the eBookManual.pdf located on your cd. If you need further assistance, contact Humana Press eBook Support by e-mail at ebooksupport@humanapr.com or by phone at 973-256-1699.

*Adobe and Reader are either registered trademarks or trademarks of Adobe Systems Incorporated in the United States and/or other countries.

xvii

Chapter 1

History and Development of Clinical Forensic Medicine

Jason Payne-James

1. INTRODUCTION

Forensic medicine, forensic pathology, and legal medicine are terms used interchangeably throughout the world. Forensic medicine is now commonly used to describe all aspects of forensic work rather than just forensic pathology, which is the branch of medicine that investigates death. Clinical forensic medicine refers to that branch of medicine that involves an interaction among law, judiciary, and police officials, generally involving living persons. Clinical forensic medicine is a term that has become widely used only in the last two or so decades, although the phrase has been in use at least since 1951 when the Association of Police Surgeons, now known as the Association of Forensic Physicians—a UK-based body—was first established. The practitioners of clinical forensic medicine have been given many different names throughout the years, but the term forensic physician has become more widely accepted. In broad terms, a forensic pathologist generally does not deal with living individuals, and a forensic physician generally does not deal with the deceased. However, worldwide there are doctors who are involved in both the clinical and the pathological aspects of forensic medicine. There are many areas where both clinical and pathological aspects of forensic medicine overlap, and this is reflected in the history and development of the specialty as a whole and its current practice.

From: *Clinical Forensic Medicine: A Physician's Guide, 2nd Edition*
Edited by: M. M. Stark © Humana Press Inc., Totowa, NJ

Table 1
Typical Roles of a Forensic Physician [a]

- Determination of fitness to be detained in custody
- Determination of fitness to be released
- Determination of fitness to be charged: competent to understand charge
- Determination of fitness to transfer
- Determination of fitness to be interviewed by the police or detaining body
- Advise that an independent person is required to ensure rights for the vulnerable or mentally disordered
- Assessment of alcohol and drug intoxication and withdrawal
- Comprehensive examination to assess a person's ability to drive a motor vehicle, in general medical terms and related to alcohol and drug misuse
- Undertake intimate body searches for drugs
- Documentation and interpretation of injuries
- Take forensic samples
- Assess and treat personnel injured while on duty (e.g., police personnel), including needle-stick injuries
- Pronounce life extinct at a scene of death and undertake preliminary advisory role
- Undertake mental state examinations
- Examine adult complainants of serious sexual assault and the alleged perpetrators
- Examine alleged child victims of neglect or physical or sexual abuse
- Examine victims and assailants in alleged police assaults

Additional roles

- Expert opinion in courts and tribunals
- Death in custody investigation
- Pressure group and independent investigators in ethical and moral issues
  - Victims of torture
  - War crimes
  - Female genital mutilation
- Refugee medicine (medical and forensic issues)
- Asylum-seeker medicine (medical and forensic issues)
- Implement principles of immediate management in biological or chemical incidents

For all these examinations, a forensic physician must accurately document findings and, when needed, produce these as written reports for appropriate civil, criminal, or other agencies and courts. The forensic physician must also present the information orally to a court or other tribunal or forum.

[a] Expanded and modified from ref. 22. This table illustrates the role of forensic physicians in the United Kingdom; roles vary according to geographic location.

Police surgeon, forensic medical officer, and forensic medical examiner are examples of other names or titles used to describe those who practice in the clinical forensic medicine specialty, but such names refer more to the appointed role than to the work done. Table 1 illustrates the variety of functions a forensic physician may be asked to undertake. Some clinical forensic medical practitioners may perform only some of these roles, whereas others may play a more extended role, depending on geographic location (in terms of country and state), local statute, and judicial systems. Forensic physicians must have a good knowledge of medical jurisprudence, which can be defined as the application of medical science to the law within their own jurisdiction. The extent and range of the role of a forensic physician is variable; many may limit themselves to specific aspects of clinical forensic medicine, for example, sexual assault or child abuse. Currently, the role and scope of the specialty of clinical forensic medicine globally are ill defined, unlike other well-established medical specialties, such as gastroenterology or cardiology. In many cases, doctors who are practicing clinical forensic medicine or medical jurisprudence may only take on these functions as subspecialties within their own general workload. Pediatricians, emergency medicine specialists, primary care physicians, psychiatrists, gynecologists, and genitourinary medicine specialists often have part-time roles as forensic physicians.

2. HISTORICAL REFERENCES

The origins of clinical forensic medicine go back many centuries, although Smith rightly commented that "forensic medicine [cannot be thought of] as an entity…until a stage of civilization is reached in which we have…a recognizable legal system…and an integrated body of medical knowledge and opinion" *(1)*.

The specific English terms *forensic medicine* and *medical jurisprudence* (also referred to as juridical medicine) date back to the early 19th century. In 1840, Thomas Stuart Traill *(2)*, referring to the connection between medicine and legislation, stated that: "It is known in Germany, the country in which it took its rise, by the name of State Medicine, in Italy and France it is termed Legal Medicine; and with us [in the United Kingdom] it is usually denominated Medical Jurisprudence or Forensic Medicine." However, there are many previous references to the use of medical experts to assist the legal process in many other jurisdictions; these physicians would be involved in criminal or civil cases, as well as public health, which are referred to frequently and somewhat confusingly in the 19th century as medical police. There is much dispute regarding when medical expertise in the determination of legal issues was first used. In 1975, Chinese archeologists discovered numerous bamboo pieces dating from approx 220 BC (Qin dynasty) with rules and regulations for examining injuries inscribed on them. Other historical examples of the link between medicine and the law can be found throughout the world.

Amundsen and Ferngren *(3)* concluded that forensic medicine was used by Athenian courts and other public bodies and that the testimony of physicians in medical matters was given particular credence, although this use of physicians as expert witnesses was "loose and ill-defined" *(4)*, as it was in the

Roman courts. In the Roman Republic, the *Lex Duodecim Tabularum* (laws drafted on 12 tablets and accepted as a single statute in 449 BC) had minor references to medicolegal matters, including length of gestation (to determine legitimacy), disposal of the dead, punishments dependent on the degree of injury caused by an assailant, and poisoning *(5)*. Papyri related to Roman Egypt dating from the latter part of the first to the latter part of the fourth century AD contain information about forensic medical examinations or investigations *(6)*.

The interaction between medicine and the law in these periods is undoubted, but the specific role of forensic medicine, as interpreted by historical documents, is open to dispute; the degree and extent of forensic medical input acknowledged rely on the historian undertaking the assessment.

A specific role for the medical expert as a provider of impartial opinion for the judicial system was identified clearly by the Justinian Laws between 529 and 564 AD. Traill *(2)* states that: "Medical Jurisprudence as a science cannot date farther back than the 16th century." He identifies George, Bishop of Bamberg, who proclaimed a penal code in 1507, as the originator of the first codes in which medical evidence was a necessity in certain cases. However, the *Constitutio Criminalis Carolina*, the code of law published and proclaimed in 1553 in Germany by Emperor Charles V, is considered to have originated legal medicine as a specialty: expert medical testimony became a requirement rather than an option in cases of murder, wounding, poisoning, hanging, drowning, infanticide, and abortion *(1)*. Medicolegal autopsies were well documented in parts of Italy and Germany five centuries before the use of such procedures by English coroners. The use of such expertise was not limited to deaths or to mainland Europe. Cassar *(7)*, for example, describes the earliest recorded Maltese medicolegal report (1542): medical evidence established that the male partner was incapable of sexual intercourse, and this resulted in a marriage annulment. Beck *(8)* identifies Fortunatus Fidelis as the earliest writer on medical jurisprudence, with his *De Relationibus Medicorum* being published in Palermo, Italy, in 1602. Subsequently, Paulus Zacchias wrote *Quaestiones Medico-Legales*, described by Beck as "his great work" between 1621 and 1635. Beck also refers to the Pandects of Valentini published in Germany in 1702, which he describes as "an extensive retrospect of the opinions and decisions of preceding writers on legal medicine." In France in 1796, Fodere published the first edition in three octavo volumes of his work *Les Lois eclairees par les Sciences Physique, ou Traite de Medicine Legale et d'Hygiene Publique*.

2.1. Late 18th Century Onward

Beginning in the latter part of the 18th century, several books and treatises were published in English concerning forensic medicine and medical jurisprudence. What is remarkable is that the issues addressed by many of the authors would not be out of place in a contemporary setting. It seems odd that many of these principles are restated today as though they are new.

In 1783, William Hunter *(9)* published an essay entitled, *On the Uncertainty of the Signs of Murder in the Case of Bastard Children*; this may be the first true forensic medicine publication from England. The first larger work was published in 1788 by Samuel Farr. John Gordon Smith writes in 1821 in the preface to his own book *(10)*: "The earliest production in this country, professing to treat of Medical Jurisprudence *generaliter,* was an abstract from a foreign work, comprised in a very small space. It bears the name of 'Dr. Farr's Elements,' and first appeared above thirty years ago." In fact, it was translated from the 1767 publication *Elemental Medicinae Forensis* by Fazelius of Geneva. Davis *(11)* refers to these and to *Remarks on Medical Jurisprudence* by William Dease of Dublin, as well as the *Treatise on Forensic Medicine or Medical Jurisprudence* by O. W. Bartley of Bristol. Davis considers the latter two works of poor quality, stating that the: "First original and satisfactory work" was George Male's *Epitome of Juridical or Forensic Medicine*, published in 1816 (second edition, 1821). Male was a physician at Birmingham General Hospital and is often considered the father of English medical jurisprudence. Smith refers also to Male's book but also comments: "To which if I may add a *Treatise on Medical Police*, by John Roberton, MD."

Texts on forensic medicine began to appear more rapidly and with much broader content. John Gordon Smith *(9)* stated in *The Principles of Forensic Medicine Systematically Arranged and Applied to British Practice* (1821) that: "Forensic Medicine—Legal, Judiciary or Juridical Medicine—and Medical Jurisprudence are synonymous terms." Having referred in the preface to the earlier books, he notes, "It is but justice to mention that the American schools have outstripped us in attention to Forensic Medicine;" he may have been referring to the work of Theodric Romeyn Beck and others. Beck published the first American textbook 2 years later in 1823 and a third edition (London) had been published by 1829 *(8)*. Before this, in 1804, J. A. Stringham, who was trained in Edinburgh and awarded an MD in 1799, was appointed as a Professor in Medical Jurisprudence at the College of Physicians and Surgeons of New York and given a Chair in 1813 *(11)*.

John Gordon Smith *(9)* wrote that "Every medical practitioner being liable to a subpoena, should make it his business to know the relations of physiological and pathological principles to the facts on which he is likely to be interrogated, and likewise the principal judiciary bearings of the case. The former of these are to be found in works on Forensic Medicine; the latter in those on Jurisprudence." Alfred Taylor *(12)* in his *A Manual of Medical Juris-*

Table 2
Chapter Contents of Guy's 1884 Text, Principles of Forensic Medicine [a]

1. Medical evidence	7. Persons found dead
2. Personal identity	Real & apparent death
Identity	Sudden dath
Age	Survivorship
Sex	8. Death by drowning
3. Impotence	Death by hanging
Rape	Death by strangulation
Pregnancy	Death by suffocation
Delivery	9. Wounds
4. Foeticide or criminal abortion	10. Death by fire
Infanticide	Spontaneous combustion
Legitimacy	Death by lightning
5. Life assurance	Death from cold
Feigned diseases	Death from starvation
6. Unsoundness of mind	11. Toxicology
	Specific poisons

[a] Adapted from ref. *16*.

prudence defined medical jurisprudence as: "That science, which teaches the application of every branch of medical knowledge to the purpose of the law"

There was a clear demand for such books, and Traill's *(2)* *Outlines of a Course of Lectures on Medical Jurisprudence*, published in 1840 when Traill was Regius Professor of Jurisprudence and Medical Police at Edinburgh, was the second edition of a book initially published in 1834 *(13)*. The first Chair of Forensic Medicine had been established in the United Kingdom in Edinburgh in 1803—the appointee being Andrew Duncan, Jr. [although Andrew Duncan Sr. had lectured there on forensic medicine topics since 1789 *(14)*]. Subsequent nonprofessorial academic forensic medicine posts were established at Guy's Hospital and Charing Cross Hospital, London. In 1839 and 1875, respectively, academic chairs of medical jurisprudence were created in Glasgow and Aberdeen *(15)*.

The relevant areas of interest to forensic medicine and medical jurisprudence were gradually becoming better defined. Table 2 summarizes the chapter contents of *Principles of Forensic Medicine* by William Guy *(16)*, Professor of Forensic Medicine at King's College, London, in 1844. Much of this material is relevant to forensic physicians and forensic pathologists working today.

Thus, by the end of the 19th century, a framework of forensic medicine that persists today had been established in Europe, the United Kingdom, America, and related jurisdictions.

3. CONTEMPORARY CLINICAL FORENSIC MEDICINE

The following working definition has been suggested: "Clinical forensic medicine includes all medical [healthcare] fields which may relate to legal, judicial, and police systems" *(17)*. Even though medicine and law interact more frequently in cases of living individuals, forensic pathology has long been established as the academic basis for forensic medicine. It is only in the last two decades that research and academic interest in clinical forensic medicine have become an area of more focused research.

The recent growth in awareness of abuses of human rights and civil liberties has directed attention to the conditions of detention of prisoners and to the application of justice to both victim and suspect. Examples of injustice and failure to observe basic human rights or rights enshrined in statute in which the input of medical professionals may be considered at least of poor quality and at worst criminally negligent have occurred and continue to occur worldwide. The death of Steve Biko in South Africa, the conviction of Carole Richardson in England, and the deaths of native Australians in prison are widely publicized instances of such problems. Reports from the European Committee for the Prevention of Torture and Inhuman and Degrading Treatment in the early 1990s drew attention to the problem of lack of independence of some police doctors. The conflicting needs and duties of those involved in the judicial system are clear, and it is sometimes believed that recognition of such conflicts is comparatively recent, which would be naïve and wrong. In England and Wales, the Human Rights Act 1998, whose purpose is to make it unlawful for any public authority to act in a manner incompatible with a right defined by the European Convention of Human Rights, reinforces the need for doctors to be aware of those human rights issues that touch on prisoners and that doctors can influence. It is worth noting that this law was enacted almost 50 years after publication of the *European Convention of Human Rights and Fundamental Freedoms*. The future role of the forensic physician within bodies, such as the recently established International Criminal Court, is likely to expand.

The forensic physician has several roles that may interplay when assessing a prisoner or someone detained by the state or other statutory body. Three medical care facets that may conflict have been identified: first, the role of medicolegal expert for a law enforcement agency; second, the role of a treating doctor; and third, the examination and treatment of detainees who allege that they have been mistreated by the police during their arrest, interrogation, or the various stages of police custody *(18)*. This conflict is well-recognized and not new for forensic physicians. Grant *(19)*, a police surgeon appointed to the Metropolitan Police in the East End of London just more than a century ago, records the following incident: "One night I was called to Shadwell [police] station to see a man charged with being drunk and disorderly, who had a number of wounds on the top of his head...I dressed them...and when I finished he whispered 'Doctor, you might come with me to the cell door'...I went with him. We were just passing the door of an empty cell, when a police constable with a mop slipped out and struck the man a blow over the head...Boiling over with indignation I hurried to the Inspector's Office [and] told him what had occurred." Dr. Grant records that the offender was dealt with immediately. Dr. Grant rightly recognized that he had moral, ethical, and medical duties to his patient, the prisoner. Dr. Grant was one of the earliest "police surgeons" in England, the first Superintending Surgeon having been appointed to the Metropolitan Police Force on April 30, 1830. The Metropolitan Police Surgeons Association was formed in 1888 with 156 members. In 1951, the association was reconstituted as a national body under the leadership of Ralph Summers, so that improvements in the education and training for clinical forensic medicine could be made. The Association of Forensic Physicians, formerly the Association of Police Surgeons, remains the leading professional body of forensic physicians worldwide, with more 1000 members.

4. GLOBAL CLINICAL FORENSIC MEDICINE

Table 3 is a summary of responses to a questionnaire on various aspects of clinical forensic medicine sent in early 2003 to specialists in different countries. The selection of countries was intended to be broad and nonselective. It shows how clinical forensic medicine operates in a variety of countries and jurisdictions and also addresses key questions regarding how important aspects of such work, including forensic assessment of victims and investigations of police complaints and deaths in custody, are undertaken. The questionnaire responses were all from individuals who were familiar with the forensic medical issues within their own country or state, and the responses reflect practices of that time. The sample is small, but numerous key points emerge, which are compared to the responses from an earlier similar study in 1997 *(20)*. In the previous edition of this book, the following comments were made about clinical forensic medicine, the italicized comments represent apparent changes since that last survey.

- No clear repeatable patterns of clinical forensic medicine practice may be seen on an international basis—*but there appears to be an increase in recognition of the need to have appropriate personnel to undertake the roles required.*
- Several countries have informal/ad hoc arrangements to deal with medical and forensic care of detainees and victims—*this still remains the case—often with*

large centers having physicians specially trained or appointed while rural or outlying areas are reliant on nonspecialists.

- The emphasis in several countries appears to be on the alleged victim rather than the alleged suspect—*this remains the case, although there are suggestions that this approach is being modified.*
- The standard of medical care of detainees in police custody is variable—*there appears to be more recognition of the human rights aspects of care of those in police custody.*
- There are no international standards of practice or training—*international standards are still lacking—but more countries appear to be developing national standards.*
- There are apparent gaps in the investigation of police complaints in some countries—*this remains the case.*
- Death-in-custody statistics are not always in the public domain—*this remains the case—and the investigation of deaths in police custody may still not be independently undertaken.*

There appears to be wider recognition of the interrelationship of the roles of forensic physician and forensic pathology, and, indeed, in many jurisdictions, both clinical and pathological aspects of forensic medicine are undertaken by the same individual. The use of general practitioners (primary care physicians) with a special interest in clinical forensic medicine is common; England, Wales, Northern Ireland, Scotland, Australasia, and the Netherlands all remain heavily dependent on such professionals.

Academic appointments are being created, but these are often honorary, and until governments and states recognize the importance of the work by fully funding full-time academic posts and support these with funds for research, then the growth of the discipline will be slow. In the United Kingdom and Europe much effort has gone into trying to establish a monospecialty of legal medicine, but the process has many obstacles, laborious, and, as yet, unsuccessful. The Diplomas of Medical Jurisprudence and the Diploma of Forensic Medicine (Society of Apothecaries, London, England) are internationally recognized qualifications with centers being developed worldwide to teach and examine them. The Mastership of Medical Jurisprudence represents the highest qualification in the subject in the United Kingdom. Further diploma and degree courses are being established and developed in the United Kingdom but have not yet had first graduates. Monash University in Victoria, Australia, introduced a course leading to a Graduate Diploma in Forensic Medicine, and the Department of Forensic Medicine has also pioneered a distance-learning Internet-based continuing-education program that previously has been serialized in the international peer-reviewed *Journal of Clinical Forensic Medicine.*

Many forensic physicians undertake higher training in law or medical ethics in addition to their basic medical qualifications. In addition to medical professionals, other healthcare professionals may have a direct involvement in matters of a clinical forensic medical nature, particularly when the number of medical professionals with a specific interest is limited. Undoubtedly, the multiprofessional approach can, as in all areas of medicine, have some benefits.

5. CONCLUSIONS

As with the previous edition of the book, key areas still need to be addressed in clinical forensic medicine:

1. It needs to be recognized globally as a distinct subspecialty with its own full-time career posts, with an understanding that it will be appropriate for those undertaking the work part-time to receive appropriate training and postgraduate education.
2. Forensic physicians and other forensic healthcare professionals must ensure that the term *clinical forensic medicine* is recognized as synonymous with knowledge, fairness, independence, impartiality, and the upholding of basic human rights.
3. Forensic physicians and others practicing clinical forensic medicine must be of an acceptable and measurable standard *(20)*.

Some of these issues have been partly addressed in some countries and states, and this may be because the overlap between the pathological and clinical aspects of forensic medicine has grown. Many forensic pathologists undertake work involved in the clinical aspects of medicine, and, increasingly, forensic physicians become involved in death investigation *(21)*. Forensic work is now truly multiprofessional, and an awareness of what other specialties can contribute is an essential part of basic forensic education, work, and continuing professional development. Those involved in the academic aspects of forensic medicine and related specialties will be aware of the relative lack of funding for research. This lack of funding research is often made worse by lack of trained or qualified personnel to undertake day-to-day service work. This contrasts more mainstream specialties (e.g., cardiology and gastroenterology), where the pharmaceutical industry underpins and supports research and development. However, clinical forensic medicine continues to develop to support and enhance judicial systems in the proper, safe, and impartial dispensation of justice. A worldwide upsurge in the need for and appropriate implementation of human rights policies is one of the drivers for this development, and it is to be hoped that responsible governments and other world bodies will continue to raise the profile of, invest in, and recognize the absolute necessity for independent, impartial skilled practitioners of clinical forensic medicine.

Table 3
Clinical Forensic Medicine: Its Practice Around the World Questions and Responses January 2003

Question A	Is there a formal system in your country (or state) by which the police and judicial system can get immediate access to medical and/or forensic assessment of individuals detained in police custody (prisoners)?
Response	
Australia	Yes (within the state). Two-tiered system addressing general health issues and forensic medical services.
England and Wales	Yes. Police surgeons (forensic medical examiners/forensic physicians) are contracted (but not generally employed) by both police and courts to undertake this. The Police & Criminal Evidence Act (PACE) 1984 made particular provision for this and for prisoners to request to see a doctor. Police surgeons do not necessarily have specific forensic training or qualifications.
Germany	Yes, only after a court order has been granted.
Hong Kong	Yes. The formal and generic mechanism is for the individual to be taken to an emergency department of a nearby hospital. Rarely he or she may be sent for a specific purpose to a specialist forensic doctor.
India	Yes. Under a Section of the Criminal Procedure Code, a police officer can immediately bring an arrested person to a doctor for examination. If the arrested person is a female, only a female registered medical practitioner can examine her. The accused/detained person can contact the doctor and have himself or herself examined.
Israel	Yes
Malaysia	No organized forensic clinical services available. Subjecting the detainees for examination is at the discretion of the agencies. If the need arises, usually doctors who have no training in clinical forensic medicine (CFM) undertake such examinations. In larger institutions, senior doctors and, at times, forensic pathologists may examine them.
The Netherlands	Yes
Nigeria	Yes (for medical reasons) dependent on the availability of the physician.
Scotland	Yes. Police retain services of doctors not all necessarily qualified in CFM.
Serbia	Yes, via the public health system. Generally for treatment purposes. Also, if considered necessary for evidence collection (by the investigator appointed under the Criminal Procedure Act (CPA) the police will refer to prosecutor in charge seeking for his or her permission to call a forensic doctor.
South Africa	Yes, but not in all parts of the country.
Spain	Yes, any individual detained in police custody has the right to be examined by a doctor. In certain cases, one has the right to have a forensic assessment (by the Forensic Surgeon Corps of the Ministry of Justice).
Sweden	Yes
Switzerland	Yes

11

Question B	*Who examines or assesses individuals who are detained in police custody to determine whether they are medically fit to stay in police custody?*
Response	
Australia	Nurses or medical practitioners who are employed or retained by police.
England and Wales	Police surgeons. Recent changes to statutory Codes of Practice suggest that an appropriate health care professional may be called.
Germany	Normally a police surgeon; if not, then any qualified doctor.
Hong Kong	Currently, the duty police officer looks and asks if medical attention is required. Most duty officers are quite liberal in referring the individuals to the emergency department.
India	A government doctor.
Israel	Police surgeons.
Malaysia	Generally not unless they become ill. Any government doctor in the nearest hospital may undertake such an examination.
The Netherlands	Generally speaking: Public health officers, who are qualified in clinical forensic medicine.
Nigeria	Any doctor attached to prison services, the police or doctors in the local hospitals, depending on who is available.
Scotland	Police surgeons—these doctors are not employees. Nursing schemes have been mooted but not yet been implemented.
Serbia	If there is an obvious health problem or if they have certain diseases that need medical attention, police will take them to a public healthcare facility or, in the case of emergency, call an ambulance.
South Africa	Not always; psychiatrist in some cases.
Spain	When a person is under arrest (without having being put under regulation), he asks to be examined by a doctor, he is usually transferred to the Spanish Health Public System doctors. The forensic surgeon takes part exceptionally.
Sweden	So-called "police doctors," who usually are general practitioners.
Switzerland	The "prison doctor": either a doctor of internal medicine of university hospital or in rural regions the district physician (acute cases). A forensic doctor of the Institute of Legal Medicine of the University of Zurich (not urgent cases, "chronic cases").

Question C	If a prisoner is suspected of being under the influence of drugs or alcohol in police custody, is it usual for him or her to be examined by a doctor (or other health care professional) to determine whether they are fit to remain in custody?
Response	
Australia	Yes, but it will largely depend on any health concerns (e.g., abusive, intoxicated person—unlikely to access medical attention, but impaired conscious state—always access medical attention).
England and Wales	Yes, if there are associated health concerns, or if there is a specific need to determine fitness to interview when either intoxication or withdrawal may render an interview invalid. Specific guidelines are published on care of substance misuse detainees in police custody.
Germany	Yes
Hong Kong	Yes, they will most certainly be sent to the emergency department. Registered addicts will occasionally be taken to a methadone clinic if they are suffering from withdrawal.
India	Yes
Israel	Yes
Malaysia	Not routinely.
The Netherlands	Yes
Nigeria	No
Scotland	Only when a need is established or the prisoner requests medical assistance. Profound intoxication or suspicion of head injury would be an indication for examination.
Serbia	Intoxicated detainees may be requested to provide a blood or other appropriate samples for analysis. The request can be refused. Samples are arranged outside police premises, usually in the public health institutions.
South Africa	Yes, but not common practice.
Spain	Yes, he or she is often examined and even blood samples are extracted (with his or her previous consent) if the prisoner is involved in some aggression, homicide or car driving, for example.
Sweden	Yes. In most custody suites, a nurse is employed nurse who will call a doctor.
Switzerland	Yes, *see* previous answer to question B.

13

Question D	*Does your country/state have specific codes/laws/statutes or regulations that make provision for the welfare of individuals in police custody?*
Response	
Australia	Yes
England and Wales	Yes
Germany	Yes
Hong Kong	There are generic guidelines for all in custody; none specific to the police.
India	The Protection of Human Rights Act 1993 stipulates detailed provisions regarding this.
Israel	Yes
Malaysia	Yes. Inspector General's Standing Order.
The Netherlands	Yes
Nigeria	Not aware of any.
Scotland	Local procedures for each police force based on central guidance, but there is no statute.
Serbia	No
South Africa	Yes
Spain	Yes, there are specific rules in Constitution and in the Penal Code.
Sweden	Not known.
Switzerland	Yes

Question E	Who undertakes the forensic medical examination and assessment of alleged victims of sexual assault?
Response	
Australia	Forensic medical officers.
England and Wales	Police surgeons or sexual offense examiners or doctors employed within specialist sexual offenses units.
Germany	Either a gynecologist or a medicolegal doctor.
Hong Kong	Forensic pathologists/doctors mainly. Accident and emergency doctors occasionally and family planning doctors. The latter when the victims do not wish to report the incident to police.
India	Different centers have different protocols (e.g., in this institution, gynecologists—mainly females).
Israel	Forensic pathologists.
Malaysia	In major hospitals, there may be fixed protocols. Some forensic physicians, primary care physicians, emergency medicine physicians, and gynecologists undertake such examinations. In smaller hospitals, nonspecialist physicians do the examinations. In some cases, forensic pathologists.
The Netherlands	Generally public health officers, qualified in clinical forensic medicine.
Nigeria	Primary care physicians and medical officers in local hospitals.
Scotland	Usually police surgeon, some may be admitted to hospital and be examined by hospital staff.
Serbia	There is no standard procedure for the examination of alleged victims of sexual assault. There are no protocols for the examination of victims, or for collection of forensic samples.
South Africa	Medical practitioner.
Spain	A forensic surgeon (*médico forense*) and a gynecologist (if the victim is female) or a proctologist (if the victim is male).
Sweden	The police are free to engage any doctor to do this. In cases of assault on adults, the examination is undertaken by specialists in FM in a small fraction of the cases. A specialist in pediatric medicine or surgery always examines children, often, but not always, with a specialist in forensic medicine.
Switzerland	Physicians of Institute of Legal Medicine of University of Zurich (District Physician); Physicians of University Department of Gynecology, University Hospital Zurich.

Question F	*Who undertakes the forensic medical examination and assessment of alleged perpetrators of sexual assault?*
Response	
Australia	Forensic medical officers.
England and Wales	Police surgeons.
Germany	Medicolegal doctor.
Hong Kong	Forensic pathologists/doctors mainly.
India	Different centers have different protocols (in this institution, forensic medicine specialists). A bizarre situation, where the victim goes to the gynecology department, whereas the accused in the same case comes to us.
Israel	Forensic pathologists.
Malaysia	Same as for alleged victims of sexual assault. *See* previous answer to question E.
The Netherlands	Generally speaking, public health officers who are qualified in clinical forensic medicine.
Nigeria	Same as for alleged victims of sexual assault. *See* previous answer to question E.
Scotland	Police surgeon (although experienced police surgeons are not readily available in some sparsely populated areas, and the inexperienced are often reluctant to embark on such an examination).
Serbia	In practical terms, rarely done although the Criminal Procedure Act allows examination of alleged perpetrators of any crime (including sexual assault) for forensic purposes even without their consent if the examination itself is not considered harmful to them.
South Africa	Medical practitioner.
Spain	A forensic surgeon.
Sweden	Similar to the procedures of adult victims.
Switzerland	Physicians of Institute of Legal Medicine of University of Zurich (District Physician).

16

Question G	In cases of sexual assault is it always possible for victim, perpetrator, or both to be examined by a doctor of the same gender if that is requested?
Response	
Australia	Generally, yes.
England and Wales	Generally, yes, but not always possible.
Germany	Yes
Hong Kong	No, there is currently only one full-time female forensic doctor able to do this.
India	Yes, if requested, a doctor of the same gender would be arranged. This would generally apply only to the victim (female gynecologists examine the victim anyway). The wishes of the accused are not always observed. It is highly unusual for a female to examine a male accused.
Israel	Not always.
Malaysia	It may be accommodated if possible.
The Netherlands	Usually but not always.
Nigeria	No
Scotland	Not always, but every effort is made to comply with an examinee's wishes.
Serbia	There is no statutory provision that regulates free choice of either the victim or the perpetrator to be examined by a doctor of preferred (same) gender.
South Africa	Yes
Spain	No. It depends on the doctor on duty.
Sweden	No
Switzerland	Yes

17

Question H	*Who undertakes the forensic medical examination and assessment of alleged child victims of sexual assault?*
Response	
Australia	Forensic medical officers *or* pediatricians.
England and Wales	Police surgeons and/or pediatricians. Ideally joint examinations (guidelines for the assessment have been issued).
Germany	Either pediatrician gynecologist or medicolegal specialist.
Hong Kong	Forensic pathologists/physicians, pediatricians, obstetricians, and gynecologists, sometimes jointly.
India	Female children—gynecologist, preferably female (which is generally the case anyway). Male children—forensic personnel of either sex.
Israel	Forensic pathologists and pediatricians.
Malaysia	Wherever possible, by pediatricians or gynecologists. Smaller hospitals by nonspecialist physicians.
The Netherlands	Generally speaking, public health officers qualified in clinical forensic medicine.
Nigeria	Same as for alleged victims of sexual assault. *See* previous answer to question E.
Scotland	In the larger centers, joint pediatric/police surgeon examinations are common. For other centers, it varies.
Serbia	Physicians with forensic training are rarely involved in initial examination and assessment. Forensic physicians tend to get involved at a later stage of investigation.
South Africa	Medical practitioner.
Spain	A forensic surgeon and a pediatrician.
Sweden	Same as for adults. *See* previous answer to question E.
Switzerland	Younger than 16 yr: female gynecologist at University Children Hospital. Older than 16 yr: examined as adult.

18

Question I	*Who undertakes the forensic medical examination and assessment of alleged child victims of physical assault?*
Response	
Australia	Forensic medical officers *or* pediatricians.
England and Wales	Police surgeons and/or pediatricians.
Germany	Pediatrician or medicolegal specialist.
Hong Kong	Pediatricians. Sometimes forensic pathologists/physicians. Sometimes jointly.
India	Forensic medicine departments.
Israel	Forensic pathologists and pediatricians.
Malaysia	Pediatricians in smaller hospitals by nonspecialist physicians.
The Netherlands	Generally speaking, public health officers qualified in clinical forensic medicine.
Nigeria	Same as for alleged victims of sexual assault. *See* previous answer to question E.
Scotland	Mostly pediatricians but some evidence is based on findings of family physicians.
Serbia	Formerly, few forensic pathologists were involved. Situation is somewhat improved, but still poor cooperation between clinicians and forensic doctors.
South Africa	Medical practitioner.
Spain	Forensic surgeon and a forensic pediatrician.
Sweden	Same as for an adult. *See* previous answer to question E.
Switzerland	Younger than 16 yr: doctors at University Children Hospital (Trauma-X group). Older than 16 yr: doctors of Institute of Legal Medicine of University of Zurich (District Physician).

Question J	Is there a system in your country/state whereby individuals detained in police custody who appear to have (or do have) psychiatric disorder or mental health problems or learning disability may be assessed?
Response	
Australia	Yes
England and Wales	Yes
Germany	Yes
Hong Kong	Yes. They are likely to be referred to psychiatrists or, in the case of learning disability, to social workers and/or clinical psychologists.
India	Yes, in theory. This may not be strictly observed until and unless there is a court order that may need to be obtained by relatives.
Israel	Yes
Malaysia	Yes
The Netherlands	Yes
Nigeria	Yes
Scotland	Variable picture. Screening by police surgeons. On-call psychiatrist or mental health team in some areas. Some courts have regular pretrial psychiatric attendance.
Serbia	Not when in police custody (within 48 h after arrest). If suspect is detained on the order of the investigative judge, then may be examined by psychiatrist and/or psychologist when need.
South Africa	Yes
Spain	Yes. If mental health problems are apparent, case is remitted to a judge and detainee is examined by a forensic surgeon and a psychiatrist.
Sweden	It's part of the "police doctors" duties, but many custodies do have access to psychiatric consultants.
Switzerland	Those who have known disorders are followed by a specialized forensic psychiatric/psychological service; others are reported by the guards.

Question K	In your country/state are there specialized units or locations where victims of sexual assault are examined or assessed?
Response	
Australia	Yes
England and Wales	Yes, but not full geographical coverage; tends to be in urban centers.
Germany	No
Hong Kong	There are purpose-built video interview and medical examination suites. These tend to be used only when there is a strong likelihood of prosecution. Often done in pediatric wards.
India	No
Israel	Yes
Malaysia	Some major hospitals have "one-stop centers" with protocols for managements, both short- and long-term.
The Netherlands	Sometimes, but not always.
Nigeria	No
Scotland	Specialized units widely available, often on police premises. Children usually in hospital.
Serbia	No
South Africa	Yes
Spain	Victims of sexual assault are examined in gynecology or pediatric units of large hospitals.
Sweden	No
Switzerland	Yes, but only in some cities.

Question L	In cases of alleged assault by police, who examines the police personnel?
Response	
Australia	Forensic medical officers (report and documentation of injuries). Police medical officers (for any occupational health and safety issues).
England and Wales	Police surgeons.
Germany	An independent medical doctor.
Hong Kong	The majority are examined by emergency medicine physicians. Some are examined by forensic pathologists/physicians.
India	No experience with this. If needed, probably forensic pathologist.
Israel	Forensic pathologist.
Malaysia	Any available physician.
The Netherlands	Generally speaking, public health officers qualified in clinical forensic medicine.
Nigeria	Physician attached to the police service, could be a uniformed officer.
Scotland	Police surgeon (unless urgent transfer to hospital).
Serbia	Physicians working for public healthcare system.
South Africa	Medical practitioner.
Spain	A forensic surgeon as member of the Ministry of Justice (completely independent of the police).
Sweden	Advised that a specialist in forensic medicine should do it.
Switzerland	Physicians of Institute of Legal Medicine, University of Zurich (District Physician).

Question M   *In cases of alleged assault by police, who examines the complainant?*

Response

Australia   Forensic medical officers (report and documentation of injuries).

England and Wales   Police surgeons.

Germany   An independent medical doctor.

Hong Kong   The majority are examined by emergency medicine specialists. Some are examined by forensic pathologists/physicians.

India   Forensic pathologist.

Israel   Forensic pathologist.

Malaysia   *See* answer to question L.

The Netherlands   Generally speaking, public health officers qualified in clinical forensic medicine.

Nigeria   Medical officer in the local hospital; (if he is lucky to have the opportunity and guts to complain).

Scotland   Police surgeon (unless urgent transfer to hospital).

Serbia   *See* answer to question L.

South Africa   Medical practitioner.

Spain   A forensic surgeon and a gynecologist or a urologist.

Sweden   *See* answer to question L.

Switzerland   Physicians of Institute of Legal Medicine, University of Zurich (District Physician).

23

Question N	In your country/state, is there a person, body, or organization that investigates complaints against the police?
Response	
Australia	Yes
England and Wales	Yes. The Police Complaints Authority, which was replaced by the Independent Police Complaints Commission (IPCC) in 2004.
Germany	State prosecutor.
Hong Kong	Yes. All complaints are handled by the Complaints Against Police Office (part of the police), but all cases are then reviewed by a statutory board the IPCC.
India	Yes. Via the police commissioner or to the magistrate. Probably rarely used.
Israel	Yes
Malaysia	There are human rights groups. Police also conduct investigations against their own staff.
The Netherlands	Yes
Nigeria	A tribunal would be set up if the issue is considered to be of significant national interest.
Scotland	The procurator fiscal (public prosecutor, legally qualified civil servants). Complaints must be referred by police where any criminality is alleged.
Serbia	There is a Commission for Complaints within the police services as a first tier. Within the Ministry of Interior there is a second tier. Victims of police assault can also report directly to the court of law in accordance with the penal code, and Criminal Procedure Act.
South Africa	Independent Complaint Directorate.
Spain	The correspondent court of first instance (the one on duty at the moment when the facts are reported).
Sweden	Yes
Switzerland	Yes

IPCC, Independent Police Complaints Commission.

Question O	If your country has a person, body, or organization that investigates complaints against the police, (a) is it completely independent of the police? and (b) who funds it?	
Response		
Australia	(a) Two bodies: police—Internal Investigations and government body—Ombudsman's Office.	(b) Government funded.
England and Wales	(a) The Police Complaints Authority is independent of the police and was replaced by the IPCC.	(b) The government.
Germany	(a) Yes	(b) Judicial system.
Hong Kong	(a) Complaints Against Police Office—No. police establishment.	(b) IPCC—Yes. Funded by taxpayer.
India	(a) Police commissioner is from the police stream itself. Magistrates are completely independent of the police.	(b) Government.
Israel	(a) Yes	(b) Ministry of Justice.
Malaysia	(a) No	(b) There are nongovernmental organizations who back the victims and provide support. Police conducts their own investigations.
The Netherlands	(a) Yes (directly under the national prosecutor's office).	(b) Ministry of Justice.
Nigeria	(a) No	(b) Government funded.
Scotland	(a) No. Complaints are investigated by police unless criminality is suspected, when immediate report to regional PF is mandatory.	(b) Cases taken by the PF are centrally funded.
Serbia	(a) No. As part of the police and Ministry of Interior, the Commission, on both tiers, is not independent from the police.	(b) Government
South Africa	(a) Yes (seemingly).	(b) International organizations.
Spain	(a) Yes. The police are subordinate to the Court of First Instance.	(b) The judge, the judicial secretary, the district attorney, and the forensic surgeon.
Sweden	(a) No. It's a special unit within the police.	(b) State funded.
Switzerland	(a) Yes	(b) The state of Zurich.

IPCC, Independent Police Complaints Commission; PF, procurator fiscal.

Question P	In your country/state, is there person, body, or organization that investigates deaths of individuals while in police custody?
Response	
Australia	Yes
England and Wales	Yes, the Police Complaints Authority.
Germany	State prosecutor and forensic legal medicine.
Hong Kong	Yes, the coroner with a mandatory inquest held in public and with a jury. However, the investigations are conducted by the police.
India	Yes, the magistrate does it. Police cannot investigate such deaths.
Israel	Yes
Malaysia	All deaths in custody are subjected to inquest by the magistrate according to Malaysian criminal procedure code.
The Netherlands	Yes
Nigeria	A uniformed police pathologist, rarely a hospital pathologist, and, in some cases, a medical officer.
Scotland	All investigations are under the supervision of procurator fiscal; there is always a public "fatal accident inquiry" before a judge.
Serbia	In the case of death in police custody, but also during the police action or allegedly as a result of police action, or while person is in penitentiary, district court that has territorial jurisdiction should order full postmortem, as well as other investigations.
South Africa	Both the Independent Complaint Directorate and forensic pathologist/medical practitioner.
Spain	Yes. The Court of First Instance (of criminal investigation).
Sweden	Yes
Switzerland	Yes, the district attorney and the Institute of Legal Medicine.

Question Q	*If the answer to the previous question is yes: (a) is that person, body, or organization independent of the police, and (b) who funds that organization?*
Response	
Australia	(a) Three bodies police—homicide squad and internal investigations, coroner's office, and Ombudsman's Office. (b) Government.
England a nd Wales	(a) Yes (b) Government.
Germany	(a) Yes (b) State.
Hong Kong	(a) Yes (b) The judiciary.
India	(a) Yes (b) Government pays the salary.
Israel	(a) Yes (b) Ministry of Justice.
Malaysia	(a) Magistrate is independent. (b) There is no full-time coroner; magistrate acts as the coroner in normal deaths, except custodial deaths, where the magistrate acts directly. Most of the deaths are investigated by the police; the coroner does not play a visible role. Inquest system needs improvement.
The Netherlands	(a) Yes
Nigeria	(a) It depends on who does the case. (b) Government funded.
Scotland	All investigations are under supervision of PF; there is always a public fatal accident inquiry before a judge.
Serbia	(a) Yes, it is a court of law. (b) State and government.
South Africa	(a) Yes (b) International organization.
Spain	(a) Yes. Doctors who assist individuals detained and prisoners are specialists totally independent of police. (b) It is funded by health system doctors (Health Public National System), forensic surgeons (Ministry of Justice), and prison doctors (Ministry of Justice).
Sweden	(a) Yes (b) The Department of Justice.
Switzerland	(a) Yes, the Department of Justice. (b) The state of Zurich.

27

Question R	*In your country/state are statistics published about deaths that have occurred in police custody?*
Response	
Australia	Yes
England and Wales	Yes
Germany	Yes
Hong Kong	Yes, in the Coroners Annual Report.
India	Yes, a publication called *Crime Statistics*, published by the Natonal Crime Records Bureau.
Israel	No
Malaysia	Police Headquarters maintains all data.
The Netherlands	Yes
Nigeria	No
Scotland	No
Serbia	Not aware of any statistics.
South Africa	Not aware of any statistics.
Spain	No
Sweden	No
Switzerland	No

Question 5	*If the answer to the previous question is yes, where, when, and how often are those statistics published and do they include an analysis of cause of death (e.g., self-harm, drugs, or other violence)?*
Response	
Australia	Coroners report includes all cases. Australian Institute of Criminology publishes it annually. Complete analysis in all cases.
England ard Wales	Annual report of the Police Complaints Authority with breakdown of causes and circumstances of death.
Germany	Granzow, Püschel. *Arch. Kriminol.* 1998 J201:1–10. Includes an analysis of cause of death.
Hong Kong	The number of occurrences, the custodian department, and the verdicts of the inquests are summarized but no details of death itself are presented.
India	Yearly publication. The figures may be inaccurate or incomplete.
Israel	No.
Malaysia	Not known whether it is regularly published, but data available.
The Netherlands	The prosecutor receives complete autopsy results.
Nigeria	Not applicable.
Scotland	Not applicable.
Serbia	Not applicable.
South Africa	Not applicable.
Spain	Not applicable.
Sweden	Not applicable.
Switzerland	In the state of Zurich, all cases are investigated by the Institute of Legal Medicine to establish the cause and manner of death.

Question T	Does your country/state have a recognized (recognized by your medical professional body) specialty or subspecialty of medicine for those working in (a) clinical forensic medicine (CFM) or (b) forensic pathology (FP)?	
Response		
Australia	(a) No	(b) Yes
England and Wales	(a) No	(b) Yes, as part of the discipline of pathology.
Germany	(a) No, only in some states in Germany.	(b) Yes
Hong Kong	(a) Yes and no.	(b) Yes. There is laid-out training for FP under the Hong Kong College of Pathologists, which includes CFM aspects. There is also statutory specialty registration but again, only in FP.
India	(a) There is just one superspecialty called FM, which caters to both (a) CFM, as well as (b) FP.	
Israel	(a) Yes	(b) Yes
Malaysia	(a) No	(b) No
The Netherlands	(a) No	(b) No
Nigeria	(a) Yes	(b) Yes. Recognition (by the Nigerian Medical Council and Postgraduate Medical College) is strictly as a subspecialty of pathology.
Scotland	(a) As for England and Wales—only that the craft is recognized by British Medical Association.	(b) Yes, as part of pathology.
Serbia	(a) Yes	(b) Yes. Specialization is designated as FM, covering both issues. There are no separate specializations. The model was imported from Germany and France at the beginning of the last century when the first medical faculties were founded in the country.
South Africa	(a) Yes—using a diploma or master's degree.	(b) Yes, recognized registered specialty.
Spain	(a) Yes and no. Each forensic surgeon has undertaken a competitive examination in the Supreme Court–Ministry of Justice. Some also are specialists in legal and FM granted by the Ministry of Education. The Ministry of Justice has recognized both for forensic surgeons working in Institutes of Legal Medicine.	
Sweden	(a) Yes	(b) Yes
Switzerland	(a) Yes	(b) Yes. The specialist title of Legal Medicine covers both subspecialties.

FM, forensic medicine

Question U	Can you supply the details (a) of the main organization that represents the interests of such practitioners and (b) the number of practitioners represented?
Response	
Australia	(a) Australian College of Pathologists. (b) Approximately 50.
England and Wales	(a) Association of Forensic Physicians (formerly the Association of Police Surgeons (approx 1000). (b) British Association in Forensic Medicine (approx 300; only 40 or so full-time).
Germany	(a) German Society of Legal Medicine. (b) Approximately 400.
Hong Kong	(a) N/A (b) Hong Kong College of Pathologists, Forensic Pathology.
India	(a) Indian Academy of Forensic Medicine. (b) Approximately 500 people are represented. For more information on IAFM, please visit its website at (http://www.fortunecity.com/campus/electrical/314/iafm.html).
Israel	(a) Israel Association of Pathologists. (b) 12
Malaysia	(a) Hospital forensic pathologists come under the Ministry of Health. Others are in the University Departments of Pathology. Forensic Unit comes under pathology. Clinical forensic medicine is mostly a neglected subject. (b) Not available.
The Netherlands	(a) Not available. (b) Not available.
Nigeria	(a) There is no professional body that represents these few specialists. (b) There are two diploma of medical jurisprudence clinical graduates. There is no forensic pathologist (including the author) in Nigeria.

IAFM, Indian Academy of Forensic Medicine.

(*Continued on next page*)

Question U (Continued)	Can you supply the details (a) of the main organization that represents the interests of such practitioners and (b) the number of practitioners represented?

Response

Scotland
(a) APS and BMA for clinical forensic medicine in UK. Pathologists by BAFM and BMA—BMA has Forensic Medicine Committee.
(b) APS, 1000; BAFM, 100.

Serbia
(a) Yugoslav Association of FM.
(b) Approximately 40–50 members.

South Africa
(a) Department of Health in collaboration with international organizations
(b) About 80 practitioners.

Spain
(a) Forensic surgeons form groups in some professional associations nationwide, such as the Asociación Nacional de Médicos Forenses, Asociación Andaluza de Médicos Forenses, Asociación Estatal de Médicos Forenses, Asociación Gallega de Médicos Forenses., etc.
(b) About 300 forensic surgeons are represented by those associations. The number of licensed medicolegal experts in Spain is currently 450, and acting medicolegal experts about 150.

Sweden
(a) The National Forensic Board, under the Department of Justice, is responsible for all examinations in the fields of forensic pathology (death investigations), forensic psychiatry, FM, and forensic genetics. All specialists who are active in these fields are employed by this organization. Competition in these fields is free but does not, with the exception for investigations of living victims and perpetrators, occur.
(b) There are approx 25 specialists in FM in Sweden today.

Switzerland
(a) Swiss Society of Legal Medicine, Website: (www.legalmed.ch).
(b) 40.

APS, Association of Forensic Physicians; BAFM, British Association in Forensic Medicine; BMA, British Medical Association; CFM, clinical forensic medicine; FM, forensic medicine.

32

Question V Can you give a rough estimate of (a) the population of your country/state, the number of medical practitioners working in (b) CFM, and (c) FP?

Response

	(a)	(b)	(c)
Australia	(a) State: 5 million.	(b) Approximately 50.	(c) Approximately 10.
England and Wales	(a) 60 million.	(b) Approximately 2000.	(c) Approximately 40.
Germany	(a) Germany: 80 million/ North Rhine–Westphalia state: 16 million.	(b) Germany: 150 /state: 50.	(c) Germany: 250/state: 50.
Hong Kong	(a) 6.5 million.	(b) None full-time. More than 1000 in different ways.	(c) 18: this group does most of the criminal cases relating to CFM.
India	(a) 1.05 billion.	(b) There are no data available on it. In peripheral regions, such as small towns and villages, even general duty doctors fulfill the work of CFM and FP.	(c) Same as (b).
Israel	(a) Six million.	(b) Eight.	(c) Same eight.
Malaysia	(a) 20 million.	(b) One trained forensic physician.	(c) Approximately 20 forensic pathologists
The Netherlands	(a) 16 million.	(b) Approximately 350.	(c) Approximately 5.
Nigeria	(a) Approximately 120 million.	(b) One part-time (a uniformed police officer).	(c) Six—all currently outside Nigeria; one of the six has retired.
Scotland	(a) Approximately 5.25 million.	(b) Approximately 150.	(c) Approximately 12 (these are mainly university staff).
Serbia	(a) 7.5 million.	(b) Approximately 40–50.	(c) Approximately 40–50.
South Africa	(a) 42 million.	(b) Approximately 180 (majority of them are part-time basis).	(c) Approximately 25.
Spain	(a) 0.5 million.	(b) Approximately 9.	(c) Approximately 9.
Sweden	(a) 9 million.	(b) 35 (10 nonspecialists in training).	(c) FM = FP in Sweden.
Switzerland	(a) 7.2 million.	(b,c) 70 (most do both CFM and FP).	

CFM, clinical forensic medicine; FP, forensic pathology.

33

Question W	Are specific qualifications available for (a) CFM or (b) FP?	
Response		
Australia	(a) Yes	(b) Yes
England and Wales	(a) DMJ (Clin), DFM, MMJ.	(b) MRCPath, DFM, DMJ, (Path).
Germany	(a,b) Yes, but they are the same.	
Hong Kong	(a) DMJ (Clin)(Lond.).	(b) DMJ (Path)(Lond.), FHKCPath, FHKAM.
India	(a) Yes, 3-yr postgraduate course in forensic medicine, which can only be done by a graduate in medicine and surgery. There is an entrance test for this course.	(b) Same as (a).
Israel	(a) No	(b) Yes
Malaysia	(a) No	(b) Master of Pathology (Forensic)—4-yr course.
The Netherlands	(a) Yes	(b) Yes
Nigeria	(a) All trained in the United Kingdom, Germany, and United States. There are no local training programs.	(b) Same as (a).
Scotland	(a,b) All UK qualifications, e.g., DMJ, DFM (not compulsory); pathologists MRCPath, DFM, DMJ, and one available from the RCP (Ed).	
Serbia	(a,b) No qualifications but training program.	
South Africa	(a) No, but being established.	(b) Yes
Spain	(a,b) There are national test (competitive examinations on supreme court-Ministry of Justice) to be admitted in the National Corps of Forensic surgeons (Cuerpo Nacional de Médicos Forenses). The professionals are the ones who conduct both CFM and FP.	
Sweden	(a) Yes	(b) Yes
Switzerland	(a,b) Yes, qualifications that cover both fields.	

CFM, clinical forensic medicine; FP, forensic pathology.

Question X	Are such qualifications mandatory to practice in (a) clinical forensic medicine or (b) forensic pathology?	
Response		
Australia	(a) Yes, in full-time practice only.	(b) Yes
England and Wales	(a) No	(b) Yes
Germany	(a) Yes	(b) Yes
Hong Kong	(a) No	(b) Yes
India	(a) No, as stated above, they are not mandatory. Although a great prestige is accorded to the report of people who have such a qualification.	(b) Same as (a).
Israel	(a) No	(b) Yes
Malaysia	(a) Ordinary doctors undertake a large part of routine autopsies and clinical cases. Depending on the availability, difficult or complicated cases are handled by specialists.	(b) Same as (a).
The Netherlands	(a) Not yet.	(b) Not officially.
Nigeria	(a) No	(b) Locally trained histopathologists and medical officers unfortunately often assume this role.
Scotland	(a) No	(b) Yes
Serbia	(a) No	(b) Yes
South Africa	(a) No	(b) Yes, but still unqualified are working.
Spain	(a) Yes	(b) Yes
Sweden	(a) Yes	(b) Yes
Switzerland	(a) Yes (but only at university institutes).	(b) Yes (but only at university institutes).

35

REFERENCES

1. Smith, S. The history and development of forensic medicine. Br. Med. J. 599–607, 1951.
2. Traill, T. S. Outlines of a course of lectures on medical jurisprudence, 2nd ed. Adam & Charles Black, Edinburgh, Scotland, 1840.
3. Amundsen, D. W., Ferngren, G. B. The physician as an expert witness in Athenian law. Bull. Hist. Med. 51:202–213, 1977.
4. Amundsen, D. W., Ferngren, G. B. Forensic role of physicians in Roman law. Bull. Hist. Med. 53:39–56, 1979.
5. Brittain, R. P. Origins of legal medicine. Roman law: Lex Duodecim Tabularum. Medico-Legal J. 35:71–72, 1967.
6. Amundsen, D. W., Ferngren, G. B. The forensic role of physicians in Ptolemaic and Roman Egypt. Bull. Hist. Med. 52:336–353, 1978.
7. Cassar, P. A medicolegal report of the sixteenth century from Malta. Med. Hist. 18:354–359, 1974.
8. Beck T. R., Darwall, J. Elements of medical jurisprudence, 3rd ed. Longman, London, UK, 1829.
9. Hunter, W. On the uncertainty of the signs of murder in the case of bastard children. London, UK, 1783.
10. Smith, J. G. The principles of forensic medicine systematically arranged and applied to British practice. Thomas & George Underwood, London, UK, 1821.
11. Davis, B. T. George Edward Male, M. D., the father of English medical jurisprudence. Proc. Royal Soc. Med. 67:117–120, 1974.
12. Taylor, A. S. A manual of medical jurisprudence. John Churchill, London, UK, 1844.
13. Traill, T. S. Outlines of a course of lectures on medical jurisprudence. Adam & Charles Black, Edinburgh, Scotland, 1834.
14. Cordner, S. M., Ranson, D. L., Singh, B. The practice of forensic medicine in Australasia: a review. Aust. N. Z. J. Med. 22:477–485, 1992.
15. Gee, D. J., Mason, J. K. The courts & the doctor. Oxford University Press, Oxford, UK, 1990.
16. Guy, W. A. Principles of forensic medicine. Henry Renshaw, London, UK, 1844.
17. Payne-James, J. J. Clinical forensic medicine. J. Clin. Forensic Med. 1:1, 1994.
18. Three-faced practice: doctors and police custody [editorial]. Lancet. 341:1245–1247, 1993.
19. Grant, G. The diary of a police surgeon. C. Arthur Pearson, London, UK, 1920.
20. Payne-James, J. J. Questionnaire on "Global Clinical Forensic Medicine," 4th Annual Clinical Forensic Medicine Postgraduate Conference, Louisville, KY, 1997.
21. Payne-James, J. J., Busuttil, A., Smock, W. Forensic medicine: clinical and pathological aspects. Greenwich Medical Media, London, UK, 2003.
22. Herring, J., Stark, M. M. The role of the independent forensic physician. Education & Research Committee of the Association of Forensic Physicians. Association of Forensic Physicians, East Kilbride, Glasgow, UK, 2003.

Chapter 2

Fundamental Principles

Roy N. Palmer

1. INTRODUCTION

Although medicine is an international discipline, practiced in much the same way throughout the English-speaking world, laws vary considerably from country to country. Much of the law applicable in the United States and in the countries of the Commonwealth derives from the English common law, but medical practitioners should not assume that the laws of their own countries or states will necessarily apply in other countries or states even if medical practices are indistinguishable. In this chapter, the author attempts to establish principles of general applicability; however, it is written from the perspective of the law applicable in England and Wales and should be read with that in mind.

Recently in the United Kingdom and elsewhere, many statutes relevant to medical practice have been enacted. Ignorance of the law is no defense, and today's doctors are at risk of prosecution for breaches of the law as no previous generation has been. Yet the teaching at undergraduate level of forensic (or legal) medicine is now patchy and variable, so today's doctors are seldom well informed about laws that govern their daily practices. It is hoped that this chapter will help redress that position, but only a brief outline of some relevant law can be offered here. Doctors are advised to continue to subscribe to one of the traditional medical defense organizations (Medical Defence Union [MDU], Medical Protection Society [MPS], or Medical and Dental Defence Union of Scotland [MDDUS] in the United Kingdom, Canadian Medical Protective Association [CMPA] in Canada, or

From: *Clinical Forensic Medicine: A Physician's Guide, 2nd Edition*
Edited by: M. M. Stark © Humana Press Inc., Totowa, NJ

one of the Australian defense bodies) or an equivalent organization or to take out adequate insurance to ensure that they have access to advice and legal representation for medicolegal problems arising from their professional work, and, of course, indemnity for any adverse awards of costs and damages for professional negligence.

1.1. Ethical Principles

Doctors who practice as forensic physicians (forensic medical examiners [FMEs], forensic medical officers, or police surgeons) have a special responsibility toward detainees, subjects whose liberty is already infringed and who are at serious risk of future curtailment of their liberty. Although enactments in Europe, such as the Human Rights Act of 1998, have afforded better protection of the rights and liberties of citizens, the forensic physician has a real part to play in acting honorably by ensuring that the rights of the detainee are upheld in accordance with medical professional codes of ethics. A forensic physician who believes that the rights of the detainee are being ignored or abused may have a duty to report the concern to an authoritative person or body.

It is not always appreciated that forensic physicians have two roles. First, they are independent medical assessors of victims and/or alleged perpetrators of crimes and, as such, no conventional therapeutic relationship exists. It is most important that this be made clear to the victims or detainees by the doctor, so that properly informed consent is secured for the proposed examination. Second, a therapeutic relationship may arise when advice or treatment or other therapeutic intervention is offered, but the nature of the therapeutic relationship will be constrained by the circumstances and by the forensic physician's duty to pass information to police officers who will be responsible for observing the detainee or victim. Great care is necessary concerning issues of consent and confidentiality in such circumstances.

Some ethical codes are national, drawn up by such bodies as national medical associations and medical boards or councils set up by the state (such as the British Medical Association and the General Medical Council [GMC] in the United Kingdom). Other codes of ethics are regional (e.g., the European Convention on Human Rights), whereas still others are international, such as the many codes and declarations prepared and published by the World Medical Association (*see* Appendix 1).

Most of the ethical principles will be familiar to doctors who practice in countries that derive their laws from the Anglo-American common law system, but the detail of local rules and regulations will vary from nation to nation and state to state.

2. CONSENT

Even when his or her life depends on receiving medical treatment, an adult of sound mind is entitled to refuse it. This reflects the autonomy of each individual and the right of self-determination. Lest reiteration may diminish the impact of this principle, it is valuable to recognise the force of the language used when the right of self determination was most recently considered in the House of Lords (1).

It is well established English law that it is unlawful, so as to constitute both a tort (a civil wrong) and the crime of battery, to administer medical treatment to an adult who is conscious and of sound mind without his consent. Such a person is completely at liberty to decline to undergo treatment even if the result of his doing so will be that he will die (2).

The principle of self-determination requires that respect must be given to the wishes of the patient, so that if an adult patient of sound mind refuses, however unreasonably, to consent to treatment or to care by which his life would or might be prolonged, the doctors responsible for his care must give effect to his wishes, even though they do not consider it to be in his best interests to do so...To this extent, the principle of the sanctity of human life must yield to the principle of self-determination ...and, for present purposes perhaps more important, the doctor's duty to act in the best interests of his patient must likewise be qualified (3).

Any treatment given by a doctor to a patient which involves any interference with the physical integrity of the patient is unlawful unless done with the consent of the patient: it constitutes the crime of battery and the tort of trespass to the person (4).

A doctor has no right to proceed in the face of objection, even if it is plain to all, including the patient, that adverse consequences and even death will or may ensue (5).

The author can do no better than to open a discussion of the topic of consent by quoting the powerful and unambiguous language of the law lords in a leading case. The underlying reason for this position:

...is that English law goes to great lengths to protect a person of full age and capacity from interference with his personal liberty. We have too often seen freedom disappear in other countries not only by coups d'etat but by gradual erosion; and often it is the first step that counts. So it would be unwise to make even minor concessions (6).

The foregoing applies to all adults who are mentally competent; when a patient lacks the capacity to make decisions about whether to consent to treatment (e.g., when he or she is unconscious or suffering from mental disability), the medical practitioners who are responsible for his or her treatment must act in the patient's best interests and, if appropriate, may conduct major invasive treatments without expressed consent *(7)*.

2.1. Requisites for Consent

To intervene without consent may give rise to criminal proceedings (for alleged trespass to the person) and may also give rise to tortious liability (a civil claim for damages). To protect against such proceedings, the medical practitioner should ensure that the patient is capable of giving consent, has been sufficiently well informed to understand and therefore to give a true consent, and has then expressly and voluntarily consented to the proposed investigation, procedure, or treatment. In the United Kingdom, the GMC has produced a booklet *(8)* outlining guidance for doctors about seeking patients' consent with which any doctor who practices in the United Kingdom must comply.

2.1.1. Capacity

If there is serious doubt about the patient's capacity to give consent, it should be assessed as a matter of priority. The patient's general practitioner or other responsible doctor may be sufficiently qualified to make the assessment, but in serious or complex cases involving difficult issues about the future health and well-being, or even the life of the patient, the issue of capacity to consent should be assessed by an independent psychiatrist (in England, ideally, but not necessarily, one approved under section 12 of the Mental Health Act of 1983) *(9)*. If after assessment serious doubts still remain about the patient's competence (e.g., the patient is incapable by reason of mental disorder of managing his or her property or affairs), it may be necessary to seek the involvement of the courts.

2.1.2. Understanding Risks and Warnings

A signature on a form is not, of itself, a valid consent. For a valid, true, or real consent in law, the patient must be sufficiently well informed to understand that to which he or she is asked to give consent. The doctor must be satisfied that the patient is capable of the following:

1. He or she can comprehend and retain the relevant information.
2. He or she believes the information.
3. He or she can weigh the pros and cons to arrive at a choice *(10)*.

To defend a doctor against a civil claim alleging lack of consent based on a failure to warn adequately, it is necessary to have more than a signature on a standard consent form. Increasingly, in medical negligence actions, it is alleged that risks were not explained nor warnings given about possible adverse outcomes. Therefore, it is essential for the doctor or any other healthcare professional to spend adequate time explaining the nature and purpose of the intended investigation, procedure, or treatment in terms that the patient can understand. Risks and adverse outcomes should be discussed. The patient's direct questions must be answered frankly and truthfully, as was made clear in the Sidaway case *(11)*, and thus the discussions should be undertaken by those with adequate knowledge and experience to deal with them; ideally, the clinician who is to perform the operation or procedure.

English law differs from the law in other common-law jurisdictions (e.g., Australia, Canada, and the United States) regarding the nature of the information that must be imparted for the consent to be "informed" and, therefore, valid. Increasingly, worldwide the courts will decide what the doctor should warn a patient about—applying objective tests, such as what a "prudent patient" would wish to know before agreeing. For example, in the leading Australian case *(12)*, the court imposed a duty to warn about risks of remote (1 in 14,000) but serious complications of elective eye surgery, even though professional opinion in Australia at the time gave evidence that they would not have warned of so remote a risk.

In the United States and Canada, the law about the duty to warn of risks and adverse outcomes has long been much more stringent. Many (but not all) US courts recognize a duty on a doctor to warn a patient of the risks inherent in the treatment proposed. In the leading case *(13)*, the District of Columbia appeals court imposed an objective "prudent patient" test and enunciated the following four principles:

1. Every human being of adult years and sound mind has a right to determine what shall happen to his or her body.
2. Consent is the informed exercise of choice and that entails an opportunity to evaluate knowledgeably the options available and their attendant risks.
3. The doctor must therefore disclose all "material risks."
4. The doctor must retain a "therapeutic privilege."

A "material risk" was held to be one that a reasonable person, in what the doctor knows or should know to be the patient's position, would likely attach significance to in deciding whether to forego the proposed treatment—this test is known as the "prudent patient test." However, the court held that a doctor has a therapeutic privilege by which he or she is entitled to withhold from the patient information about risk if full disclosure would pose a serious threat of psychological detriment to the patient. In the leading Canadian case *(14)*, broad agreement was expressed with the propositions expressed in the American case.

English law continues to allow the doctor discretion in deciding what information is to be imparted to the particular patient being advised. The practitioner is not required to make an assessment based on the information to be given to an abstract "prudent patient;" rather, the actual patient being consulted must be assessed to determine what that patient should be told. However, the Sidaway and Bolitho *(15)* cases make clear that doctors must be supported by a body of professional opinion that is not only responsible but also scientifically and soundly based as determined by the court.

The message for the medical and allied health care professions is that medical paternalism has no place where consent to treatment is concerned; patients' rights to self-determination and personal autonomy based on full disclosure of relevant information is the legal requirement for consent.

2.1.3. Voluntary Agreement

Consent obtained by fraud or duress is not valid. A doctor must be satisfied that the patient is giving a free, voluntary agreement to the proposed investigation, procedure, or treatment.

Consent may then be given expressly or by implication. Express consent is given when the patient agrees in clear terms, verbally or in writing. A verbal consent is legitimate, but because disputes may arise about the nature and extent of the explanation and warnings about risks, often months or years after the event, it is strongly recommended that, except for minor matters, consent be recorded in written form. In the absence of a contemporaneous note of the discussions leading to the giving of consent, any disputed recollections will fall to be decided by a lengthy, expensive legal process. The matter then becomes one of evidence, with the likelihood that the patient's claimed "perfect recall" will be persuasive to the court in circumstances in which the doctor's truthful concession is that he or she has no clear recollection of what was said to this particular patient in one of hundreds of consultations undertaken.

A contemporaneous note should be made by the doctor of the explanation given to the patient and of warnings about risks and possible adverse outcomes. It is helpful to supplement but not to substitute the verbal explanation with a printed information leaflet or booklet about the procedure or treatment. The explanation should be given by the clinician who is to undertake the procedure—it is not acceptable to "send the nurse or junior hospital doctor" to "consent the patient."

For more complex and elective procedures, it is wise to give the patient some time to reflect on the advice and on the choices, offering to meet him or her again before a final decision is made and to respond to any interim questions that the patient might wish to pose. For simple procedures (e.g., taking blood pressure and performing a venepuncture), it may be sufficient for consent to be implied—by the patient proffering an arm for the purpose. However, in circumstances in which the procedure has a forensic rather than a therapeutic content and the doctor is not the patient's usual medical attendant but may be carrying out tasks that affect the liberty of the individual (e.g., as a forensic physician or as an assessor in a civil claim), it is prudent to err on the side of caution. If no assumptions are made by the doctor and express agreement is invariably sought from the patient—and documented contemporaneously—there is less chance of misunderstandings and allegations of duress or of misleading the individual.

2.2. Adult Patients Who Are Incompetent

Since the implementation of the 1983 Mental Health Act in England and Wales (and the equivalent in Scotland) no parent, relative, guardian, or court can give consent to the treatment of an adult patient who is mentally incompetent *(16)*. The House of Lords had to consider a request to sterilize a 36-yr-old woman with permanent mental incapacity and a mental age of 5 years who had formed a sexual relationship with a fellow patient. The court held that no one, not even the courts, could give consent on behalf of an adult who was incompetent. (This is because the 1983 act removed the *parens patriae* jurisdiction of the courts in England and Wales; those jurisdictions in which courts retain *parens patriae* powers retain the ability to provide consent in such circumstances.) However, the House of Lords made clear that doctors could act in the best interests of their adult patients who are incompetent by treating them in accordance with a responsible body of professional opinion (i.e., in accord with the Bolam principle, ref. *17*).

2.3. Age of Consent

In England, section 8 of the Family Law Reform Act 1969 provides that any person of sound mind who has attained 16 year of age may give a valid consent to surgical, medical, or dental treatments. The consent of a parent or guardian is not required. For those under 16 years of age the House of Lords decided *(18)* that valid consent could be given by minors, provided that they understood the issues. The case concerned the provision of contraceptive advice to girls younger than 16 years in circumstances in which a parent objected. The House of Lords held that parental rights to determine whether a child younger than 16 years received treatment terminated if and when the child achieved a sufficient understanding and intelligence to enable him or her to comprehend the issues involved. It is the capacity to understand, regardless of age or status, that is the determinant factor.

2.4. Intimate Samples and Intimate Searches

Section 62 of the Police and Criminal Evidence Act of 1984 (and the equivalent statute in Scotland) provides that intimate samples can only be taken from an individual if authorized by a police inspector (or higher ranking police officer) and if consent is obtained. For this purpose the age of consent is 17 (not 16) years. For those between 14 and 17 years of age, the consent of both the detainee and the parent or guardian is required, and for those younger than 14 years of age, only the consent of the parent or guardian is statutorily required.

Section 55 of the Police and Criminal Evidence Act (and an equivalent provision in Scotland) provides that an intimate search of an individual may be conducted on the authority of a police officer of at least the rank of inspector only if there are grounds for suspecting that an individual is hiding on himself or herself either an object that might be used to cause physical injury while he is detained or a class A controlled drug. A doctor called on to conduct an intimate search will be wise to consider carefully whether a detainee is likely to be able to give a free and voluntary consent in such circumstances; an intimate search should not be conducted unless the doctor is thoroughly satisfied that the individual has given valid consent. An intimate search may, exceptionally, be conducted by a doctor if he or she believes it necessary to remove a concealed object that is an immediate danger to the life or personal safety of those responsible for the detainee's supervision.

2.5. Video and Audio Recordings

The GMC has issued guidance *(19)* requiring doctors to inform patients before making a video or audio recording and, except in situations in which consent may be understood from a patient's cooperation with a procedure (e.g., radiographic investigation), to obtain his or her explicit consent. Doctors may make recordings without consent in exceptional circumstances, such as when it is believed that a child has been the victim of abuse.

If a recording has been made in the course of investigation or treatment of a patient but the doctor now wishes to use it for another purpose, the patient's consent must be obtained. Recordings are not to be published or broadcast in any form without the explicit, written consent of the patient. Consent is required before recordings are published in textbooks or journals or before the public is allowed access to them.

If patients can be identified from recordings, a doctor must ensure that the interests and well-being of the patient take precedence over all other considerations. This is especially so for patients who are mentally ill or disabled, seriously ill, or children or other vulnerable people. When disability prevents patients from giving informed consent, the GMC advises the doctor to obtain agreement from a close relative or caregiver; where children lack the understanding to consent, the permission of the parent or guardian is recommended.

2.6. Recording Telephone Calls

Many countries have laws or regulations that govern the electronic recording of telephone conversations, which are designed to protect individuals' rights. Commonly, a provision will be included stating that persons whose telephone calls are being recorded must be informed of the fact—the details vary from country to country. In the United Kingdom, for example, the Telecommunications Act of 1984 requires that the person making a recording shall make "every reasonable effort to inform the parties" of doing so. "Every reasonable effort" is not defined statutorily, but the Office of Telecommunications , which is a government-appointed regulatory body, now subsumed within OfCom (Website: www.ofcom.org.uk), has issued guidance. Reasonable effort may be achieved by the use of warning tones, prerecorded messages, verbal warnings given by a telephone operator, or written warnings in publicity material.

A recording may be an invaluable aid for forensic evidence or to help refute a complaint or claim for compensation, but practitioners who make electronic recordings of telephone calls must ensure that they comply with local laws and practice codes.

2.7. Emergencies

Before leaving the topic of consent, it is necessary to state clearly that in a medical emergency in which a patient is unconscious and thus unable to give or withhold consent and there is no clear instruction to the contrary in the form of a valid, extant advance directive made by the patient, treatment that is clearly essential to save life or prevent serious harm may and indeed should be given. However, nonurgent treatment should be deferred until the patient is able to give consent.

3. CONFIDENTIALITY

"And whatsoever I shall see or hear in the course of my profession, as well as outside my profession in my intercourse with men, if it be what should not be published abroad, I will never divulge, holding such things to be holy secrets..." (20).

"...I will respect the secrets which are confided in me, even after the patient has died ..." (21).

"...A physician shall preserve absolute confidentiality on all he knows about his patient even after the patient has died ..." (22).

Information acquired by a medical practitioner from or about a patient in the course of his or her professional work is confidential and must never be disclosed to others without either the consent of the patient or other proper justification.

Confidentiality is primarily a professional conduct matter for the medical practitioner, but patients also have a legal right to confidentiality, protected by law. The GMC in the United Kingdom and other medical councils and medical boards worldwide have published guidance to doctors, making it clear that a breach of confidentiality is a serious professional offense. The GMC's current guidance *(23)* requires doctors to:

"Treat information about patients as confidential. If in exceptional circumstances there are good reasons why you should pass on information without a patient's consent, or against a patient's wishes, you must follow our guidance "Confidentiality: Protecting and Providing Information" *and be prepared to justify your decision to the patient, if appropriate, and to the GMC and the courts, if called upon to do so."*

A separate GMC booklet *(24)* sets out more detailed guidance, including the principles of confidentiality and exceptions to the general rule.

Doctors are responsible for the safekeeping of confidential information against improper disclosure when it is stored, transmitted to others, or discarded. If a doctor plans to disclose information about a patient to others, he or she must first inform the patient of that intention and make clear that the patient has an opportunity to withhold permission for its disclosure. Patients' requests for confidentiality must be respected, except for exceptional circumstances, such as where the health or safety of others would otherwise be at serious risk.

If confidential information is disclosed, the doctor should release only as much as is necessary for the purpose and must always be ready and willing to justify the disclosure—for example, to the relevant medical council or board or to the courts. Where confidential information is to be shared with healthcare workers or others, the doctor must ensure that they, too, respect confidentiality.

3.1. Death and Confidentiality

The duty of confidentiality extends beyond the death of the patient. The extent to which information may properly be disclosed after the death of a patient depends on the circumstances. In general, it is prudent to seek the permission of all the personal representatives of the deceased patient's estate, such as the executors or administrators, before any information is disclosed. They, in turn, should be advised of the foreseeable consequences of disclosure. A doctor with any doubt should take advice from a professional advisory organization, such as a protection or defense organization.

3.2. Detention and Confidentiality

A forensic physician (or equivalent) should exercise particular care over confidentiality when examining persons who are detained in custody. When taking the medical history and examining the detainee, it is common for a police or other detaining official to be in attendance, perhaps as a "chaperone" or simply as a person in attendance, nearby to overhear the conversation. Such officials will not owe to the detainee the same duty of confidentiality that is owed by a medical or nurse practitioner nor be subject to similar professional sanctions for a breach of confidentiality.

The doctor called on to examine a detainee must take great care to ensure that the person being examined clearly understands the role of the forensic physician and the implications for confidentiality. The detainee must understand and agree to the terms of the consultation before any medical information is gathered, preferably giving written consent.

The examining doctor should do everything possible to maintain the confidentiality of the consultation. An accused person's right of silence, the presumption of innocence, rights under human rights legislation, and so forth may produce areas of conflicting principle. The doctor's code of professional conduct may conflict with statutory codes to which custody officials are bound (e.g., the duty on a police officer to record events). It may be essential to take the medical history in strict confidence, commensurate with adequate safeguards against violent behavior by the prisoner, and insist on a neutral chaperone for a physical examination. In the rest of this chapter, it is possible only to highlight the issues; their resolution will vary according to local rules and circumstances. In the United Kingdom, guidance for forensic physicians is available from their professional bodies *(25)*.

3.3. Exceptions to the General Duty of Confidentiality

Under several circumstances the doctor may legitimately disclose information gained about a patient during his or her professional work. For a full consideration, refer to the GMC guidance *(24)* or equivalent locally relevant guidance. In summary, the main exceptions are listed in Subheadings 3.3.1. to 3.3.5.

3.3.1. The Patient's Permission

The confidences are those of the patient, not those of the doctor, so if a patient requests or consents to their disclosure, the information may be perfectly and properly disclosed within the terms of the patient's permissions.

Consent to disclose confidential information may be given by the patient in a range of circumstances. These include employment and insurance purposes, housing and welfare, testimonials and references, or legal proceedings (whether civil or criminal or family law matters, etc.). However, care must be taken to ensure that disclosure is limited strictly to the terms of the patient's permission and that there is no disclosure to parties with whom the patient may be in contention unless the patient expressly agrees to it. (The classic pitfalls are disclosure to the advisers of the other spouse or other party in contested divorce, child custody, or personal injury cases.)

3.3.2. The Patient's Best Interests

In circumstances in which a patient is incapable of giving consent because of incapacity, immaturity, etc., and has refused to allow the doctor to speak to other appropriate persons, the doctor may disclose information to other appropriate persons if convinced that it is in the patient's best medical interests. If a doctor believes that a patient is the victim of physical or sexual abuse or neglect, he or she may disclose relevant information to an appropriate person or statutory agency in an attempt to prevent further harm to the patient.

Another example of this exception is when a doctor believes that seeking permission for the disclosure would be damaging to the patient but that a close relative should know about the patient's condition (e.g., terminal or some psychiatric illnesses).

The doctor must always act in the patient's best medical interests and be prepared to justify his or her decision. Advice may be taken from appropriate colleagues and/or from a protection or defense organization or other professional body.

3.3.3. The Public Interest, Interest of Others, or Patients Who Are Violent or Dangerous

Disclosure in the interests of others may be legitimate when they are at risk because a patient refuses to follow medical advice. Examples include patients who continue to drive when unfit to do so and against medical advice or who place others at risk by failing to disclose a serious communicable disease. Each case demands careful consideration, and doctors who have any doubt regarding how best to proceed should not hesitate to seek appropriate counsel.

Doctors may also be approached by the police for information to assist them in apprehending the alleged perpetrator of a serious crime. A balance must be struck between the doctor's duty to preserve the confidences of a patient and his or her duty as a citizen to assist in solving a serious crime where he or she has information that may be crucial to a police inquiry. In cases of murder, serious assaults, and rape in which the alleged assailant is still at large, the doctor may be persuaded that there is a duty to assist in the apprehension of the assailant by providing information, acquired professionally, that will be likely to assist the police in identifying and apprehending the prime suspect or suspects. However, where the accused person is already in custody, the doctor would be wise not to disclose confidential information without the agreement of the patient or legal advisers or an order from the court. Each case must be weighed on its own facts and merits, and the doctor may wish to seek advice from an appropriate source, such as a protection or defense organization. Guidance about gunshot wounds is given in Subheading 3.3.6.

A patient who is violent or dangerous poses particular dilemmas for the doctor. In the course of a consultation, a patient may tell a doctor that he or she intends to perpetrate some serious harm on another person—perhaps a close relative or friend or someone with whom there is a perceived need to "settle an old score." Each case must be carefully assessed on its own facts and merits, and careful clinical judgement exercised; however, under some circumstances, a doctor may feel obligated to override the duty of confidentiality to the individual and to disclose confidential information to the intended victim, the police, or another person in authority with the power to take appropriate action. Indeed, a failure to act in such circumstances has led to adverse judicial rulings, as in the Tarasoff *(26)* case in California, in which a specialist psychologist failed to give a warning to the girlfriend of a patient who was later murdered by the patient. The court decided that although no general common law duty exists to protect or warn third parties, a special relationship may impose such a duty.

In the United Kingdom, a psychiatrist was sued because he had released, without the consent of a patient who was violent, a report prepared at the request of the patient's solicitors in connection with an application for release from detention.

The psychiatrist advised against release, and the solicitors decided not to make use of the report. The psychiatrist was so concerned about his findings that he released a copy of the report to the relevant authorities and, as a consequence, the patient's application for release was refused. The patient's subsequent civil claim for compensation was rejected by the courts *(27)*, which held that the psychiatrist was entitled, under the circumstances, to put his duty to the public above the patient's right to confidentiality.

3.3.4. Medical Teaching, Research, and Audit

In general, data should be made anonymous. Every reasonable effort must be made to inform the concerned patients and to obtain their permission to disclose or publish case histories, photographs, and other information. Where consent cannot be obtained, the matter should be referred to a research ethics committee for guidance. The GMC and similar bodies give guidance *(8,23)*, and reputable medical journals have strict codes of practice, requiring that appropriate consent be obtained before even anonymous data are published, but the topic is not discussed in this chapter.

3.3.5. Judicial and Statutory Exceptions

Statutory provisions may require a doctor to disclose information about patients. In the United Kingdom they include, for example, notifications of births, miscarriages, and deaths; notifications of infectious diseases; notifications of industrial diseases and poisonings; and notifications under the provisions of the Abortion Act of 1967.

A doctor may be required to attend court and to answer questions if ordered to do so by the presiding judge, magistrate, or sheriff. When in the witness box, the doctor may explain that he or she does not have the consent of the patient to disclose the information (or indeed that the patient has expressly forbidden the doctor to disclose it), but the court may rule that the interests of justice require that the information held by the doctor about the patient be disclosed to the court. The doctor must then answer or risk being charged with contempt of court.

However, disclosure should only be made in judicial proceedings in one of two situations: first, when the presiding judge directs the doctor to answer, or second, when the patient has given free and informed consent. A request by any other person (whether police officer, court official, or lawyer) should be politely but firmly declined. As always, the doctor's protection or defense organization will be pleased to advise in any case of doubt.

Other statutory provisions of forensic relevance exist, but they are peculiar to individual countries or states and are not included here.

3.3.6. Reporting Gunshot Wounds

In September 2003, the GMC published new guidance, *Reporting Gunshot Wounds Guidance for Doctors Working in Accident and Emergency*

Departments, developed in conjunction with the Association of Chief Police Officers. The guidance may be obtained from the GMC and viewed on its Website at www.gmc-uk.org.

In summary, it states that: "The police should be told whenever a person has arrived at a hospital with a gun shot wound," but "at this stage identifying details, such as the patient's name and address, should not usually be disclosed." The doctor with clinical responsibility for the patient should ensure that the police are notified but may delegate the task to any member of the accident and emergency staff. Ordinarily, the patient's consent to disclose his or her name and other information must be sought and the treatment and care of the patient must be the doctor's first concern. If the patient's consent is refused, information may be disclosed only when the doctor judges that disclosure would prevent others from suffering serious harm or would help prevent, detect, or prosecute a serious crime. In short, the usual principles of confidentiality apply, and any doctor who breaches confidentiality must be prepared to justify his or her decision.

4. NOTEKEEPING

All doctors should keep objective, factual records of their consultations with patients and of other professional work. Not only is this desirable *per se*, but also it is now a professional requirement. Current GMC guidance *(23)* states that in providing care doctors must keep clear, accurate, and contemporaneous patient records that record the relevant findings, decisions made, information given to the patient, and any drugs or other treatment provided.

Good notes assist in the care of the patient, especially when doctors work in teams or partnership and share the care of patients with colleagues. Notes then help to keep colleagues well informed. Good notes are invaluable for forensic purposes, when the doctor faces a complaint, a claim for compensation, or an allegation of serious professional misconduct or poor performance. The medical protection and defense organizations have long explained that an absence of notes may render indefensible that which may otherwise have been defensible. The existence of good notes is often the key factor in preparing and mounting a successful defense to allegations against a doctor or the institution in which he or she works.

Notes should record facts objectively and dispassionately; they must be devoid of pejorative comment, wit, invective, or defamatory comments. Patients and their advisers now have increasing rights of access to their records and rights to request corrections of inaccurate or inappropriate information.

5. ACCESS TO HEALTH RECORDS

Access to medical and other health records, which is provided for by statute law, varies considerably from one jurisdiction to another. In English law, patients have enjoyed some rights of access to their medical records since the passage of the Administration of Justice Act of 1970. The relevant law is now contained in the Data Protection Act of 1998, which came into effect on March 1, 2000, and repealed previous statutory provisions relating to living individuals, governing access to health data, such as the Data Protection Act of 1984 and the Access to Health Records Act of 1990. However, the Access to Medical Reports Act of 1988 remains fully in force. Unfortunately, space considerations do not permit an explanation of the detailed statutory provisions; readers are respectfully referred to local legal provisions in their country of practice.

The Data Protection Act of 1998 implements the requirements of the European Union Data Protection Directive, designed to protect people's privacy by preventing unauthorized or inappropriate use of their personal details. The Act, which is wide ranging, extended data protection controls to manual and computerized records and provided for more stringent conditions on processing personal data. The law applies to medical records, regardless of whether they are part of a relevant filing system. As well as the primary legislation (the Act itself), secondary or subordinate legislation has been enacted, such as the Data Protection (Subject Access Modification) (Health) Order of 2000, which allows information to be withheld if it is likely to cause serious harm to the mental or physical health of any person.

Guidance notes about the operation of the legislation are available from professional bodies, such as the medical protection and defense organizations. In the United Kingdom, compliance with the requirements of the data protection legislation requires that the practitioner adhere to the following:

- Is properly registered as a data controller.
- Holds no more information about patients than is needed for their medical care and uses it only for that purpose.
- Stores records securely and restricts access to authorized personnel only.
- Complies with patients' legitimate requests for access to their health records.

6. PREPARATION OF REPORTS

Doctors are frequently asked to prepare reports for medicolegal reasons. It is important to understand the nature of the request and what is required—a simple report of fact, a report on present condition and prognosis after a medical examination, an expert opinion, or a combination of these. Because a doctor possesses expertise does not necessarily make him or her an expert witness every time a report is requested.

A report may be required for a variety of reasons, and its nature and content must be directed to the purpose for which it is sought. Is it a report of the history and findings on previous examination because there is now a criminal prosecution or civil claim? Is an expert opinion being requested based on the clinical notes made by others? Is it a request to examine the patient and to prepare a report on present condition and prognosis? Is it a request for an expert opinion on the management of another practitioner for the purposes of a medical negligence claim?

The request should be studied carefully to ascertain what is required and clarification sought where necessary in the case of any ambiguity. The fee or at least the basis on which it is to be set should also be agreed in advance of the preparation of the report. If necessary, the appropriate consents should be obtained and issues of confidentiality addressed.

Care must be taken in the preparation of any report. A medicolegal report may affect an individual's liberty in a criminal case or compensation in a personal injury or negligence action. A condemnatory report about a professional colleague may cause great distress and a loss of reputation; prosecuting authorities may even rely on it to decide whether to bring homicide charges for murder ("euthanasia") or manslaughter (by gross negligence). Reports must be fair and balanced; the doctor is not an advocate for a cause but should see his or her role as providing assistance to the lawyers and to the court in their attempt to do justice to the parties. It must always be conisdered that a report may be disclosed in the course of legal proceedings and that the author may be cross-examined about its content, on oath, in court, and in public.

A negligently prepared report may lead to proceedings against the author and perhaps even criminal proceedings in exceptional cases. Certainly a civil claim can be brought if a plaintiff's action is settled on disadvantageous terms as a result of a poorly prepared opinion. There is also the attendant risk of adverse judicial comment and press publicity.

The form and content of the report will vary according to circumstances, but it should always be well presented on professional notepaper with relevant dates and details carefully documented in objective terms. Care should be taken to address the questions posed in the letter of instructions from those who commissioned it. If necessary, the report may be submitted in draft before it is finalized, but the doctor must always ensure that the final text represents his or her own professional views and must avoid being persuaded by counsel or solicitors to make amendments with which he or she is not content: it is the doctor who will have to answer questions in the witness box, and this may be a most harrowing experience if he or she makes claims outside the area of expertise or in any way fails to "come up to proof" (i.e., departs from the original statement).

In civil proceedings in England and Wales, matters are now governed by the Civil Procedure Rules and by a Code of Practice approved by the head of civil justice. Any practitioner who provides a report in civil proceedings must make a declaration of truth and ensure that his or her report complies with the rules.

7. ATTENDANCE AT COURT

Courts broadly consist of two types: criminal and civil. Additionally, the doctor will encounter the Coroners Court (or the Procurators Fiscal and Sheriffs in Scotland), which is, exceptionally, inquisitorial and not adversarial in its proceedings. A range of other special courts and tribunals exists, from ecclesiastical courts to social security tribunals; these are not described here.

A doctor may be called to any court to give evidence. The type of court to which he or she is called is likely to depend on the doctor's practice, specialty, and seniority. The doctor may be called to give purely factual evidence of the findings when he or she examined a patient, in which case the doctor is simply a professional witness of fact, or to give an opinion on some matter, in which case the doctor is an expert witness. Sometimes, a doctor will be called to give both factual and expert evidence.

Usually the doctor will receive fair warning that attendance in court is required and he or she may be able to negotiate with those calling him or her concerning suitable dates and times. Many requests to attend court will be made relatively informally, but more commonly a witness summons will be served. A doctor who shows any marked reluctance to attend court may well receive a formal summons, which compels him or her to attend or to face arrest and proceedings for contempt of court if he or she refuses.

If the doctor adopts a reasonable and responsible attitude, he or she will usually receive the sympathetic understanding and cooperation of the lawyers and the court in arranging a time to give evidence that least disrupts his or her practice. However, any exhibition of belligerence by the doctor can induce a rigid inflexibility in lawyers and court officials—who always have the ability to "trump" the doctor by the issuance of a summons, so be warned and be reasonable.

Evidence in court is given on oath or affirmation. A doctor will usually be allowed to refer to any notes made contemporaneously to "refresh his memory," although it is courteous to seek the court's agreement.

7.1. Demeanor in Court

In the space available, it is not possible to do more than to outline good practice when giving evidence. Court appearances are serious matters; an individual's liberty may be at risk or large awards of damages and costs may rely on the evidence given. The doctor's dress and demeanor should be appropriate to the occasion, and he or she should speak clearly and audibly.

As with an oral examination for medical finals or the defense of a written thesis, listen carefully to the questions posed. Think carefully about the reply before opening your mouth and allowing words to pour forth. Answer the question asked (not the one you would like it to have been) concisely and carefully, and then wait for the next question. There is no need to fill all silences with words; the judge and others will be making notes, and it is wise to keep an eye on the judge's pen and adjust the speed of your words accordingly. Pauses between questions allow the judge to finish writing or counsel to think up his or her next question. If anything you have said is unclear or more is wanted from you, be assured that you will be asked more questions.

Be calm and patient, and never show a loss of temper or control regardless of how provoking counsel may be. An angry or flustered witness is a gift to any competent and experienced counsel, as is a garrulous or evasive witness.

Try to use simple language devoid of jargon, abbreviations, and acronyms. Stay well within your area of skill and expertise, and do not be slow to admit that you do not know the answer. Your frankness will be appreciated, whereas an attempt to bluff or obfuscate or overreach yourself will almost certainly be detrimental to your position.

Doctors usually seek consensus and try to avoid confrontation (at least in a clinical setting). They should remember that lawyers thrive on the adversarial process and are out to win their case, not to engage on a search for truth. Thus, lawyers will wish to extract from witnesses answers that best support the case of the party by whom they are retained. However, the medical witness is not in court to "take sides" but rather to assist the court, to the best of the expert witness' ability, to do justice in the case. Therefore, the witness should adhere to his or her evidence where it is right to do so but must be prepared to be flexible and to make concessions if appropriate, for example, because further evidence has emerged since the original statement was prepared, making it appropriate to cede points. The doctor should also recall the terms of the oath or affirmation—to tell the truth, the whole truth, and nothing but the truth—and give evidence accordingly.

8. THE DUTIES OF EXPERT WITNESSES

Some medical practitioners have made a career from giving expert opinions, and a few have brought the profession into disrepute by being demonstrably partisan or by giving opinion evidence that is scientifically unsupportable. The courts have now laid down guidance *(28)* for expert witnesses, and the UK Expert Witness Institute has prepared a code of practice *(29)* for experts.

The essential requirements for experts are as follows:

- Expert evidence presented to the court should be seen as the independent product of the expert, uninfluenced regarding form or content by the exigencies of litigation *(30)*.
- Independent assistance should be provided to the court by way of objective unbiased opinion regarding matters within the expertise of the expert witness *(31)*. An expert witness in the court should never assume the role of advocate.
- Facts or assumptions on which the opinion was based should be stated together with material facts that could detract from the concluded opinion.
- An expert witness should make clear when a question or issue falls outside his or her expertise.
- If the opinion was not properly researched because it was believed that insufficient data were available, that should be stated with an indication that the opinion is provisional. If the expert cannot assert that the report contains the truth, the whole truth, and nothing but the truth, that qualification should be stated on the report *(32)*.
- If after an exchange of reports an expert witness changes an opinion, the change of view/opinion should be communicated to the other parties through legal representatives without delay and, when appropriate, to the court.

The Expert Witness Institute (EWI) *(33)* has also produced an declaration for use by experts that follows the form recommended by Lord Woolf, the Chief Justice of England and Wales, in his review of civil justice procedures and that incorporates the legal principles just set out. The EWI Website (www.ewi.org.uk) provides an easy route to access several important documents.

In England and Wales, new Civil Procedure Rules for all courts came into force on April 16, 1999 *(34)*, and Part 35 establishes rules governing experts. The expert has an overriding duty to the court, overriding any obligation to the person who calls or pays him or her. An expert report in a civil case must end with a statement that the expert understands and has complied with the expert's duty to the court. The expert must answer questions of clarification at the request of the other party and now has a right to ask the court for directions to assist him in conducting the function as an expert. The new rules make radical changes to the previous use of expert opinion in civil actions.

9. PITFALLS

The potential pitfalls of forensic medical practice are many. Most pitfalls may be avoided by an understanding of the legal principles and forensic processes—a topic of postgraduate rather than undergraduate education now. The normal "doctor–patient" relationship does not apply; the forensic physician–detained person relationship requires that the latter understands the role of the former and that the former takes time to explain it to the latter.

Meticulous attention to detail and a careful documentation of facts are required at all times. You will never know when a major trial will turn on a small detail that you once recorded (or, regrettably, failed to record). Your work will have a real and immediate effect on the liberty of the individual and may be highly influential in assisting the prosecuting authorities to decide whether to charge the detained person with a criminal offense.

You may be the only person who can retrieve a medical emergency in the cells—picking up a subdural hematoma, diabetic ketoacidosis, or coronary thrombosis that the detaining authority has misinterpreted as drunkenness, indigestion, or simply "obstructive behavior." Get it right, and you will assist in the proper administration of the judicial process, with proper regard for human rights and individual's liberty. Get it wrong, and you may not only fail to prevent an avoidable death but also may lay yourself open to criminal, civil, and disciplinary proceedings.

You clearly owe a duty of care to those who engage your services, for that is well-established law. The issue of whether a forensic physician owes a wider duty to the victims of alleged crime was decided in the English Court of Appeal during 1999 *(35)*. A doctor working as an FME examined the victim of an alleged offense of rape and buggery (sodomy). The trial of the accused offender was fixed, and all prosecution witnesses were warned and fully bound, including the FME.

The trial was scheduled to begin on December 7, and on December 6, the FME was warned that she would not be required to attend on the first day of trial but would be needed some time after that. The trial commenced on December 7, and the accused pleaded not guilty. On Friday, December 8, the FME was told that she would not be needed that day but would be required the following week. She did not state that this would cause any problem. However, on December 11, the FME left the country for a vacation. On December 14, the police officer in charge of the case spoke by telephone with the FME. She said she could not return to give evidence before December 19. The remainder of the prosecution case was finished on December 14. The trial judge refused to adjourn the case until December 19. On December 20, the judge accepted a defense submission of no case to answer and directed the jury to return a verdict of not guilty. A few weeks later, the FME was convicted of contempt of court for failing to attend court to give evidence, and she was fined.

The female victim commenced civil proceedings against the FME, alleging negligent conduct in failing to attend, as warned, to give evidence. In her claim, the claimant asserted that if the FME had given evidence (presumably in accordance with her witness statement), the trial judge would have refused the defense submission of no case to answer. The claimant also contended that on the balance of probability, the accused would have been convicted because the FME's evidence would have undermined the credibility of the accused's defense that no anal interference had occurred. The claimant claimed that the FME owed her a duty of care to take all reasonable steps to provide evidence of the FME's examination in furtherance of the contemplated prosecution and to attend the trial of the accused as a prosecution witness when required. She claimed to suffer persistent stress and other psychological sequelae from failing to secure the conviction of her alleged assailant and knowing that he is still at large in the vicinity.

The claimant did not contend that there was any general duty of care on the part of a witness actionable in damages at the suit of another witness who may suffer loss and damage through the failure of the first witness to attend and give evidence in accordance with his or her witness statement.

When the case came before the Court of Appeal, Lord Justice Stuart-Smith stated that the attempt to formulate a duty of care as pleaded,

> *"is wholly misconceived. If a duty of care exists at all, it is a duty to prevent the plaintiff from suffering injury, loss or damage of the type in question, in this case psychiatric injury. A failure to attend to give evidence could be a breach of such duty, but it is not the duty itself."*

Later, Lord Justice Stuart-Smith stated:

> *"it is quite plain in my judgment that the defendant, in carrying out an examination at the behest of the police of Crown Prosecution Service, did not assume any responsibility for the plaintiff's psychiatric welfare; the doctor/patient relationship did not arise."*

He concluded his judgment:

> *"it is of no assistance to the plaintiff here in trying to construct a duty of care to attend court to give evidence which, as I have already pointed out, could amount to breach of a wider duty which is not alleged and could not be supported."*

The other two Lords Justice of Appeal agreed. Lord Justice Clarke observed that:

> *"In (the circumstances of the case) any duty of care owed (by the FME) must be very restricted. It seems to me that she must have owed a duty of care to carry out any examination with reasonable care, and thus, for example, not to make matters worse by causing injury to the plaintiff. It also seems to me to be at least arguable that where an FME carries out an examination and discovers that the person being examined has, say, a serious condition which needs immediate treatment, he or she owes a duty to that person to inform him or her of the position."*

The plaintiff's claim against the FME for damages was dismissed, and it was confirmed that there was no duty of care owed by the FME to the victim to attend the trial as a prosecution witness when required.

REFERENCES

1. *St George's Healthcare NHS Trust v S* [1998] 3WLR 936, 950E per Judge LJ.
2. *Airedale NHS Trust v Bland* [1993] AC789, 857 per Lord Keith of Kinkel.
3. Ibid. per Lord Goff of Chieveley, 864.
4. Ibid. per Lord Browne-Wilkinson, 882.
5. Ibid. per Lord Mustill, 891.
6. S. v McC and M; *W v W* [1972] AC 24 per Lord Reid, 43.
7. St George's Healthcare NHS Trust case [ibid.], 951G.
8. General Medical Council. Seeking patients' consent: the ethical considerations. The General Medical Council, London, UK, 1998.
9. St George's Healthcare NHS Trust case [ibid], 969C.
10. In re C [1994] 1WLR 290.
11. *Sidaway v Board of Governors of the Bethlem Royal and Maudsley Hospitals* [1985] AC 871; [1985] 1 AllER 643.
12. *Rogers v Whitaker* [1992] 175 CLR 479; [1992] AMLD 6993; 16 BMLR, 148 (Australian High Court).
13. *Canterbury v Spence* [1972] 464 F2d 772 (US App DC).
14. *Reibl v Hughes* 114 DLR 3d 1 (Canadian Supreme Court 1980); [1980] 2 SCR 880.
15. *Bolitho v City & Hackney Health Authority* [1998] AC 232 ; [1998] 1 Lloyd's Rep. Med. 26.
16. In re F [1990] 2.AC 1.
17. *Bolam v Friern Hospital Management Committee* [1957] 2 AllER 118; [1957] 1 WLR 582.
18. *Gillick v West Norfolk & Wisbech Area Health Authority* [1984] AC 112.
19. General Medical Council. Making and using visual and audio recordings of patients. General Medical Council, London, UK, 2002.
20. Extract from the Hippocratic Oath. 5th century BC. ·

21. Extract from The Declaration of Geneva. World Medical Association, 1948, restated 1983.
22. Extract from The International Code of Medical Ethics. World Medical Association, Geneva, Switzerland, 1983.
23. General Medical Council. Good medical practice. General Medical Council, London, UK, 2001.
24. General Medical Council. Confidentiality. General Medical Council, London, 2000.
25. Association of Police Surgeons and British Medical Association. Revised interim guidelines on confidentiality for police surgeons in England, Wales and Northern Ireland. Association of Police Surgeons (now the Association of Forensic Physicians), East Kilbride. British Medical Association, London, UK, 1998.
26. *Tarasoff v Regents of the University of California* [1976] P 551 2d 334 (Cal. Sup. Ct. 1976).
27. *W v Egdell* [1990] Ch. 359 ; [1990] 1 All ER 835 .
28. *National Justice Compania Naviera SA v Prudential Assurance Co. Ltd.* ("The Ikarian Reefer"); (The Times, March 5, 1993); [1993] 2 Lloyd's Rep. 68 (High Court 1993); [1995] 1 Lloyd's Rep. 455 (CA 1995).
29. Expert Witness Institute. Newsletter. EWI, London, UK, 1998.
30. *Whitehouse v Jordan* [1981] 1WLR 246, 256 per Lord Wilberforce.
31. *Polivitte Ltd v Commercial Union Assurance Co.* [1987] plc 1 Lloyd's Rep. 379, 386 per Garland J.
32. *Derby & Co. Ltd. and Others v Weldon and Others* (No. 9) The Times, November 9, 1990 per Staughton LJ.
33. Expert Witness Institute.
34. Civil Procedure Rules. The Stationery Office, London, 1999; and on the Department of Constitutional Affairs (formerly Lord Chancellor's Department). Available at Website: (www.dca.gov/uk).
35. Re N [1999] Lloyds Law Reports (Medical) 257; [1999] EWCA Civ 1452.

Chapter 3

Sexual Assault Examination

Deborah Rogers and Mary Newton

1. INTRODUCTION

Sexual assaults create significant health and legislative problems for every society. All health professionals who have the potential to encounter victims of sexual assaults should have some understanding of the acute and chronic health problems that may ensue from an assault. However, the primary clinical forensic assessment of complainants and suspects of sexual assault should only be conducted by doctors and nurses who have acquired specialist knowledge, skills, and attitudes during theoretical and practical training.

There are many types of sexual assault, only some of which involve penetration of a body cavity. This chapter encourages the practitioner to undertake an evidence-based forensic medical examination and to consider the nature of the allegation, persistence data, and any available intelligence.

The chapter commences by addressing the basic principles of the medical examination for both complainants and suspects of sexual assault. Although the first concern of the forensic practitioner is always the medical care of the patient, thereafter the retrieval and preservation of forensic evidence is paramount because this material may be critical for the elimination of a suspect, identification of the assailant, and the prosecution of the case. Thus, it is imperative that all forensic practitioners understand the basic principles of the forensic analysis.

Thereafter, the text is divided into sections covering the relevant body areas and fluids. Each body cavity section commences with information regard-

From: *Clinical Forensic Medicine: A Physician's Guide, 2nd Edition*
Edited by: M. M. Stark © Humana Press Inc., Totowa, NJ

ing the range and frequency of normal sexual practices and the relevant anatomy, development, and physiology. This specialist knowledge is mandatory for the reliable documentation and interpretation of any medical findings. The practical aspects—which samples to obtain, how to obtain them, and the clinical details required by the forensic scientist—are then addressed, because this takes priority over the clinical forensic assessment.

The medical findings in cases of sexual assault should always be addressed in the context of the injuries and other medical problems associated with consensual sexual practices. Therefore, each section summarizes the information that is available in the literature regarding the noninfectious medical complications of consensual sexual practices and possible nonsexual explanations for the findings. The type, site, and frequency of the injuries described in association with sexual assaults that relate to each body area are then discussed. Unfortunately, space does not allow for a critical appraisal of all the chronic medical findings purported to be associated with child sexual abuse, and the reader should refer to more substantive texts and review papers for this information *(1–3)*.

Throughout all the stages of the clinical forensic assessment, the forensic practitioner must avoid partisanship while remaining sensitive to the immense psychological and physical trauma that a complainant may have incurred. Although presented at the end of the chapter, the continuing care of the complainant is essentially an ongoing process throughout and beyond the primary clinical forensic assessment.

2. BASIC PRINCIPLES OF THE MEDICAL EXAMINATION

2.1. Immediate Care

The first health care professional to encounter the patient must give urgent attention to any immediate medical needs that are apparent, e.g., substance overdose, head injury, or serious wounds. This care takes precedence over any forensic concerns. Nonetheless, it may be possible to have a health care worker retain any clothing or sanitary wear that is removed from a complainant until this can be handed to someone with specialist knowledge of forensic packaging.

2.2. Timing of the Examination

Although in general terms the clinical forensic assessment should occur as soon as possible, reference to the persistence data given under the relevant sections will help the forensic practitioner determine whether the examination of a complainant should be conducted during out-of-office hours or deferred until the next day. Even when the nature of the assault suggests there is unlikely to be any forensic evidence, the timing of the examination should be influenced by the speed with which clinical signs, such as reddening, will fade.

2.3. Place of the Examination

Specially designed facilities used exclusively for the examination of complainants of sexual offenses are available in many countries. The complainant may wish to have a friend or relative present for all or part of the examination, and this wish should be accommodated. Suspects are usually examined in the medical room of the police station and may wish to have a legal representative present.

During the examinations of both complainants and suspects, the local ethical guidance regarding the conduct of intimate examinations should be followed *(4)*.

2.4. Consent

Informed consent must be sought for each stage of the clinical forensic assessment, including the use of any specialist techniques or equipment (e.g., colposcope) and obtaining the relevant forensic samples. When obtaining this consent, the patient and/or parent should be advised that the practitioner is unable to guarantee confidentiality of the material gleaned during the medical examination because a judge or other presiding court officer can rule that the practitioner should breach medical confidentiality. If photo documentation is to form part of the medical examination, the patient should be advised in advance of the means of storage and its potential uses (*see* Subheading 2.8.); specific written consent should then be sought for this procedure. The patient must be advised that he or she can stop the examination at any time.

2.5. Details of the Allegation

If the complainant has already provided the details of the allegation to another professional, for example, a police officer, it is not necessary for him or her to repeat the details to the forensic practitioner. Indeed, Hicks *(5)* notes that attempts to obtain too detailed a history of the incident from the complainant may jeopardize the case at trial because at the time of the medical examination the patient may be disturbed and, consequently, the details of the incident may be confused and conflict subsequent statements. The details of the allegation can be provided to the forensic practitioner by the third party and then clarified, if necessary, with the complainant. It may be difficult for the complainant to describe oral and anal penetrative sexual assaults, and the forensic practitioner may need to ask direct questions regarding these acts sensitively *(6)*.

2.6. Medical and Sexual History

The purpose of obtaining the medical and sexual history is essentially twofold: first, to identify any behavior or medical conditions that may cause the doctor to misinterpret the clinical findings, for example, menstrual bleeding; and second, to identify any medical problems that may be attributable to the sexual assault, for example, bleeding, pain, or discharge. Other specific details may be required if emergency contraception is being considered.

When children are examined, the parent or caregiver should provide comprehensive details of the past medical history. When adults are examined, only relevant medical and sexual history should be sought because confidentiality cannot be guaranteed. What constitutes relevant medical history must be determined on a case-by-case basis by considering the differential causes for any medical findings and the persistence data for the different sexual acts.

Forensic practitioners should not ask suspects about the alleged incident or their sexual history.

2.7. Nature of the Examination

2.7.1. General Examination

In all cases, a complete general medical examination should be conducted to document injuries and to note any disease that may affect the interpretation of the medical findings.

2.7.2. Anogenital Examination

Whenever there is a clear account of the alleged incident, the anogenital examination should be tailored to the individual case (e.g., if an adult complainant only describes being made to perform fellatio, there is usually no indication to examine the external genitalia). However, in some cases, the complainant may not be aware of the nature of the sexual assault. Furthermore, children and some adults may not have the language skills or may feel unable to provide a detailed account of the sexual acts at the initial interview. In such cases, a comprehensive anogenital examination should be undertaken if the patient or the person with legal authority to consent on behalf of the patient gives his or her consent.

2.8. Ownership and Handling of Photo Documentation

Any video or photographic material should be retained as part of the practitioner's confidential medical notes and stored in a locked cabinet a locked premises. To preserve anonymity, the material should be labeled both on the casing and within the video/photograph itself (by holding a card within the frame) using either a unique identification code or the patient's initials and the date of the examination. With the specific consent of the patient, the video/ photograph can be shown to other colleagues for second opinions, viewed by a named doctor providing expert testimony for the defense, and used for teaching purposes. The material should not be released to nonmedical parties except on the directions of the court.

3. BASIC PRINCIPLES OF THE FORENSIC ANALYSIS

The scientific examination at the forensic laboratory can provide information regarding:
- What sexual acts have occurred.
- The gender and possible identification of the assailant.
- Potential links with any other offenses.

3.1. Prevention of Contamination

To ensure that there is no accidental transfer of body fluids or fibers between the parties who have been involved in a sexual act, each complainant and each suspect should be transported in separate vehicles and examined in different locations by different forensic practitioners.

Because of the sensitivity of the techniques used to extract and analyze DNA, forensic practitioners should take all possible steps to ensure that their own cellular material does not contaminate the samples they obtain. Therefore, gloves must be worn throughout the forensic examination and changed when sampling different body areas. Some jurisdictions require that all used gloves should be retained and exhibited. In addition, the forensic physician should avoid talking, coughing, or sneezing over unsealed samples and should handle all samples as little as possible. If a doctor believes that there is a possibility that he or she will cough or sneeze over an unsheathed swab, a face mask should be worn when the sample is being obtained.

3.2. Collection of Forensic Samples

The swabs and containers used to collect forensic evidence differ from those used in clinical tests. The swabs should be made of fibers that readily release absorbed material *(7)*. The quality and integrity of any swab or container used to obtain a forensic sample must be ensured. The provision of sealed, standardized clinical forensic examination kits or modules ensures that these requirements can be guaranteed *(8,9)*.

Forensic swabs should be placed in plastic sheaths that do not contain transport media or in specially designed boxes that allow the swabs to air-dry. Blood and urine samples for drug and alcohol analysis should be placed in containers with a preservative that prevents decomposition and fermentation (e.g., sodium fluoride), and the container for the blood sample should also contain an anticoagulant (e.g., potassium oxalate). The blood sample for DNA analysis and, where still applicable, conventional grouping, should be placed in a container with the appropriate preservative (e.g., ethylene diaminetetra-acetic acid). Because many of the samples are subsequently frozen, all the containers should be shatterproof.

Only sealed, disposable instruments (e.g., proctoscopes, specula, scissors, and forceps) should be used to retrieve forensic samples. All instruments used in the sampling process should be retained. However, if storage space is restricted, then any used proctoscopes or specula may be swabbed and only the swabs retained for later forensic sampling.

Sterile water may be used to moisten the proctoscope/speculum to facilitate its insertion into a body orifice. Other lubricants should not be used when body fluid analysis or lubricant identification may be pertinent to the case (*see* Heading 11 on Lubricants).

3.3. Controls

An unopened swab from each batch should be retained and sent with the samples as a control for that batch of swabs.

If any water is used in the sampling process, the remaining water in the ampule or an unused swab moistened with some of the water should be retained as a control sample for the water.

3.4. Packaging and Continuity

Any retrieved items must be packaged quickly and efficiently to prevent accidental loss of material and minimize decomposition of the sample. The use of bags with integral tamper-evident seals is recommended to prove that the sample has not been contaminated with exogenous substances since it was sealed. The exhibit should be labeled with the site of the sample, the date and time (24-h clock) it was obtained, and the name of the examinee. Again, the use of bags with integral labels will prevent accidental detachment of this vital information (*see* Fig. 1). Each exhibit is also labeled with an exhibit identification code, usually formed by the forensic practitioner's initials and a number reflecting the order in which the samples were obtained. The latter is particularly important when more than one sample has been obtained from the same site *(7)*. Every exhibit should be signed by the person who first handled

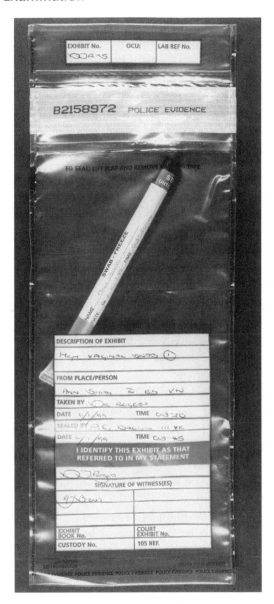

Fig. 1. Exhibit bag with integral label and tamper-evident seal.

the sample and by the person who sealed the package (this may be the same person). It is good practice for others who subsequently handle the exhibit to sign the label also, so that, if necessary, they can be called to court to explain their part in collection, transport, and storage *(10)*.

The clothing worn by the complainant during or after the incident may be an invaluable source of information in terms of the nature of the assault (e.g., damage to clothing and body fluid stains) and the identification of the assailant. Even stains on clothing that has been washed have been found to contain sufficient spermatozoa to produce a DNA profile *(11)*. Clothing should be placed in bags made of material, such as paper, that prevents the accumulation of condensation, which could accelerate decomposition of body fluids. Submitted clothing should be sealed and labeled as described previously. When the clothing is overtly wet or possibly contaminated with accelerants, the forensic science laboratory should be asked for advice on packaging and storage. The following additional information should then be recorded on the appropriate label:

- Which items were worn during the offense.
- Which items were removed and not replaced.
- Which items were removed and replaced.
- Which new items were worn after the offense.

The forensic scientist must be provided with salient information regarding the incident and subsequent actions of the complainant in order to determine the type of forensic analysis required. A useful means of transmitting this information is via a pro forma (*see* Fig. 2).

3.5. Analysis

Identification microscopy (e.g., spermatozoa), comparison microscopy (e.g., hairs and fibers), serological analyses (e.g., conventional ABO grouping or species identification), and biochemical analyses (e.g., phosphoglucomutase) have played a fundamental role in the investigation of crime for many years and are still used today in some circumstances. However, discovery of the specificity of an individual's DNA profile has considerably enhanced the information that can be provided by a forensic science service for connecting a person to an offense and linking offenses to each other. Although a detailed consideration of current DNA techniques is beyond the scope of this chapter, a general understanding of the terms and techniques will benefit the forensic practitioner.

Except for identical twins, each person's nuclear DNA is unique. An individual's gender and DNA profile may be obtained from any of his or her body fluids or tissues (e.g., blood, semen, and bones). The current technical process employed for DNA profiling is termed short tandem repeat (STR) analysis. STR loci are a class of polymorphic markers consisting of simple repeated sequences of 1–6 base pairs in length. STRs are present throughout the human genome (DNA), occurring, on average, every 6–10 kb along the

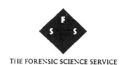

MEDX1B

THE FORENSIC SCIENCE SERVICE

All sections of this form must be completed and a copy forwarded to the laboratory
Please print in capitals using ball-point pen and tick the appropriate boxes.

INFORMATION FORM for the examination of Complainant
Use for submission with sexual offences samples (1 per person)

GENERAL INFORMATION		FME case reference:

Name of Medical Examiner:

Contact telephone number:

Name of Subject:

Age	Sex	M	F	Weight

Date & time of incident: Date & time of examination:
(Please use 24 hour clock)

Date & time of other <u>relevant</u> sexual activity within previous 10 days.

Items used in previous intercourse.   Sheath   Spermicide   Lubricant

Other (Specify)

SPECIFIC INFORMATION RELATING TO THE ALLEGED OFFENCE

Penile/Oral penetration	No	Yes
Penile/Vaginal penetration	No	Yes
Penile/Anal penetration	No	Yes
Object penetration	No	Yes (specify)
Ejaculation onto skin/hair	No	Yes (site)
Kissed /licked /bitten (circle relevant action)	No	Yes (site)
Condom / lubricant /spermicide used	No	Yes (specify)
Menstrual bleeding	No	Yes
Bleeding due to genital/anal injury	No	Yes (specify)
The following removed / inserted:	Pad	Tampon Sponge Diaphragm
Other relevant injuries	No	Yes (specify)
Showered/washed/bathed/douched	No	Yes (specify)
Genital/anal/relevant skin area wiped	No	Yes (how)
Anal intercourse: defaecated since offence	No	Yes
Oral intercourse: mouth cleansed since offence	No	Yes
	Drink	Mouth wash Toothbrush

TOXICOLOGY INFORMATION
Was alcohol consumed?   No   Yes   Not known
If Yes please specify   prior   during   after   offence

Start time of drinking: End time of drinking:

Quantity and type of alcoholic beverage consumed:

If known, please specify the time of previous urination (i.e. time of urination prior to the specimen provided in this examination)

Date: Time:

Have any drugs (prescribed or otherwise) been used by/administered to the subject within 4 days of the examination?

No   Yes   Not known   If Yes please specify   prior   during   after   offence

Give details:

Are other substances suspected of having been used/administered, which could be relevant to the offence?

No   Yes   Not known   If Yes please specify   prior   during   after   offence

Give details:

FURTHER INFORMATION (Continue on MEDX1C if necessary)

Signature of Medical Examiner	Date

Fig. 2. Proforma used to relay relevant information to forensic scientist. (Reproduced with permission of the members of the Joint Working Party [A.C.P.O., A.P.S., F.S.S., and M.P.S.] for the design of an examination kit for sexual offenses).

DNA and may exhibit a high degree of length variation resulting from differences in the number of repeat units displayed by individuals. Their abundance and hypervariability make them ideal markers for the identification of an individual. When a DNA STR analysis is performed, the specific areas of interest on the molecule are initially targeted. Multiple copies of these areas are then produced using polymerase chain reaction (PCR) techniques, which amplify minute amounts of DNA. The DNA pieces are then sorted according to their size, producing the individual's DNA STR profile *(12)*.

DNA STR analysis, including a DNA sex test *(13)*, is now part of the routine forensic assessment of biological samples in Europe and is replacing both traditional serological analysis of blood groups and classical single- and multi-locus DNA fingerprinting *(12)*. The formation of the European DNA Profiling Group has led to standardization of DNA analysis procedures used in the European community and associated western European countries. The current standard system focuses on analysis of 10 STR loci and is known as AMPflSTR® SGMPlus™. This system contains all of the Interpol and European Networks Forensic Science International (ENFSI)-recommended European loci, which provides points of comparison for DNA intelligence purposes outside of the United Kingdom *(14–21)*. When DNA profiling was first applied to forensic science, large amounts of nucleated material were required. However, the use of PCR technology has enabled much smaller amounts of material to be analyzed. Furthermore, when there are only small amounts of DNA, a technique termed low copy number (LCN) may be used to obtain an STR profile. LCN is a handcrafted, highly sensitive extension of the AMPflSTR® SGMPlus™ that has led to an increase in the sample types suitable for DNA testing, which, in turn, can provide valuable intelligence to the police *(22)*. Because DNA is physically much more resistant to degradation than proteins, it is even possible to analyze degraded samples *(23)*.

Fluorescence *in situ* hybridization (FISH) is a new technology that uses a Y-specific DNA probe to label male epithelial cells. Once identified, the cells may be separated from the rest of the sample and submitted for DNA profiling. Without separation, the profile may be dominated by the DNA from the examinee, making it difficult to interpret. As yet, it is unclear how useful this tool will be in the forensic setting (*see* Subheadings 5.1.2.3. and 8.5.2.2.).

Mitochondrial DNA analysis has been used in forensic casework. This technique examines the DNA contained within mitochondria and obviates the need for nuclear material. Because mitochondrial DNA is only passed from mother to child (unlike nuclear DNA, there is no contribution from the father), all the descendants along the maternal line will have the same mitochondrial DNA. The technique is best suited to discrete samples, such as hairs without roots and fecal material, and is not ideal for mixtures of body fluids, particularly when the complainant's body fluid is likely to be present in larger quantities than that of the assailant (Tully, G., personal communication, 1998). Therefore, in sexual offenses, the selection of material to be analyzed by this technique is limited and its use needs careful consideration.

The forensic science laboratory must be notified when it is alleged that people who are closely related have been involved in a sexual offense, because their profiles will have greater similarity than profiles from individuals picked at random, and further differentiating tests may need to be performed.

4. Skin

The comments in this section refer to nongenital skin. For genital and perianal skin, *see* Headings 8–10.

4.1. Forensic Evidence

4.1.1. Method of Sampling

All areas of unwashed skin that have been licked, kissed, sucked, bitten, or ejaculated on by either the assailant or the complainant must be sampled. Cellular material, amenable to DNA profiling techniques, has also been identified where there has been skin-to-skin contact (e.g., manual strangulation or gripping the arm) (*[24]* and Burgess, Z., personal communication, 2001). Therefore, when dealing with an assault conducted by an unknown assailant, consideration should be given to sampling marks or injuries on the skin that the complainant attributes to direct contact by the offender. However, the problem with this type of sampling is there is considerable lack of understanding about issues of transfer and persistence *(24)*. Consequently, speculative skin swabbing in the absence of visible marks or injuries is not recommended.

Although several techniques, including the use of surgical gauze pads *(25)* and cigarette papers *(26)*, have been employed to recover saliva and other trace evidence from the skin with variable success, the use of sterile swabs is the most widely used technique that has received international endorsement *(27)*. If the skin appears moist, the stain should be retrieved on dry swabs, which are then placed in sheaths without transport medium. The double-swab technique, described by Sweet et al., is the recommended method to recover dried stains or possible cellular material from skin *(28)*. When using this technique, sterile water is used to wet completely the cotton tip of the first swab. The tip of the swab is then rolled over the area of skin using circular motions while rotating the swab on its long axis to ensure maximum contact between the skin and the swab. Then, a second dry swab is rolled over the same area to absorb the water left on the skin by the initial swab and collect any remaining cells. Minimal pressure should be applied to prevent exfoliation of the patient's own epithelial cells. The forensic practitioner should use as many swabs as necessary to remove any visible stain (repeating wet swab followed by dry swab). If no stain is visible, two swabs will suffice (the first wet; the second dry). The swabs are then placed in sheaths without transport medium.

Some authors comment that ultraviolet (UV) light causes fluorescence of semen and saliva and advocate its use in determining the areas of skin to be swabbed (29,30). This advice must be interpreted cautiously, because a study by Santucci and colleagues found that although many creams and ointments fluoresced when exposed to a Wood's lamp (wavelength 360 nm), none of the 28 semen samples examined did (31). In addition, other authors have commented that detergents, lubricants (particularly those that contain petroleum jelly), and milk also fluoresce (32).

However, when semen stains are exposed to a high-intensity light source of variable wavelengths (e.g., the Polilight®) and viewed using goggles to block the strong excitation light, then semen may be detectable, even when the background surface is fluorescent (33). Furthermore, the location of the stain may be recorded using photography.

A recent experiment by Marshall and colleagues found that semen from a single donor could be detected on skin using several excitation wavelengths (emitted by a Poliray®) and emission filter combinations (34). Optimal results were obtained using 415 nm ± 40 nm band-pass filter and a 475 high-pass and 505 band-pass ± 40 nm interference filter. More research must be conducted using semen from multiple donors and isolating semen from other fluorescing contaminants, such as oils.

Furthermore, Nelson and Santucci have recently described training forensic physicians to use an alternative light source (the Bluemaxx BM500) to identify semen (100% sensitivity) and to differentiate it from other products (35).

4.1.2. Forensic Analysis

The most common reason for forensic analysis of skin swabs is after licking, kissing, or biting of the skin. Forensic analysis for other body fluids or exogenous substances is considered elsewhere in the chapter.

4.1.2.1. Detection of Saliva

The only means of confirming the presence of saliva on the skin is by detecting the enzyme amylase. However, in practice, this enzyme is not usually found in high enough concentrations in samples removed from the skin (Austin, C., personal communication, 2002).

4.1.2.2. Identification of the Assailant

The preferred method for the forensic assessment of a possible saliva sample is the use of DNA STR analysis. Although it may be possible to determine the ABO-secretor status of the sample submitted, the test is only relevant if the saliva originates from one of the 80% of the population who secrete their ABO blood group in their body fluids.

4.1.3. Persistence Data

There is only limited information available regarding the persistence of body fluids and cellular material on the skin of the living. A DNA STR profile matching the assailant has been obtained from a swab of unwashed facial skin 6 hours after an assault where it was alleged that the assailant salivated over the complainant's skin (Austin, C., personal communication, 2002). Rutty studied the transference and survivability of human DNA after simulated manual strangulation. Although this study found that when using the LCN technique DNA was recoverable from either the victim's neck or the offender's fingers for at least 10 days after the contact, the author stressed that this apparent persistence may have resulted from secondary or tertiary transfer from other individuals or objects (the study subjects worked in the same building and shared the same bathroom and kitchen facilities during the period of the study) *(24)*.

Sweet and colleagues have shown that it is possible to obtain a DNA profile from saliva stains (corresponding to a bite mark) on cadaver skin when the saliva was deposited up to 48 hours earlier *(*Austin, C., personal communication, and ref. *36)*. This study showed that the amount of recoverable material diminished with time; hence, it is prudent to sample the relevant body areas as soon as possible after the offense.

4.2. Medical Evidence

On average, 40% of complainants of sexual assaults will have no general injuries *(37–41)*. Of those who are injured, most will have only minor injuries, which will fade rapidly or heal without a trace *(37,38)*. Nonetheless, the whole body must be thoroughly inspected for stains (e.g., dirt and blood), injuries (including signs of substance use), skin disease, and scars (including self-inflicted injuries). All injuries must be described using the recognized nomenclature described in Chapter 4 and recorded in terms of site (measured, if possible, from a fixed bony point), two-dimensional size, covering surface (e.g., scabbing, bleeding, or swelling), and color. The body surfaces should then be palpated and a note made of the site and approximate size of any tender areas. More credence will be given to a finding of tenderness if it is verified later in the consultation (ideally while the patient is distracted) or at a follow-up assessment, particularly if a bruise becomes apparent. All negative observations should also be recorded.

If the person can identify an injury that he or she believes was caused by a true bite, as opposed to a suction or "love-bite," or if the examination reveals an injury that has features that are suggestive of a bite, arrangements must be made for the area to be professionally photographed so that the injury can be considered by a forensic odontologist. Several studies have reported that the female breasts are bitten in 7–19% of sexual offenses *(42,43)*.

Preprinted body diagrams are useful for recording injuries. Although the original diagram is part of the forensic practitioner's contemporaneous record, copies may be appended to the statement or to the forms sent to the forensic scientist. The latter may use the diagrams to direct the forensic assessment (e.g., if the patient was bitten, the scientist will refer to the diagram to determine where to commence the search for saliva on any clothing that may have been contaminated concurrently).

5. HAIR: HEAD AND PUBIC

5.1. Forensic Evidence

Hair is most commonly sampled to detect body fluids or retrieve foreign hairs or particles. It has been known for many decades that numerous ingested, prescribed, and illicit drugs (e.g., barbiturates, amphetamines, opiates, cocaine, benzodiazepines, γ-hydroxy butyrate, and cannabis) are deposited in the hair *(44)*. Although toxicology of hair was originally used to detect drugs that had been repeatedly ingested, recent advances in analytical techniques have meant that toxicology may be useful after single-dose ingestion as would occur in a substance-facilitated sexual assault *(45,46)*. This is particularly pertinent because complainants of possible drug-facilitated sexual assaults frequently do not report the incident expeditiously because of amnesia and/or doubt about what might have happened, and drugs may be accessible to analysis for longer periods in hair compared to blood or urine *(47)*. In addition, it may be used as a reference sample for DNA analysis.

5.1.1. Method of Sampling

5.1.1.1. Cutting

Hairs should be sampled by cutting if they appear to be contaminated by material that has the potential to have forensic significance (e.g., semen). If the patient does not consent to having the contaminated hairs cut or if it is not practical to cut them because of the extent of foreign material contamination, then the relevant areas can be swabbed (follow method of sampling given under Subheading 4.1.1.).

For drug analysis, approx 50 hairs should be cut close to the scalp at least 7 days after the substance-facilitated sexual assault *(48)*. The ideal site for sampling is the crown of the head, although this may not be acceptable to the complainant. The hairs must be kept in line, with the cut end demarcated by a rubber band. The sampled hairs are then wrapped in aluminum foil.

5.1.1.2. Combing

Any foreign particles or hairs identified on the head or pubic hair should be collected with forceps and submitted for analysis. It is no longer considered necessary to comb the head hair routinely, because these samples are infrequently examined by forensic scientists (Lewington, F., personal communication, 1994) or are rarely pivotal to the case *(49,50)*. However, if a balaclava or other article was worn on the head during the assault, the hair should be sampled with low-adhesive tape, which is then attached to acetate *(51)*.

Pubic hairs may be transferred between individuals during sexual inter-course. Exline et al. *(52)* studied volunteer heterosexual couples who combed their pubic hairs immediately after sexual intercourse in the "missionary" posi-tion. Even under such optimal collection conditions, pubic hair transfers were only observed 17.3% of the time using macroscopic and microscopic compari-sons. Pubic hair transfer to males (23.6%) was more common than transfer to females (10.9%).

Some studies on sexual offense case material have shown lower rates of pubic hair transfer between complainant and assailant. Mann *(53)* reported that only 4% of female complainants and no male complainants were identified as having pubic hairs consistent with the assailant hairs isolated from combings of the pubic hair, and Stone *(54)* identified foreign pubic hairs among the pubic hair combings of 2% of the complainants studied. However, a survey of sexual offense case material submitted to laboratories throughout the United States *(55)* found pubic hairs that associated the complainant and the assailant in 15% of cases. Therefore, the authors advocate that the complainant's/suspect's pubic hairs should routinely be combed onto a piece of uncontaminated paper (A4 size), with the complainant in the semilithotomy position; the paper enclosing the comb should be folded inward and submitted for analysis. Other loose pubic hairs on the complainant that are macroscopically different from his or her own pubic hairs can be collected with sterile forceps and submitted for forensic analysis.

5.1.1.3. Reference Sample for DNA Analysis

If it is not possible to obtain buccal cells or a blood sample, then one can seek the examinee's consent to obtain 10–25 head hairs with attached roots (plucked individually while wearing gloves) for use as the reference sample. It is never necessary to pluck pubic hair.

5.1.2. Forensic Analysis

5.1.2.1. Chemical Analysis

Chemical analysis may be relevant if the hair has been dyed or contaminated with exogenous substances, such as a lubricant or hairspray.

5.1.2.2. Comparison Microscopy

Although this was the standard method of hair analysis, discrimination of hairs by microscopic means alone yields limited information in terms of assailant identification. Therefore, although retrieved foreign hairs and pubic hair combings should be saved, it is no longer necessary to obtain control samples routinely from the complainant, although they may be required from a defendant in custody. In the rare circumstance that it should become necessary to perform comparison microscopy, a control sample from the complainant can be obtained later.

5.1.2.3. DNA Analysis

Because of the improved sensitivity provided by PCR techniques and the development of mitochondrial DNA analysis, stronger, more objective conclusions in terms of assailant identification can be reached from hairs both with and without roots (56).

Research has recently been undertaken to determine if FISH technology could be used to identify the gender of retrieved hair. The research has demonstrated that there is a potential forensic application in sexual offense cases where microscopy cannot determine the source of the hair (57).

5.1.2.4. Drug Analysis

Only specialist laboratories offer hair analysis because hair specimens are not suitable for comprehensive drug screens and the sample is quickly consumed in testing for a few drugs (58–60). It must be noted that hair cannot be tested for alcohol.

5.1.3. Persistence Data

There are no data on how long after the assault foreign pubic hairs have been retrieved from a complainant. Although spermatozoa have been recovered from head hair that was washed (61), there are no detailed data regarding the persistence of spermatozoa on the hair regarding time since assault.

Hair grows at a rate of 0.7–1.5 cm/30 d (48). Cutting the hair will eventually remove the section of hair where the drugs have been deposited.

5.2. Medical Evidence

Occasionally, head or pubic hairs may have been accidentally or deliberately pulled out during a sexual assault; the identification of bleeding hair follicles and/or broken hairs would support this complaint.

6. NAILS

6.1. Forensic Evidence

During the course of a sexual assault, trace materials, such as skin, body fluids, hairs, fibers, and soil, can collect under the fingernails of both the complainant and the assailant. The latter deserve particular attention because digital vaginal penetration is alleged to have occurred in nearly one in five (18%) of the sexual assault cases submitted for analysis to the Forensic Science Service (FSS); frequently, this is a precursor to another penetrative act (Newton, M., personal communication, 2003). A study undertaken by Neville in a forensic laboratory found that 38% of individuals have DNA from someone other than themselves under their fingernails and several cases submitted to the FSS have produced a DNA match between the complainant and the assailant from the material recovered from the fingernails (Moore, E., and Harris, E., personal communication, 1998; Neville, S., personal communication, 2002).

Therefore, fingernail samples should be obtained from the complainant if the circumstances of the offense suggest that trace material may be present; for example, if there has been a struggle or if the details of the assault are uncertain and the forensic practitioner, in observing the complainant's hands, notices material of interest under or on the surface of the nails. They should also be considered if a fingernail broke during the offense and the broken section may be recovered from the scene. Samples should be obtained from the suspect if it is alleged that his or her hands had direct contact with the female genitalia or if he or she scratched the complainant.

6.1.1. Method of Sampling

The optimal sample is clippings of the whole fingernail as these are more practical to handle. However, in some cases, the fingernails may be too short to cut or the complainant may withhold consent for the sample; complainants who cherish their well manicured nails may find the proposal distressing, and the examiner must be sensitive to this. In such cases, scrapings of the material under the nails should be taken using a tapered stick or both sides of the fingernails should be swabbed using the double-swab technique (*see* Subheading 4.1.1.). When obtaining fingernail scrapings, the forensic practitioner should try not to disturb the nail bed (Clayton, T., personal communication, 2003).

Each hand should be sampled and specimens packaged separately enclosing the stick (enveloped in a piece of folded paper), if used.

On the rare occasions when a nail has broken during the incident and the broken fragment of nail is recovered, the residual nail on the relevant finger should be clipped within 24 hours to enable comparison of nail striations *(62)*. If it is not clear which finger the broken nail came from, then it may be necessary to clip and submit all the macroscopically broken nails, as the fingernail striations are individual to a particular finger.

6.1.2. Forensic Analysis

The fingernail samples may be examined microscopically for any visible staining. The nails would then be swabbed to remove any possible body fluids and the material submitted for DNA analysis.

6.1.3. Persistence

Lederer reported recovery of DNA matching the complainant from a suspect's fingernails 2 days after the alleged digital penetration occurred; the suspect denied any form of contact and claimed to have washed his hands several times during the elapsed period *(63)*.

6.2. Medical Examination

The length and any damage to fingernails should be noted.

7. ORAL CAVITY

Although the oral cavity may be injured in several ways during a sexual assault, the specific sexual acts that may result in forensic or medical evidence are fellatio, cunnilingus, and anilingus.

7.1. Fellatio

7.1.1. Definition

Fellatio (also referred to as irrumation) is a sexual activity in which the penis is placed in the mouth; sexual stimulation is achieved by sucking on the penis while it moves in and out of the oral cavity. Ejaculation may or may not occur.

7.1.2. Frequency

7.1.2.1. Consensual

Fellatio is part of the sexual repertoire of heterosexual and male homo-sexual couples. A study of 1025 women attending a genitourinary clinic found that 55% practiced fellatio occasionally and 15% practiced fellatio often *(64)*.

7.1.2.2. Nonconsensual

Fellatio is not an infrequent component of a sexual assault sometimes occurring in isolation but occurring more frequently in conjunction with other sexual acts *(6)*. Among the 1507 (1403 females, 104 males) sexual assault cases submitted to the Metropolitan Police Laboratory, London, during 1988 and 1989, 17% of the females and 14% of the males described performing fellatio and 31% of the males had fellatio performed on them during the sexual assault *(65)*.

7.1.3. Legal Implications

The legal definitions of many jurisdictions, including England and Wales, consider nonconsensual fellatio to be analogous to nonconsensual penile penetration of the vagina and anus *(66,67)*.

7.1.4. Forensic Evidence

7.1.4.1. Method of Sampling

1. After oral–penile contact, the oral cavity should be sampled when fellatio was performed during the sexual assault or in circumstances in which the details of the incident are unknown. There is no current worldwide consensus as to which is the best sampling method.

    Possible techniques include saliva collection (ideally 10 mL), application of swabs, gauze pads *(68)*, or filter paper *(69)*, and oral rinses using 10 mL of distilled water (Newman, J., personal communication, 1998). Willott and Crosse *(70)* reported that spermatozoa are found more often in the saliva sample compared with mouth swabs, but also highlight several cases in which spermatozoa were recovered from swabs taken from specific areas of the oral cavity (e.g., under the tongue, the roof of the mouth, and the lips).

    Although no studies have investigated the order in which the samples should be taken, the authors' practice is to obtain 10 mL of saliva as the first sample. Then two swabs in sequence are rubbed over the inner and outer gum margins (with particular attention to the margins around the teeth); over the hard and, where tolerated, soft palate; on the inside of the cheeks and lips; and over both surfaces of the tongue. The mouth is then rinsed with 10 mL of sterile water, which is retained in a bottle as the final sample. The samples can be obtained by a police officer or other attending professional before the arrival of the forensic practitioner, minimizing any delay.

Spermatozoa have also been recovered from dentures and other fixtures that have remained *in situ* during fellatio. Although the optimum exhibit for the forensic scientist would be the dental fixture itself but, understandably, this may not be acceptable to the complainant. A compromise would be to swab the dental fixture. Interestingly, sufficient spermatozoa for a DNA profile have also been recovered using standard extraction techniques from chewing gum that was retained in the mouth during nonconsensual fellatio *(68)*. In this case, the gauze pad obtained at the scene of the incident and the oral swabs obtained subsequently during the medical were negative.

2. DNA reference sample: Buccal cells are the preferred DNA reference sample from both suspect and complainant. The buccal cells are obtained by firmly rubbing a special swab over the inside of the cheek.
3. Determination of the secretor status: A sample of saliva is used as the reference sample for the secretor status. This sample is no longer a requirement in the United Kingdom.

7.1.4.2. Forensic Analysis

After actual or possible oral ejaculation, the sample is initially examined microscopically to identify spermatozoa (*see* Subheading 8.5.2.1.) followed by DNA analysis.

7.1.4.3. Persistence Data

Rapid retrieval of the forensic samples from the oral cavity is of paramount importance because of the limited period that spermatozoa remain in this orifice. Even though the maximum persistence of spermatozoa in the oral cavity is recorded as 28–31 hours, only a few spermatozoa are detected unless the sample is taken within a few hours of ejaculation *(71)*. Consequently, the forensic exhibits must be collected as soon as an allegation of nonconsensual fellatio is made, and law enforcement agencies should be instructed accordingly. In the United Kingdom, an early evidence kit is available for use by the first response police officer; this is particularly beneficial in cases where there may be a time delay before a medical examination can occur.

Although rinsing of the mouth, drinking, and brushing of teeth do not necessarily remove all traces of spermatozoa *(72)*, such activities should be discouraged until the samples have been obtained. Spermatozoa have also been recovered from toothbrushes used by complainants to cleanse the mouth after fellatio (forensic scientists, personal communication, 1998). The use of interdental toothbrushes may enhance the retrieval of spermatozoa from the interdental spaces, and research in this area is currently underway in the United Kingdom.

In acts of fellatio, it is common for the semen to be spat or vomited onto clothing where it will remain until washed. Therefore, any potentially contaminated clothing or scene samples should be submitted for forensic examination.

7.1.5. Medical Evidence

Because a significant proportion of the population performs consensual fellatio, anecdotal accounts from oral surgeons suggest that palatal lesions consequent to such acts are rarely identified during routine casework, although this may be a result of the rapid resolution of the injuries. Nevertheless, several case reports have documented palatal lesions after fellatio. Areas of petechial hemorrhage and confluent bruising have been described on the soft palate and at the junction between the hard and soft palates after consensual fellatio (73–75). These areas of bruising vary from discrete single or bilateral lesions of 1.0–1.5 cm in diameter, located on or either side of the midline (74), to larger bands of bruising that cross the midline (73,75). The bruises are painless and resolve in 7–10 days (73,74), although they may reappear with repeated fellatio (74).

A forensic practitioner may be asked to explain to the court why these bruises occur. Although the precise mechanism is unknown, the following hypotheses have been proffered:

1. Repeated contraction of the palatal muscles: As the penis touches the palatal mucosa, the gag reflex is activated, with resultant contraction of the soft palate and other constrictor muscles of the pharynx. It is suggested that the combination of retching and repeated palatal movements causes rupture of the blood vessels in the highly vascular palatal mucosa (73).
2. Sucking: Sucking on the penis produces a negative intraoral pressure, which is postulated to cause rupture of the blood vessels in the palatal mucosa. This theory is supported by the anecdotal accounts of oral surgeons who found petechial hemorrhages on the palates of children who "made a habit of forceful sucking into a drinking glass" (74).
3. Blunt trauma: Case reports describe palatal bruises subsequent to sexual assaults wherein a digit or digits have been forced into the mouth (76). However, there is no specific evidence to support the hypothesis that direct blunt trauma from a penis can cause palatal bruising.

Erythema and an erosion of the hard palate have also been described after fellatio (74,75), but the reliability of such findings is questionable. Indeed, in one such case, the mucositis was eventually diagnosed as oral candidiasis contracted from direct contact with an infected penis (75).

Other nonsexual causes for similar palatal lesions include infectious mononucleosis; local trauma (e.g., hard food stuffs or ill-fitting dentures); paroxysms of vomiting, coughing, or sneezing; playing a wind instrument; tumors; and bleeding diatheses *(77)*. Therefore, whenever palatal bruising, erythema, or erosions are identified during the examination of a complainant who may have been subjected to fellatio, alternative explanations should be excluded by taking a detailed medical, dental, and social history; conducting a comprehensive general examination; and, where necessary, undertaking relevant special investigations.

Whenever a complaint of nonconsensual fellatio is made, the head and face must be carefully examined because there may be other injuries around the oral cavity that support the allegation, such as bruises on the face and neck or lacerations of the frenula *(78)*.

7.2. Cunnilingus and Anilingus

7.2.1. Definitions

Cunnilingus (*cunnilinctus*) is the sexual activity in which the female genitalia are licked, sucked, or rubbed by the lips and/or tongue.

Anilingus (analingus or "rimming") is the sexual activity in which the anus is licked, sucked, or rubbed by the lips and/or tongue.

7.2.2. Frequency

7.2.2.1. Consensual

Interviews with 18,876 individuals (44% male) aged 16–59 years in the United Kingdom revealed that 66–72% had experienced cunnilingus *(79)*. Although it is not known how many heterosexual and homosexual couples engage in consensual anilingus, 15% of the women questioned in one study acknowledged erotic feelings with anal stimulation, which, for the majority, included anilingus *(80)*.

7.2.2.2. Nonconsensual

Cunnilingus is alleged to have occurred in only 3–9% of reported sexual assaults *(6,81)*. There are no published reports regarding the number of incidents involving anilingus; anecdotal case material suggests that it is rare.

7.2.3. Legal Implications

In some jurisdictions, penetration of the vagina or anus with the tongue during nonconsensual cunnilingus or anilingus is considered to be legally analogous to nonconsensual penile penetration of the vagina and anus (South Carolina and Rhode Island) *(66,67)*. The British Parliament has recently created a new offense of "assault by penetration," which is defined as nonconsensual penetration of the anus or genitalia by an object or a body part. This new offense attracts the same maximum penalty as rape.

7.2.4. Forensic Evidence

7.2.4.1. Method of Sampling

See Headings 8 and 10 for more detailed information.

7.2.4.2. Forensic Analysis and Persistence Data

Traditionally, the detection of the enzyme amylase on vulval and vaginal swabs was considered confirmatory evidence of the presence of saliva. However, in 1992, a study conducted at the Metropolitan Police Laboratory, London, using vaginal swabs from volunteer female donors who had not participated in cunnilingus revealed high levels of endogenous amylase *(82)*. Furthermore, amylase has been specifically isolated from cervical mucus *(83)*. Therefore, the FSS in London no longer routinely tests for amylase in such cases. Instead, DNA analysis is undertaken on the vulval and/or vaginal swabs. If the assailant's DNA profile is obtained, it can be used to support an allegation of cunnilingus, although, obviously, the precise interpretation will depend on whether the complainant was subjected to other sexual acts that could account for the presence of the DNA (e.g., ejaculation). There are no published persistence data regarding the maximum time it is possible to obtain the assailant's DNA pattern from the female genitalia after cunnilingus/anilingus.

There are no published data regarding the possibility of obtaining the complainant's DNA STR profile from a swab or saliva sample taken from the assailant's oral cavity or lips after an allegation of cunnilingus or anilingus. Correspondence with numerous forensic biologists has not revealed any cases in which this has been undertaken, and the general consensus among these experts is that it is unlikely that such samples would isolate sufficient material for forensic analysis because of the usual time delay between the sexual act and the obtaining of the samples from the suspect and the limited number of vaginal cells that are likely to be present. Indeed, this presumption appears to be supported by the work of Banaschak et al. *(84)*, who found mixed DNA STR patterns in five samples obtained from five couples who had kissed for 2 minutes. However, in all cases, the kissing partner's DNA STR pattern was only identifiable in the samples immediately after kissing (maximum 60 seconds), and no mixed DNA STR patterns were identified when the volunteers were retested at 5 minutes.

7.2.5. Medical Evidence

Repeated thrusting of the tongue over the edges of the mandibular incisors during cunnilingus or anilingus may cause ulceration of the lingual frenulum, which completely heals within 7 days *(85)*. Such lesions should be specifically sought during the examination of the suspect's oral cavity when such an act has been described by the complainant or when the precise details of the assault are unknown.

8. FEMALE GENITALIA

8.1. Frequency

Penile–vaginal intercourse is the most common sexual act performed between heterosexuals. A UK survey of the sexual practices of 10,492 females aged between 16 and 59 years found that only 5.7% of them had never experienced heterosexual penile–vaginal intercourse *(86)*. A more recent survey of sexual attitudes and lifestyles undertaken between 1999 and 2001 found that 30% of the men and 26% of the women reported first heterosexual intercourse before the legal age of consent (16 years in the United Kingdom) *(87)*.

8.2. Legal Implications

Although in English law the legal definition of "rape" relates to nonconsensual penile penetration of the mouth, anus, or vagina, a new offense of assault by penetration has been recently created to cover nonconsensual penetration of the anus or the genitalia by an object or a body part; this new offense has the same maximum sentence as rape. In Scotland, nonconsensual penile–vaginal penetration is defined by common law as "carnal knowledge of a female by a male against her will" *(88)*. Other jurisdictions, such as some American states, define all penetrative acts as sexual assaults subcategorized by the degree of force and coercion used. In many jurisdictions, the legal interpretation of "vaginal penetration" refers to penetration of the labia and does not require that the penis actually enter the vagina *(89)*.

The age at which a female can legally give consent for penile–vaginal intercourse varies from country to country; for example, in England, the age of consent is 16 years, whereas in California, it is 18 years *(90)*.

8.3. Anatomy

The external female genitalia (vulva) includes the mons pubis, the labia majora, the labia minora, the clitoris, and the vestibule (which incorporates the openings of the urethra and the vagina).

The hymen is the tissue that partially or completely surrounds the opening of the vagina. It appears that all females have hymenal tissue present at birth (91). The hymen may be annular (encircling the vaginal opening), crescentic (present at the lateral and posterior margins), fimbriated (frilly edged), or, usually after childbirth, present only as interrupted tags or remnants. It is important that the reader refer to atlases that illustrate these variations (2,92). There is usually a single opening in the hymen. Uncommon congenital variants include two or more hymenal openings, referred to as septate or cribriform, respectively, and, rarely, complete absence of an opening (imperforate hymen).

Indentations or splits in the hymenal rim have been variously described as deficits, concavities, transections, clefts, notches, and, when clearly of recent origin, tears or lacerations (fresh and healed). In this text, the term *notch* will be used to describe divisions or splits in the hymenal rim. Superficial notches have been defined as notches that are less than or equal to half the width of the hymenal rim at the location of the notch, and deep notches have been defined as notches that are more than half the width of the hymenal rim at the location of the notch (93). Superficial notches of all aspects of the hymen have been described in both prepubertal (0–8 years) and postpubertal females (9.5–28 years) who have no history of sexual activity (93–96). Notches ranging from 0.5 mm to 3 mm in depth were noted in the ventral half of the hymens of 35% of newborns examined by Berenson; this study does not subcategorize the notches as superficial or deep. Deep notches of the anterior and lateral aspects of the hymen have been found in 14 of 200 postpubertal females (9.5–28 years) who denied having sexual activity (96). Deep notches of the posterior hymenal margin have not been described in prepubertal females screened for abuse. Deep notches of the hymenal margin have been described among postpubertal females who deny having sexual activity, although because these females were not screened for abuse, it is not possible to state whether these were the result of unreported sexual abuse.

The other pertinent anatomic landmarks in this area are the posterior fourchette (where the labia minora unite posteriorly), the fossa navicularis (a relatively concave area of the vestibule bounded anteriorly by the vaginal opening, posteriorly by the posterior fourchette, and laterally by the labia minora), and the anterior fourchette (where the labia minora meet anteriorly and form the clitoral hood).

The skin of the labia majora and the outer aspects of the labia minora is keratinized squamous epithelium, but only the outer aspects of the labia majora are hair bearing. The skin of the inner aspects of the labia minora and the vestibule (including the hymen) is nonkeratinized. This area is usually pink, but in the nonestrogenized child, it may appear red because the skin is thinner and consequently the blood vessels beneath its surface are more apparent *(97)*.

The forensically relevant areas of the internal female genitalia are the vagina and the cervix. The pertinent landmarks are the vaginal fornices (anterior, posterior, right, and left) and the cervical os (opening of the cervical canal).

The vagina and cervix are covered by nonkeratinized squamous epithelium that normally appears pink in the estrogenized female. Occasionally, the columnar endocervical epithelium, which appears red, may be visible around the cervical os because of physiological or iatrogenic (e.g., exogenous estrogens) eversion of the endocervical canal; these are sometimes erroneously referred to as cervical erosions.

8.4. Development

The female hypothalamic–pituitary–gonadal axis is developed at the time of birth. During the first 5 days of life, the level of gonadotrophin-releasing hormone (GnRH) rises, with a consequent transient rise in gonadal estrogen, attributable to the withdrawal of placental estrogen *(98)*. The estrogen causes prominence of the labia and clitoris and thickening and redundancy of the hymen. The neonatal vagina is purported to measure 4 cm in length *(97)*. Although after 3 months the GnRH levels gradually fall, the estrogenized appearance of the genitalia may persist for the first 2–4 years of life *(99,100)*. During this period, the external genitalia gradually become less prominent; eventually, the hymen becomes thin and translucent and the tissues appear atrophic; occasionally, the hymen remains thick and fimbriated throughout childhood. The nonestrogenized vagina has relatively few rugae and lengthens by only 0.5–1.0 cm in early childhood *(97,98)*.

The hypothalamic–pituitary–gonadal axis is reactivated in late childhood, and the breasts and external genitalia alter accordingly. These changes are classically described in terms of their Tanner stage *(101)*. Under the influence of estrogens, the vagina lengthens to 7.0–8.5 cm in late childhood, eventually reaching its adult length of 10–12 cm *(97,98)*.

The estrogenized vagina is moist because of physiological secretions. This endogenous lubrication is enhanced with ovulation and with sexual stimulation *(102)*. When the endogenous estrogen levels fall resulting from menopause, the vulva and vagina atrophy.

8.5. Forensic Evidence

Although legally it is not necessary to have evidence of ejaculation to prove that vaginal intercourse has occurred, forensic science laboratories are frequently requested to determine whether semen is present on the swabs taken from the female genitalia because semen evidence can play a central role in identification of the assailant. The female genitalia should also be sampled if a condom was used during the sexual act (*see* Heading 11) and if cunnilingus is alleged to have occurred (*see* Heading 7).

It is also important to sample the vagina, vulva, and perineum separately when only anal intercourse is alleged to exclude the possibility of leakage from the vagina to account for semen in the anal canal (*see* Heading 10).

8.5.1. Method of Sampling

The scientist is able to provide objective evidence in terms of the quantity (determined crudely) and quality of the spermatozoa present and may be asked to interpret the results in the context of the case. When providing expert evidence regarding whether vaginal penetration has occurred, the scientist must be able to rely on the forensic practitioner to obtain the samples in a manner that will refute any later suggestions by the defense that significant quantities of spermatozoa, which were only deposited on the outside of the vulva, could have been accidentally transferred to the high vaginal area during the medical examination *(7)*. It is worth noting that there has been no research to support or refute this hypothesis.

Currently, there is no internationally agreed method for obtaining the samples from the female genital area. The following method has (October 2003) been formulated by experienced forensic practitioners and forensic scientists in England to maximize the recovery of spermatozoa while considering these potential problems:

1. Any external (sanitary napkins or pads) or internal (tampons) sanitary wear is collected and submitted for analysis with a note about whether the item was in place during the sexual act and whether other sanitary wear has been in place but discarded since the incident.
2. Two swabs are then used sequentially to sample the vulva (i.e., the inner aspects of labia majora, the labia minora, and the vestibule). Particular attention must be paid to sampling the interlabial folds. Even though traditionally these swabs have been labeled "external vaginal swab," they should be labeled as "vulval swab" to clearly indicate the site of sampling.

    Moist stains should be recovered on dry swabs. However, if the vulval area or any visible staining appears dry, the double-swab technique should be used *(28)* (*see* Subheading 4.1.1.).
3. The labia are then separated, and two sequential dry swabs are used to comprehensively sample the lower vagina. These are labeled "low vaginal swabs."
4. An appropriately sized transparent speculum is then gently passed approximately two-thirds of the way into the vagina; the speculum is opened, and any foreign bodies (e.g., tampons or condoms) are removed and submitted for analysis. Then,

two dry swabs are used to comprehensively sample the vagina beyond the end of the speculum (particularly the posterior fornix where any fluid may collect). These are labeled "high vaginal swabs."

5. When relevant (*see* Subheading 8.5.3.), a single endocervical sample is then obtained. At this point, the speculum may be manipulated within the vagina to locate the cervix.

The best practice is to use only sterile water to lubricate the speculum, because research has shown that swabs contaminated by some lubricants yield significantly less DNA, and lubricants may have been used in the incident (Newton, M., personal communication, 2003). If doctors decide for clinical reasons to use a lubricant, then they should take care to apply the lubricant (from a single use sachet or tube) sparingly and must note its use on the forms returned to the forensic scientist.

In the process of sampling the vagina, the speculum may accumulate body fluids and trace evidence. Therefore, the used speculum should be retained, packaged separately, and stored in accordance with local policy. If the speculum is visibly wet on removal, swabbing may be undertaken to retrieve visible material. If storage space is restricted, swab the instrument and retain the swabs instead.

In some centers, additional methods of semen collection are employed *(5,63,103)* in the form of aspiration of any pools of fluid in the high vagina and/or placing 2–10 mL of saline or sterile water in the vagina and then aspirating the vaginal washings. However, vaginal aspirates should not be necessary if dry swabs are used to sample the vagina in the manner described. Furthermore, there are no data to confirm that vaginal washings retrieve spermatozoa more effectively than vaginal swabs.

In exceptional circumstances (e.g., genital injury or age of the examinee), it may not be possible to pass a speculum to obtain the "high vaginal" and endocervical swabs. On these occasions, two dry swabs should be inserted sequentially into the vagina under direct vision, avoiding contact with the vestibule and hymen. An attempt should then be made to comprehensively sample the vagina by gently rotating and moving each swab backward and forward. These swabs should be labeled "vaginal swabs". Unfortunately, in such circumstances, it is impossible to be certain that the high vaginal swab was not contaminated from semen in the low vagina, which could be there because of drainage from external ejaculation.

8.5.2. Forensic Analysis

8.5.2.1. Spermatozoa

Some guidelines recommend that the forensic practitioner perform an immediate microscopic examination of a wet mount of the material obtained from the vaginal fornices to identify motile spermatozoa on the basis that the presence and motility of spermatozoa may help determine whether recent vaginal ejaculation had occurred. However, a considerable body of opinion does not commend this practice *(104)*. Forensic science laboratories have specialist extraction procedures, staining techniques, and microscopic equipment to maximize spermatozoa recovery and facilitate identification. A survey of 300 cases in which spermatozoa were eventually identified found that they were only detected in four of the cases in the native preparation (before the application of specialist stains) *(105)*.

When nonconsensual penile–vaginal penetration is alleged, the samples are examined microscopically by the forensic scientist to identify spermatozoa, and a DNA analysis is performed on any spermatozoa found.

8.5.2.2. Seminal Fluid

If no spermatozoa are detected, an attempt is made to corroborate the allegation by the microscopic identification of seminal choline crystals. Seminal choline is present in high concentrations in seminal fluid, and the choline crystals can be precipitated by the addition of reagents *(106)*. There are also electrophoretic techniques by which seminal fluid can be identified *(107)*. If the assailant is a secretor, his semen, regardless of whether spermatozoa are present, will contain his ABO group antigens. However, serological analysis has been superseded by DNA STR analysis in many countries.

The FSS is currently researching the use of FISH technology to identify small amounts of male epithelial cells that subsequently can be isolated to enable STR DNA profiling to be conducted on the recovered material *(108–110)*. This will be useful where the offender is suspected to be oligospermic or aspermic or when only minimal amounts of male epithelial cells have been deposited; Y chromosome-positive cells have been isolated from vaginal swabs taken immediately after intercourse where no ejaculation had occurred.

8.5.2.3. Blood

A retrospective survey carried out at the Metropolitan Police Forensic Science Laboratory (MPFSL) found that nearly one-third of the vaginal swabs received at the laboratory were blood stained *(7)*. Whenever bleeding is noted during the medical examination, the forensic practitioner should communicate to the scientist any possible source for the bleeding. In the MPFSL study, the examining doctors believed that 22% of the blood-stained swabs were attributed to menstruation and 10% to female genital trauma. In the remaining cases, no explanation for the bleeding was given. In these cases, the presence of blood must be interpreted with caution, particularly if in small quantity, because traces of uterine blood may be present at any time of the cycle *(7)* and, currently, there is no accepted method of differentiating between traumatic or uterine blood *(111)*. Furthermore, even traumatic bleeding may result from consensual sexual acts (*see* Subheading 8.6.). On rare occasions assailants injure their penises during a sexual act, and this may be the source of blood found in the vagina.

8.5.2.4. Lubricant

See Heading 11 for detailed information.

8.5.3. Persistence Data

Research conducted at the MPFSL has found that after vaginal intercourse, spermatozoa should be found in the vagina for 24 hours, are likely to be found up to 3 days later, and occasionally, are found 7 days later *(112,113)*. Longer times for persistence are the exception rather than the rule.

The quantity of semen in the vagina will diminish progressively with time, usually as a result of drainage. The posture and activity of the complainant subsequent to the act are likely to affect this. Similarly, washing, douching, or bathing may accelerate the loss of semen. Drainage of semen from the vagina may also result in soiling of intimate clothing items worn at the time, and these can prove valuable sources of body fluids.

It has been observed that spermatozoa can be isolated for longer periods in the endocervix. Graves et al. *(114)* report that spermatozoa were isolated from the endocervix 17 days after intercourse. Studies that compared paired swabs from the vagina and cervix have found that 2 days or more after vaginal ejaculation there is a larger quantity of spermatozoa on endocervical swabs compared with the vaginal swabs *(115)*. Therefore, it is recommended that if a complainant presents 48 hours or more after alleged vaginal intercourse, an endocervical swab be taken in addition to the swabs from the vagina.

Although seminal choline has only been found on vaginal swabs up to 24 hours after vaginal ejaculation *(116)*, using FISH technology, Y-chromosome-intact cells have been identified on postcoital vaginal swabs 7 days after sexual intercourse with ejaculation *(117)*.

There is interest in the possibility of determining the timing of intercourse by changes in spermatozoa. Spermatozoa may remain motile in the vagina for up to 24 hours and longer in the cervical mucosa *(50,118,119)*, but the periods for persistence are extremely variable. For example, Rupp *(120)* observed that motile spermatozoa persisted longer in menstruating women but added that identification is hindered by the presence of red blood cells, and Paul *(121)* reported that the period of spermatozoa motility ranged from 1–2 hours at the end of the menstrual cycle to as long as 72 hours at the time of ovulation.

However, the morphology of the spermatozoa does show more consistent temporal changes. In particular, the presence of large numbers of spermatozoa with tails is indicative of recent intercourse. The longest time after intercourse that spermatozoa with tails have been found on external vaginal swabs is 33 hours and 120 hours on internal vaginal swabs *(122)*.

A full DNA STR profile matching the assailant should be obtainable from vaginal swabs taken up to 14 hours postcoitus; partial DNA STR profiles are more likely to be obtained between 24 and 48 hours postcoitus (Elliott, K., personal communication, 2002).

8.6. Medical Evidence

8.6.1. Examination Methods

The forensic practitioner should inspect the mons pubis and note the color, coarseness, and distribution (Tanner stages 1–5) of any pubic hair. A note should also be made if the pubic hair appears to have been plucked (including bleeding hair follicles), shaved, cut, or dyed.

Then the vulval area must be carefully inspected before the insertion of a speculum, because even gentle traction on the posterior fourchette or fossa navicularis during a medical examination can cause a superficial laceration at these sites. Whenever possible, the vagina and cervix should be inspected via the transparent speculum after the high vaginal samples have been obtained. Colposcopy and the application of toluidine blue dye are two specialist techniques used by some forensic practitioners during female genitalia examinations.

8.6.1.1. Colposcopy

A colposcope is a free-standing, binocular microscope on wheels that is most commonly used for direct visualization of the cervix (using a bivalve speculum) after the detection of abnormal cervical cytology. Many centers, particularly those in the United States, advocate the use of the colposcope for external and, where relevant, internal genital and/or anal assessments of complainants of sexual assault.

The colposcope undoubtedly provides considerable advantages over gross visualization. First, it provides magnification (5–30 times) and greater illumination, enabling detection of more abnormalities. Slaughter and Brown *(123)* demonstrated positive colposcopic findings in 87% of female complainants of nonconsensual penile penetration within the previous 48 h, whereas gross visualization has historically identified positive genital findings in only 10–40% of cases *(37–39,124,125)*.

Second, with the attachment of a still or video camera, the colposcope allows for a truly contemporaneous, permanent video/photographic record of the genital/anal findings without resorting to simultaneous dictation, which has the potential to distress the complainant. If a video is used, it will document the entire genital examination and will show any dynamic changes, such as reflex anal dilatation. If appropriate, the medical findings can be demonstrated to the complainant and carer; some teenagers have apparently appreciated the opportunity to have any fears of genital disfigurement allayed by the use of this equipment.

Finally, if a remote monitor is used, the whole examination can be viewed by another doctor for corroboration or teaching purposes without additional parties having to be present during the intimate examination. This facility is obviously more pertinent when video recording is not available.

Obviously, it is important that in all cases the colposcopic evidence be interpreted in the context of the limited information that is currently available regarding colposcopic assessments after consensual sexual acts *(90,126,127)*.

8.6.1.2. Toluidine Blue

Toluidine blue stains nuclei and has been used on the posterior fourchette to identify lacerations of the keratinized squamous epithelium that were not apparent on gross visualization *(128,129)*. Use of toluidine blue increased the detection rate of posterior fourchette lacerations from 4 to 58% in adult (older than 19 years) complainants of nonconsensual vaginal intercourse, from 4 to 28% in sexually abused adolescents (11–18 years old), and from 16.5 to 33% in pediatric sexually abused patients (0–10 years old) *(129,130)*.

The same frequency of posterior fourchette lacerations has been identified by use of the stain in adolescents after consensual penile penetration and nonconsensual sexual acts *(129)*. In contrast, adult complainants of nonconsensual vaginal intercourse and sexually abused children had significantly more lacerations demonstrable by toluidine blue staining than control groups *(130)*, although such staining does not identify lacerations that cannot be detected using a colposcope *(123)*. Therefore, if a colposcope is not available, toluidine blue may be an adjunct to the genital assessment of prepubertal and adult complainants of vaginal penetration *(129,130)*. Furthermore, some centers use the stain during colposcopy to provide a clear pictorial presentation of the injuries for later presentation to juries *(123)*.

Vulval swabs for forensic analysis must be taken before the stain is applied. Toluidine blue (1%) is then painted on the posterior fourchette, using a swab, before any instrumentation. After a few seconds, the residual stain is removed with lubricating jelly and gauze *(128)*. The patient may experience some stinging at the application site. The time parameters within which the use of toluidine blue is beneficial in highlighting injuries have not been identified.

8.6.2. Injuries

Little information is available regarding the incidence and type of genital injuries that result from consensual sexual acts involving the female genitalia. Although penile–vaginal penetration is the most frequent sexual act performed by heterosexual couples, anecdotal reports from doctors who regularly conduct nonforensic assessments of the female genitalia (general practitioners, gynecologists, or genitourinary physicians) suggest that injuries resultant from sexual activity are rarely identified. However, this may be explained by the nature of routine assessments, which are usually limited to naked-eye inspection or because of the rapid and complete resolution of minor injuries *(90)*. On the other hand, there are reports describing genital injuries in complainants of sexual assault, although, unfortunately, few have matched the findings with the specific complaint or the subsequent outcome in court. To date, no case-control study has compared the genital findings in complainants of sexual assault with those in a sexually active control population.

8.6.2.1. External Genitalia

For penile penetration of the vagina to occur, the penis must first pass between the labia minora and through the hymenal opening. The apposition of the penis and the posterior fourchette in the majority of sexual positions means that this area may be stretched, rubbed, or receive blunt trauma as vaginal penetration is achieved. Lacerations, abrasions, or bruises at the posterior fourchette have all been described after consensual sexual activity, although in all these cases, the examinations were enhanced by the use of toluidine blue or a colposcope *(90,128,129)*. Wilson *(131)* has also described macroscopically visible hematomata of the labia with consensual sexual activity. These injuries usually heal completely without residual scarring *(90)*.

Among 311 postpubertal females (age range 11–85 years) who made a "valid" (defined as "police investigation corroborated the victim's history and the victim did not recant") complaint of sexual assault, 200 had colposcopically detected injuries at one or more of the following sites on the external genitalia: posterior fourchette, labia minora, hymen, and fossa navicularis *(90)*. Although all categories of injuries ("tears," bruises, abrasions, redness, and swelling) were described at all sites, the predominant injuries described were site dependent; for example, tears were most frequently described on the posterior fourchette ($n = 83$) and fossa navicularis ($n = 28$), whereas abrasions were most frequently described on the labia minora ($n = 66$) and bruises were the most frequent injuries seen on the hymen ($n = 28$) *(90)*. Adams and colleagues found similar types and distributions of injuries among the adolescent complainants (14–19 years) they examined *(132)*. In this population, tears of the posterior fourchette or fossa navicularis were the most common findings (40%). The studies of macroscopic findings among complainants of sexual assault have also found that most of the injuries detected are located on the external genitalia *(133,134)*.

Healing of lacerations of the posterior fourchette is predominantly by first intention, with no residual scarring being detected at follow-up assessments *(90)*. Nonetheless, scarring may occur occasionally in these areas, but it is important not to mistake a linear vestibularis, a congenital white line identified in the fossa navicularis (present in 25% of neonates), for a scar *(135)*.

Accidental injuries of the external genitalia of female children are well documented in the literature. The site and nature of the injury will depend on the type of trauma and the conformation of any object involved *(136,137)*.

8.6.2.2. Hymen

The hymen must be examined in detail after an allegation of a nonconsensual penetrative act. When the hymen is fimbriated, this assessment may be facilitated by the gentle use of a moistened swab to visualize the hymenal edges. When the hymenal opening cannot be seen at all, application of a few drops of warm sterile water or saline onto the hymen will often reveal the hymenal edges. Foley catheters are also a useful tool to aid hymenal visualization in postpubertal females *(138)*. A small catheter is inserted through the hymenal opening, the balloon is then inflated with 10–20 mL of air, and the catheter is gently withdrawn so that the inflated balloon abuts the hymen. The balloon is deflated before removal. This procedure is well tolerated by the examinee. Obviously, in the acute setting, none of these maneuvers should be attempted until the relevant forensic samples have been retrieved.

There is little specific information available regarding the type and frequency of acute hymenal injuries after consensual sexual acts, particularly regarding the first act of sexual intercourse. Slaughter et al. *(90)* conducted colposcopic examinations of the genitalia of 75 women who had experienced "consensual" vaginal intercourse in the preceding 24 hours. They found lacerations (tears) with associated bruising at the 3-o'clock and 9-o'clock positions on the hymen of a 14-year-old and bruises at the 6-o'clock and 7-o'clock positions on the hymens of two other females (aged 13 and 33 years). No other hymenal injuries were detected. Unfortunately, no details regarding previous sexual experience are recorded on their pro forma.

In the same article, the hymen was noted to be one of the four most commonly injured genital sites among 311 postpubertal complainants of nonconsensual sexual acts. The hymenal injuries detected colposcopically were bruises ($n = 28$), lacerations ($n = 22$), abrasions ($n = 13$), swelling ($n = 10$), and redness ($n = 4$). The hymenal lacerations were either single ($n = 12$), nine of which were at the 6-o'clock position, or paired around the 6-o'clock position ($n = 10$). The authors found that hymenal lacerations were four times more common in the younger age groups. Again, there was no information regarding previous sexual experience. Bowyer and Dalton (133) described three women with hymenal lacerations (detected with the naked eye) among 83 complainants of rape who were examined within 11 days of the incident; two of the three women had not previously experienced sexual intercourse. One retrospective survey of the acute injuries noted among adolescent complainants of sexual assault (aged 14–19 years) found that hymenal tears were uncommon, even among the subgroup that denied previous sexual activity (132). Bruises, abrasions, reddening, and swelling completely disappear within a few days or weeks of the trauma (90,139). Conversely, complete hymenal lacerations do not reunite and thus will always remain apparent as partial or complete transections (123), although they may be partially concealed by the effects of estrogenization (140). However, lacerations that do not extend through both mucosal surfaces may heal completely (2). There is one case report of a 5-year-old who was subjected to penile penetration and acquired an imperforate hymen resulting from obliterative scarring (141).

On the basis of the current literature, complete transections in the lower margin of the hymen are considered to provide confirmatory evidence of previous penetration of the hymen. However, it is not possible to determine whether it was a penis, finger, or other object that caused the injury, and there is an urgent need for comprehensive research to determine whether sporting activities or tampon use can affect hymenal configuration. Although partial or complete transections of the upper hymen may represent healed partial or complete lacerations beyond the acute stage, there is no method of distinguishing them from naturally occurring anatomical variations.

Goodyear and Laidlaw (142) conclude that, "it is unlikely that a normal-looking hymen that is less than 10 mm in diameter, even in the case of an elastic hymen, has previously accommodated full penetration of an adult finger, let alone a penis." However, there is no objective evidence on which to base this conjecture, and it is not known whether measuring the hymenal opening using a digit, or other previously measured object, in the clinical setting when the practitioner is particularly anxious not to cause the patient any distress accurately reflects what the hymen could have accommodated during a sexual assault.

On the other hand, it is now generally accepted that postpubertal females can experience penile vaginal penetration without sustaining any hymenal deficits; this is attributed to hymenal elasticity *(142,143)*. Furthermore, the similarity between the dimensions of the hymenal opening among sexually active and nonsexually active postpubertal females *(96)* makes it impossible for the physician to state categorically that a person has ever had prior sexual intercourse unless there is other supportive evidence (pregnancy, spermatozoa on a high vaginal swab; *see* Subheading 8.5.; Forensic Evidence) *(96,142,144)*.

8.6.2.3. Vagina

Lacerations and ruptures (full-thickness lacerations) of the vagina have been described in the medical literature after consensual sexual acts *(145–147)*. They are most commonly located in the right fornix or extending across the posterior fornix; this configuration is attributed to the normal vaginal asymmetry whereby the cervix lies toward the left fornix, causing the penis to enter the right fornix during vaginal penetration *(147)*. Factors that predispose to such injuries include previous vaginal surgery, pregnancy, and the puerperium, postmenopause, intoxication of the female, first act of sexual intercourse, and congenital genital abnormalities (e.g., septate vagina) *(145)*. Although most vaginal lacerations are associated with penile penetration, they have also been documented after brachiovaginal intercourse ("fisting") *(147)*, vaginal instrumentation during the process of a medical assessment *(147)*, and the use of plastic tampon inserters *(148)*.

Vaginal lacerations have been documented without any direct intravaginal trauma after a fall or a sudden increase of intra-abdominal pressure (e.g., lifting a heavy object) *(147)*.

Injuries of the vagina have been noted during the examinations of complainants of sexual assault. Slaughter et al. *(90)* describe 26 colposcopically detected vaginal injuries among the 213 complainants who had genital trauma identified. These were described as "tears" ($n = 10$), bruises ($n = 12$), and abrasions ($n = 4$). Other articles that considered only macroscopically detectable lesions found vaginal "injuries" in 2–16% of complainants of nonconsensual penile vaginal penetration *(133,134)*. However, one study included "redness" as a vaginal injury when, in fact, this is a nonspecific finding with numerous causes.

When a vaginal laceration may have been caused by an object that has the potential to fragment or splinter, a careful search should be made for foreign bodies in the wound *(145)* (this may necessitate a general anesthetic), and X-rays should be taken of the pelvis (anteroposterior and lateral), including the vagina, to help localize foreign particles *(149)*. Any retrieved foreign bodies should be appropriately packaged and submitted for forensic analysis.

8.6.2.4. Cervix

Bruises and lacerations of the cervix have been described as infrequent findings after nonconsensual sexual acts *(90,150,151)*. In one article, the injuries related to penetration by a digit and by a "knife-like" object. There are no reports of cervical trauma after consensual sexual acts.

8.6.2.5. Nonspecific

Norvell et al. *(126)* have also documented areas of increased vascularity/ telangiectasia ($n = 7$), broken blood vessels ($n = 2$), and microabrasions ($n = 2$) during colposcopic assessment of the introitus, hymen, and lower 2 cm of the vagina of 18 volunteers who had participated in consensual sexual activity within the preceding 6 hours. However, the areas of increased vascularity may have been normal variants *(90)*, and the precise location of the other findings was not described. Fraser et al. *(152)* describe the macroscopic and colposcopic variations in epithelial surface of the vagina and cervix in healthy, sexually active women (age 18–35 years). They documented changes in the epithelial surface in 56 (17.8%) of the 314 inspections undertaken; six were located at the introitus, 26 in the middle or lower thirds of the vagina, eight on the fornical surfaces of the cervix, 14 in the vaginal fornices, and two involved generalized changes of the vaginal wall. The most common condition noted was petechiae. The more significant conditions noted were three microulcerations, two bruises, five abrasions, and one mucosal tear. The incidence of these conditions was highest when the inspections followed intercourse in the previous 24 hours or tampon use.

9. MALE GENITALIA

During examination of the male genitalia, the forensic practitioner is expected to document any features that could assist with subsequent identification of the assailant, to note any acquired or congenital conditions that could make an alleged sexual act impossible, to describe in detail any injuries that could relate to a sexual act, and to retrieve any forensic evidence. Although the specifics of the medicolegal assessment of the male genitalia are case dependent, the principles of the examination, whether of the complainant or the defendant, are the same.

9.1. Anatomy and Physiology

9.1.1. Penile Size

Forensic practitioners may be asked to provide evidence on the size of a defendant's penis in the flaccid state to support a hypothesis that a certain sexual act could not have occurred because of intergenital disproportion between the complainant and the defendant. However, such measurements are unhelpful because it is not possible to predict the maximum erectile size from the flaccid length, and there is "no statistical support for the 'phallic fallacy' that the larger penis increases in size with full erection to a significantly greater degree than does the smaller penis" (153). Furthermore, even when the erect penis is measured during automanipulation or active coition, the measurements are recognized to be unreliable (153).

9.1.2. Erections

Forensic practitioners may also be asked to comment on a person's ability to achieve a penile erection, particularly if the male is young or elderly. Masters and Johnson (153) note that during their research, "penile erection has been observed in males of all ages ranging from baby boys immediately after delivery to men in their late eighties;" they report that one 89-year-old study subject was able to achieve a full penile erection and ejaculate. Therefore, it is not possible to reach a conclusion regarding erectile efficiency based on age alone. When a defendant reports erectile dysfunction, the expert opinion of a urologist should be sought.

Penile erection may result from visual stimulation (including fantasy) or tactile stimulation. The penis, scrotum, and rectum are all sensitive to tactile stimulation (153), which may explain why involuntary penile erections can be experienced by a male subjected to nonconsensual anal intercourse.

9.1.3. Semen Production

Semen is not produced until the male experiences puberty, which usually begins between 9 and 14 years of age (154). Semen consists of seminal fluid (produced by the prostate) and spermatozoa. The normal volume of a single ejaculate is between 2 and 7 mL, and it will contain approx 50–120 million spermatozoa/mL. There are numerous congenital and acquired causes for impaired spermatogenesis (155), resulting in either decreased numbers (oligozoospermia) or absence of (azoospermia) spermatozoa. Both conditions may be permanent or transitory depending on the underlying cause. Permanent azoospermia (e.g., after a successful vasectomy) would be of particular forensic significance because it could lead to the elimination of a suspect from an inquiry if spermatozoa had been identified that were known to relate to the offense. It is not possible to determine whether spermatozoa are present in the ejaculate without microscopic assessment. However, analysis of a defendant's semen is not a routine part of the forensic assessment.

9.2. Forensic Evidence

After an allegation of fellatio, swabs from the complainant's penis can be examined for saliva, but, as discussed earlier in Subheading 7.2.4.2., the likelihood of definitive identification of saliva by amylase estimation is low. Nonetheless, enough material may be obtained for DNA analysis. When an allegation of vaginal or anal intercourse is made, penile swabs from the suspect can be examined for cells, feces, hairs, fibers, blood, and lubricants.

It should be noted that vaginal fluid from recent previous intercourse, unrelated to the allegation, may be detected by DNA analysis of swabs taken from the unwashed penis (Harris, E., personal communication, 1998).

9.2.1. Sampling Method

Data collected by the MPFSL between 1987 and 1995 *(122)* have shown that after vaginal intercourse, cellular material from the complainant can be recovered from the coronal sulcus (groove around the penis just below the glans) even if the suspect has washed or bathed since the offense. Swabs taken from the meatus and urethra are not suitable for microscopic assessment because some male urethral cells can be similar to vaginal cells *(7)*. Therefore, when vaginal intercourse is alleged, two swabs (the first wet, the second dry) should be obtained sequentially from the coronal sulcus, and two additional swabs (the first wet, the second dry) should be taken sequentially from the glans and the shaft together. The swabs must be labeled accordingly, and the order in which the samples were obtained must be relayed to the scientist. The same samples are also taken if it is believed that a lubricant or condom has been used during a sexual act or if the assault involved fellatio or anal intercourse.

9.2.2. Forensic Analysis

9.2.2.1. Microscopic and Biochemical Analyses

Such analyses of the penile swabs may be undertaken to identify cellular material, blood, or amylase. When the complaint is of anal intercourse, swabs that are discolored by fecal material can be analyzed for urobilinogen and examined microscopically for vegetable matter.

9.2.2.2. Assailant Identification

DNA STR profiling of body fluids on the penis is now the method of choice used to provide evidence of penile–vaginal/oral/anal contact. It has proved particularly useful when multiple assailants have had intercourse with a single complainant (forensic scientists, personal communication, 1998), because DNA STR profiles matching the other assailants may also be found on the penile swabs taken from one assailant.

Certain forensic science laboratories are now able to extract mitochondrial DNA from the degraded cellular material present in feces, although the value of this method of analysis in relation to sexual offenses must be considered in relation to the other sexual acts that are alleged to have occurred during the assault.

9.2.3. Persistence Data

Female DNA profiles have been obtained on penile swabs up to 24 hours postcoitus *(156)*. Blood and feces have been recovered from penile swabs taken 15 and 18 hours, respectively, after the incident (for saliva, *see* Subheading 7.1. and ref. *7*).

9.3. Medical Evidence

When obtaining the relevant forensic samples, the forensic practitioner should inspect the male genitalia with particular reference to the following points:

1. Pubic hair should be described in terms of its coarseness, distribution (Tanner stages 1–5), and color. A note should be made if the pubic hair appears to have been plucked (including bleeding hair follicles), shaved, cut, or dyed.
2. Congenital abnormalities, such as microphallus and cryptorchidism. Penile length in the flaccid state is said to vary from 8.5 to 10.5 cm (measured from the anterior border of the symphysis along the dorsal surface to the distal tip of the penis), with a documented range of 6–14 cm *(153)*.
3. Acquired abnormalities, such as circumcision, Peyronie's disease, balanitis xerotica obliterans, vasectomy scars, phimosis, tattoos, and piercing.
4. Signs of infection, such as warts, discharge, erythema, and vesicles.
5. Foreign bodies may be worn around the base of the penis, sometimes also encircling the scrotum, in an attempt to increase and sustain penile tumescence. Such devices may result in local and distal genital trauma (penile tourniquet syndrome) *(157)*. In several case reports, children have had human hairs wrapped around the penis; these hairs may be virtually invisible because of edema or epithelialization *(158)*. Kerry and Chapman *(159)* have described the deliberate application of such a ligature by parents who were attempting to prevent enuresis.

6. Assessment of injuries. After consensual sexual intercourse, lacerations of the foreskin and frenulum, meatitis, traumatic urethritis, penile edema, traumatic lymphangitis, paraphimosis, and penile "fractures" have all been described *(160–163)*. Accidental trauma is more common when there is a pre-existing abnormality, such as phimosis *(160)*. Skin injury may be incurred if the genitals are deliberately bitten during fellatio *(160)*. Although the precise incidence of male genital trauma after sexual activity is unknown, anecdotal accounts suggest that it is rare to find any genital injuries when examining suspects of serious sexual assaults *(164)*.

In children the genitalia may be accidentally or deliberately injured, and the latter may be associated with sexual abuse *(165)*. Bruises, abrasions, lacerations, swelling, and burns of the genitalia of prepubescent males have all been described *(165,166)*.

10. PERIANAL AREA AND ANAL CANAL

10.1. Definitions

Buggery is a lay term used to refer to penile penetration of the anus (anal intercourse) of a man, a woman, or an animal (also known as bestiality). Sodomy relates to anal intercourse between humans only.

10.2. Frequency

10.2.1. Consensual

Although anal intercourse among heterosexuals is the least common component of the sexual repertoire, it has been experienced on at least one occasion by 13–25% of heterosexual females surveyed *(64,80,167)*, and it was described as a regular means of sexual gratification for 8% of women attending one gynecologist *(80)*. Among 508 men who reported having had a same-gender sexual experience at some stage in their lives, 33.7% reported insertive anal intercourse, and 35.4% had experienced receptive anal intercourse. Interestingly, in contrast to a common perception, more men had experienced both practices than had been in exclusively receptive or insertive roles *(168)*.

10.2.2. Nonconsensual

Anal intercourse was reported by 5–16% of females who described having been sexually assaulted *(6,169)*. Although it may be the only sexual act performed, it is more frequently combined with vaginal and oral penetration *(6,169)*. Fewer data are available regarding sexual assaults on males, although Hillman et al. *(170,171)* report that penetrative anal intercourse was described by 75–89% of the male complainants they studied.

10.3. Legal Implications

Under English common law, the term *buggery* is defined as anal intercourse by a man with another man or a woman and anal or vaginal intercourse by a man or a woman with an animal (bestiality). Although the 1967 Sexual Offences Act provided that it was not an offense for two consenting men who had attained the age of 21 to commit buggery in private, it remained an offense for a man to commit buggery with a woman, even if both parties consented, until 1994.

The Criminal Justice and Public Order Act 1994 expanded the definition of rape, which had previously related to only vaginal intercourse, to include nonconsensual penile penetration of the anus independent of the gender of the recipient. The Sexual Offences (Amendment) Act 2000 reduced the minimum age at which a person, whether male or female, may lawfully consent to buggery to 16 years.

A recent change in English law has defined nonconsensual penetration of the anus by an object or a body part (excluding the penis) as "assault by penetration," this new offense has the same maximum sentence as rape. In some other jurisdictions, such as Australia, such acts are included in the legal definition of rape *(172)*.

10.4. Anatomy and Physiology

An understanding of the normal anatomy and physiology of the perianal area and anal canal is important for the reliable description and interpretation of the medical findings after allegations of anal penetrative acts. Unfortunately, varying definitions have resulted in considerable confusion, such that there is no consensus among forensic practitioners about the nomenclature that should be used in describing injuries to this area. Therefore, a brief overview of the relevant information is given in the remaining Subheadings, together with references to more substantive texts.

10.4.1. Anus

The anus refers not to an actual anatomical structure but to the external opening of the anal canal. The skin that immediately surrounds the anus is variously referred to as the *anal verge* or *anal margin (173)*. Because the anal canal can evert and invert as the anal sphincters and pelvic floor muscles relax and contract, the anal verge/margin is not a fixed, identifiable landmark.

10.4.2. Perianal Area

The perianal area is a poorly defined, approximately circular area that includes the folds of skin encircling the anus. It is covered by skin that is often hyperpigmented when compared with the skin on the buttocks, although this varies with age and ethnicity *(174)*.

10.4.3. Anal Canal

Although the anal canal has been variously defined, the definition that has practical clinical forensic value is that of the anatomical anal canal, which extends from the anus to the dentate line. The *dentate line* refers to the line formed either by the bases of the anal columns (most distinct in children) or, when these are not apparent, by the lowest visible anal sinuses *(175)*. The average length of the anatomical anal canal in adults (age range 18–90 years) is only 2.1 cm, with a range of 1.4–3.8 cm in males and 1.0–3.2 cm in females *(176)*. Between the epithelial zones of the anal canal and the rectum is the anal transitional zone, which is usually located in the region of the anal columns and is purple *(177)*.

The anal canal, as previously defined, is lined by nonkeratinized squamous epithelium and is salmon pink in the living *(174)*. It is sensitive to touch, pain, heat, and cold to just above the dentate line *(175)*. The anus and lumen of the anal canal usually appear as an asymmetric Y-shaped slit when viewed via a proctoscope (anoscope). The folds of mucosa and subcutaneous tissue (containing small convulated blood vessels surrounded by connective tissue) between the indentations of the Y are referred to as the anal cushions. Although this appearance is usually obscured externally by the folds of skin on the perianal area, it may become apparent if the patient is anesthetized or as the anus dilates.

10.4.4. Rectum

The rectum extends from the anal transitionary zone to the sigmoid colon and is 8–15 cm long. It is lined by typical intestinal mucosa and is red in the living. The rectum has only poorly defined dull sensation *(175)*.

10.4.5. Anal Sphincters and Fecal Incontinence

Although numerous muscles encircle the anal canal, the two that are forensically significant are the internal and the external anal sphincters.

10.4.5.1. Internal Anal Sphincter

This sphincter is a continuation of the circular muscle coat of the rectum and extends 8–12 mm below the dentate line. In the normal living subject, the internal anal sphincter is tonically contracted so that the anal canal is closed. The internal sphincter is supplied by autonomic nerve fibers and is not considered to be under voluntary control *(3)*. Thus, although it appears to contract during a digital assessment of voluntary anal contraction, it is presumed to result from its compression by the surrounding external sphincter fibers *(177)*.

10.4.5.2. External Anal Sphincter

This sphincter encircles the internal sphincter but extends below it, ending subcutaneously. The lower edges of the external and internal sphincters can be distinguished on digital palpation. Although this sphincter is tonically contracted in the resting state, this contraction can be overcome with firm pressure *(177)*. If the patient is asked to contract the anus during a digital assessment, the external sphincter can be felt to ensure contraction and closing of the anus tightly. However, because the muscle fibers are predominantly the slow-twitch type, a maximum contraction of the external sphincter can only be maintained for approx 1 minute*(178)*.

Fecal continence is maintained by several factors, the relative importance of which has not been fully elucidated. Currently, the most important factor is the angulation between the rectum and the anal canal, which is maintained at a mean of 92° by continuous contraction of the puborectalis muscles, located above the external sphincter. Both sphincters have supportive roles in maintaining fecal continence *(175)*, and their disruption can result in incontinence (*see* Subheading 10.6.2.).

10.5. Forensic Evidence

The presence of semen in the anus or rectum of a male complainant can be corroborative evidence of alleged anal intercourse in conjunction with the presented history and possible physical findings.

The same is only true for a female complainant if no semen is detected in the vagina, because semen has been found on rectal and anal swabs taken from women who described vaginal intercourse only. It is postulated that the presence of semen in these cases results from vaginal drainage *(49,179)*.

Swabs should also be taken if a condom or lubricant was used during the sexual assault and if anilingus is alleged (*see* Subheading 7.2. and Heading 11).

10.5.1. Method of Sampling

Two samples must first be obtained from the perianal area. Just as when sampling the skin elsewhere, if the perianal skin is moist, the stain should be retrieved on dry swabs. If there is no visible staining or the stain is dry, the double-swab technique should be used *(28)*. The forensic practitioner should use as many swabs as are necessary to remove any visible stain (repeating moistened swab followed by dry swab). If no stain is visible, two swabs will suffice (the first wet, the second dry). Although not specifically defined for forensic purposes, the perianal area should be considered as an area with a radius of 3 cm from the anus. The swabs are then placed in sheaths without transport medium. Even though traditionally these swabs have been labeled "external anal swab," they should be labeled as "perianal swab" to clearly indicate the site of sampling. The anal canal is then sampled by passing a wet swab and then a dry swab, sequentially, up to 3 cm through the anus. The proctoscope (anoscope) is then passed 2–3 cm into the anal canal, and the lower rectum is sampled using a dry swab. As the proctoscope is withdrawn, the anal canal can be sampled, again with a dry swab. As discussed previously, when examining female complainants of anal intercourse alone, swabs should also be obtained from the vagina.

The best practice is to use only sterile water to lubricate the proctoscope, because research has shown that swabs that are contaminated by some lubricants yield significantly less DNA, and lubricants may have been used in the incident (Newton, M., personal communication, 2003). In practice, this presents major difficulties. If doctors decide for clinical reasons to use a lubricant, they should apply the lubricant (from a single-use sachet or tube) sparingly, taking care not to contaminate the swabs, and must note its use on the forms returned to the forensic scientist.

In the process of sampling the rectum/anal canal, the proctoscope may accumulate body fluids and trace evidence. Therefore, the used proctoscope should be retained, packaged separately, and stored in accordance with local policy. If the proctoscope is visibly wet on removal, swabbing may be conducted to retrieve visible material. If storage space is restricted, then the instrument should be swabbed and the swabs retained instead.

Stool samples and toilet paper need not be collected routinely because the other samples described should be adequate for laboratory requirements.

10.5.2. Forensic Analysis

Microscopic examination for spermatozoa (or analysis for seminal choline if no spermatozoa are present) is initially undertaken, followed by DNA analysis if any body fluids are identified. ABO grouping is not successful with anal swabs because the complainant's own group predominates *(180)*.

Lubricant and saliva analysis are discussed in Heading 11 and Subheading 7.2., respectively.

10.5.3. Persistence Data

Under normal circumstances, the maximum recorded interval between the act of anal intercourse and the identification of spermatozoa on a rectal swab is 65 hours *(181)*. However, in one exceptional case in which a female remained prone in the hospital for several days because of injuries sustained during a sexual assault, semen was detected on anal swabs taken 113 hours after the act of anal intercourse *(181)*.

Swabs should be taken even if the complainant has defecated since the assault. An unpublished review of 36 MPFSL cases of alleged anal intercourse in which the complainant had defecated before the examination found that in six cases (four female and two male) the internal/external anal swabs were still positive for spermatozoa, although only a few were present; one of these subjects, a male, had a positive external anal swab 52 hours after the anal intercourse (Allard, J., personal communication, 1998). Anal swabs have produced a positive DNA STR analysis up to 48 hours after the incident (Elliott, K., personal communication, 2003).

10.6. Medical Evidence

When an allegation of anal penetration is made, the perianal skin, anal canal mucosa, and, when tolerated, the lower portion of the rectum should be examined with the aid of a proctoscope/anoscope. This can be done simultaneously with the retrieval of the forensic evidence.

It is generally accepted that with gradual dilatation and lubrication, consensual penile anal intercourse can be performed without any resultant injury *(80,182)*. Furthermore, it is important to emphasize that nonconsensual anal penetration can also occur in both children and adults without producing acute or chronic injury *(3)*.

Although anecdotal accounts have detailed the anal and rectal injuries that result from consensual penile/object anal penetration *(121,175)*, few peer-reviewed articles have addressed this subject. Similarly, many studies have documented the presence of anal symptoms or signs among complainants of sexual assault *(133,170)*, but few of these have described the acute injuries in any detail or related these injuries to the specific complaint and its subsequent outcome.

10.6.1. Anal Fissures, Tears, and Lacerations

The most frequent injuries that are documented after allegations of nonconsensual anal penetration are anal fissures, tears, and lacerations. Use of these different terminologies is confusing and makes comparing the different data impossible. A consensus should be reached among forensic practitioners worldwide regarding what terms should be used and what they mean.

Clinically, an anal fissure refers to a longitudinal laceration in the perianal skin and/or mucosa of the anal canal. Anal fissures may be acute (usually healing within 2–3 weeks) or chronic and single or multiple. Most fissures will heal by first intention and not leave a scar. However, after healing, the site of some fissures may be apparent as a fibrous skin tag *(183)*. Manser *(134)* described the medical findings in only 16 of 51 complainants (15 males and 36 females) of anal intercourse (21 were categorized as child sexual abuse). The majority (61%) of this study population was examined at least 72 hours after the sexual contact. Fissures were found in eight cases (16%).

A major problem in the forensic interpretation of anal fissures is that they may result from numerous other means that are unrelated to penetrative trauma, including passage of hard stools, diarrhea, inflammatory bowel disease, sexually transmitted diseases, and skin diseases *(183,184)*.

In the study by Manser *(134)*, lacerations were documented as being present in only one of the 51 complainants of anal intercourse and five of 103 females complainants of nonconsensual vaginal penetration aged between 12 and 69 years, some of whom complained of concurrent nonconsensual anal penetration with either an object or a penis (the majority of whom were examined within 24 hours of the sexual assault). It may be that these "lacerations" were long or deep anal fissures, but because the parameters of length or depth of an anal fissure have not been clinically defined, the distinction may be arbitrary. Conversely, these "lacerations" may have been horizontally or obliquely directed breaches in the epithelium *(185)*, which would immediately differentiate them from anal fissures and render them highly forensically significant because of the limited differential diagnoses of such injuries compared with fissures.

Slaughter et al. *(90)* described the gross and colposcopic findings in 311 females aged from 11 to 85 years who reported nonconsensual sexual acts, 55 of whom described anal contact. The majority (81%) of the population was examined within 72 hours of the sexual assault. They found "anal findings" in 56% of the 55 patients who reported anal contact. The anal injuries were categorized as tears in 19 of the cases. Although elsewhere Slaughter has qualified the term "tear" to mean "laceration" *(186)*, this was not done in this article and again means that interpretation of the forensic significance of these injuries may be limited.

Because a significant percentage of the heterosexual and male homosexual population has engaged in consensual anal penetration, anecdotal accounts suggest that resultant injuries, such as fissures, are rare. This could be because the injuries do not warrant medical attention or because patients are not specifically questioned about anal intercourse when the causative factors for anal abnormalities/complaints are considered. However, one study that specifically attempted to address this issue documented that among 129 women who gave a history of anal intercourse, only one patient described anal complications, namely proctitis and an anal fissure; both these signs related to a gonococcal infection *(80)*. However, because this study was limited to the medical history, it is not possible to rule out the presence of minor asymptomatic conditions or injuries in this study population.

Whether an injury heals by first or secondary intention, the latter resulting in scar formation, depends on several factors, including the width and depth of the breach in the epithelium. Manser *(134)* reported scarring in 14% of the people examined because of possible anal intercourse. The Royal College of Physicians working party stated that in children, "The only specific indicator of abuse is a fresh laceration or healed scar extending beyond the anal margin onto the perianal skin in the absence of reasonable alternative explanation, e.g., major trauma" *(173)*. Disappointingly, this report does not clarify how they differentiate between lacerations and fissures.

10.6.2. Anal Sphincter Tone

The forensic practitioner may be asked about the effects that a single episode or repeated episodes of anal penetration have on anal sphincter tone and subsequent continence of feces. In terms of single anal penetrative acts, partial tears and complete disruptions of the anal sphincters have been described after a single traumatic sexual act *(187,188)*; one case was caused by pliers and the others by brachioproctic intercourse (fisting). However, it is not clear from these case reports whether the sexual practices were consensual or nonconsensual. The two patients who were described as having complete disruption of the sphincters both developed fecal incontinence. There is a case report of "multiple ruptures" of the internal anal sphincter with resultant fecal incontinence after nonconsensual anal penetration with a penis and fist *(189)*.

Regarding repeated acts of anal penetration, the studies are conflicting. A study of 129 heterosexual women who gave a history of anal intercourse found no reports of "gross fecal incontinence" *(64)*. Similarly, Chun et al. *(190)* found that although the 14 anoreceptive homosexual males studied had significantly lower resting anal canal pressures when compared with the control group (10 nonanoreceptive heterosexual males), there were no complaints of fecal incontinence by the study subjects. In contrast, Miles et al. *(191)* found a significant increase in fecal incontinence or urgency (requiring immediate defecation to avoid incontinence) in anoreceptive individuals. In addition, they found an inverse relationship between the maximum resting sphincter pressure and the estimated number of acts of anal intercourse. Not surprisingly, they also found that the more traumatic forms of anoreceptive practices, such as brachioproctic intercourse (fisting), were more likely to result in objective sphincter dysfunction. Both the Chun and Miles studies used special equipment to measure the sphincter tone, and neither comments on whether sphincter laxity was apparent clinically in any of the subjects.

Interestingly, reflex anal dilatation (that is, dilatation of the external and internal anal sphincters when the buttocks are gently separated for 30 s), which many authors have said is associated with anal intercourse, was not seen in any of the anoreceptive subjects in the Miles' study group *(191)*.

10.6.3. Rectal Lacerations

Other, apparently rare, major complications that have been reported in adult males after penile–anal intercourse are nonperforating and, less frequently, perforating lacerations of the rectal mucosa *(187,188)*. Mucosal lacerations are also seen in association with brachioproctic intercourse and the insertion of inanimate foreign bodies *(187,188)*. On occasions, the injury may be fatal *(187,188)*. Slaughter et al. *(90)* described five rectal lacerations among eight women who underwent proctoscopy after "anal contact" during a sexual assault. The relationship between the precise sexual act and the medical findings is not described.

10.6.4. Other Injuries

The other anal injuries that have been described in complainants of anal penetration are bruises (2–4%), abrasions (4–5%), erythema (2–8%), and swelling/edema (2–6%) *(90,134)*. Slaughter et al. *(90)* described a high number of rectal injuries, in addition to the lacerations described (ecchymosis, $n = 1$; abrasions, $n = 2$; redness, $n = 1$; and swelling, $n = 6$) that were detectable among eight sexual assaults complainants who described "anal contact" *(90)*. Although bruises are indicative of blunt trauma, the other findings may have innocent explanations, for example, a superficial abrasion of the anal verge has been identified on a child who interrupted the medical to pass a motion (observation of D. Rogers). Although erythema and swelling/edema are also nonspecific findings, if they have completely resolved at a follow-up examination, it may be possible to relate them to the allegation. All these minor injuries would be expected to hcal within 2 weeks of the incident without any residual scarring.

11. LUBRICANTS

Traces of lubricant found on vaginal or internal anal swabs may provide confirmatory evidence of recent penetration of a body orifice. This has particular relevance if a condom is worn during a penetrative act. Consequently, if the forensic practitioner has used lubricant (other than sterile water) on specula, proctoscopes, or gloved digits, it must be communicated to the forensic scientist. In terms of lubricant analysis, the most frequent request received by the forensic science service is to check vaginal swabs for the presence of condom lubricant. A review of cases at the Las Vegas Metropolitan Police Department found that 19 of 80 complainants reported that either the assailant had worn a condom during the incident or they had experienced consensual intercourse with a partner wearing a condom within the 72 hours preceding the assault (Cook, Y. L., personal communication, 1993, and ref *192*). The most commonly encountered lubricants applied directly to the penis to aid penetration are Vaseline® (petroleum-based product) and KY® Jelly (water-based product) *(193)*. However, various other substances have been used to facilitate penetration during a sexual assault, including hand cream, cooking oil, and margarine, the diversity of the products apparently reflecting what is immediately at hand. Saliva is also used as a lubricant (*see* Heading 4 and Subheading 7.2.) (Keating, S. M., personal communication, 1992). The constituents of condom lubricant (e.g., silicon and polyethylene glycol) are also found in numerous other skin care products and suppositories. Therefore, when relevant, the forensic practitioner should ask if the complainant has applied anything to the genital/anal area in the preceding 2 days. This information should be noted on the paperwork that is made available to the forensic scientist so that scientist can source the relevant product to check what it contains. Dusting agents used on condoms may also be detected in the form of starch grains and lycopodium spores and can be used to correlate the finding of condom lubricant (Black, R., personal communication, 2002). The same dusting agents are used on some clinical gloves. Therefore, the forensic practitioner should wear nonpowdered gloves when sampling the genital and anal area *(194)*.

To maximize the possibility of lubricant detection, the necessary swabs should be obtained as soon as possible after the incident. The forensic science laboratory must then be told that lubricant analysis may be relevant, because this potentially requires scientists from more than one discipline to examine the same sample, e.g., when both body fluids and lubricant analysis are requested. If the forensic science laboratory is not made aware of this requirement, potential evidence could be inadvertently destroyed during laboratory processes.

Many factors may affect the length of time that a lubricant will persist on skin or in a body orifice. Condom lubricant has been detected on a swab taken from an unwashed penis 50 hours after intercourse and, in a different case, on a vaginal swab (also when the complainant had not washed or douched) taken 24 hours after intercourse, but detection after such prolonged periods would appear to be exceptional (Black, R., personal communication, 2002); water-based lubricants (e.g., those containing polyethylene glycol) have only been detected within 8 hours of the sexual act *(193,195)*.

12. Blood and Urine Analysis

12.1. Reason for Analysis

When drugs or alcohol have been consumed or possibly administered before or during a sexual assault, consideration should be given to the need to obtain samples of blood and urine for toxicological analysis. The length of time that a drug or its metabolites remain detectable in blood or urine depends on several factors, including the quantity taken, the individual's metabolism, and the sensitivity and specificity of the analytical methods employed by the laboratory *(196)*. Although the metabolites of some substances may be excreted for up to 168 hours in the urine *(196)*, many are detectable for only a few hours (*see* Subheading 12.4. on Persistence Data). In general, drugs and their metabolites will be identifiable for longer in urine than in blood.

12.2. Method of Sampling

12.2.1. Blood

It is good practice to request a sample of blood for drug/alcohol analysis when the incident has occurred in the preceding 4 days. A single sample of 10 mL of venous blood should be placed in a container with an anticoagulant (e.g., potassium oxalate) and a preservative that prevents decomposition and fermentation (e.g., sodium fluoride) for drug and alcohol analysis. If volatiles are suspected, a portion of blood must be collected into a container with an intrinsic rubber bung to enable the dead space above the blood to be analyzed.

12.2.2. Urine

It is good practice to request a sample of urine for drug/alcohol analysis when the incident has occurred in the preceding 4 days. If the allegation exceeds this time limit, contact the forensic science laboratory for advice on whether a sample is required. Ideally, 20 mL of urine should be placed in a container with a preservative that prevents decomposition and fermentation (e.g., sodium fluoride), although samples in plain bottles can be analyzed. Urine should be collected as soon as practically possible. Samples from complainants do not need to be witnessed. Complainants should be advised not to dispose of any towels, panty liners, or tampons at this stage.

Table 1
Approximate Detection Windows
for Prescribed/Illicit Substances

Prescribed/abused drugs	Blood	Urine
Diazepam/Temazepam	2 d	4 d
Methadone	1 d	2–3 d
Flunitrazepam	12–24 h	3 d
γ-Hydroxy butyrate	6 h	12 h
Barbiturates	1 or more d	2 or more d
Amphetamines	12–24 h	1–2 d
Ecstasy	12–24 h	2–3 d
Cocaine	12–24 h	2–3 d
Heroin/morphine	12–24 h	1–2 d
Cannabis—occasional user	0–4 h	12 h
Cannabis—regular user	days	weeks

From personal communications with A. Clatworthy and J. Taylor, members of the toxicology section of the Metropolitan Laboratory of Forensic Science, 2003.

12.3. Forensic Analysis

Forensic science laboratories have the capability of detecting a range of prescribed and illicit substances, but the persistence of different substances or their metabolites in the blood and urine of an individual depends on numerous factors. In some circumstances, the forensic science laboratory may undertake back calculations to estimate the blood alcohol concentration of the individual at the time of the sexual assault *(197)*.

Certain information is required to assist the forensic scientist with interpretation of the toxicological results.

- Sex, body weight, and build of the individual.
- The time that any drugs/alcohol were consumed or believed to have been administered. Was it a single dose or more?
- The exact time that the blood and urine samples were taken.
- Details of any prescribed medication or other substances normally consumed by the individual, including quantity and the date and time of most recent use.

12.4. Persistence Data

Table 1 provides the approximate detection windows for several prescribed/illicit substances. The detection windows depend on a few different factors, including the amount of substance used/administered and the frequency of use. Specialist advice is available for the toxicology section of the forensic laboratory.

13. CARE OF THE COMPLAINANT
13.1. Medical Treatment

The medical facilities should be stocked with the necessary provisions to enable minor injuries to be cleaned and dressed. Analgesia may be required. On rare occasions, a tetanus booster will be advisable.

13.2. Practical

The examination facilities should incorporate a shower or bath for the complainant to use after the medical is complete, and a change of clothing should be available (preferably the patient's own garments). Complainants should have access to a telephone so that they can contact friends or relatives and should be encouraged to spend the next few days in the company of someone that they trust. On occasions, emergency alternative accommodation will need to be organized.

13.3. Pregnancy

Consideration must be given to the patient's risk of becoming pregnant. Whenever any risk is identified, the patient should be counseled regarding the availability of hormonal and intrauterine methods of emergency contraception; the most suitable method will depend on the patient profile and the time since the assault *(198)*. When patients elect for insertion of an intrauterine contraceptive, they should be given prophylactic antibiotics *(see* Subheading 13.4.) either in advance of or at the time of the fitting. Follow-up appointments should be made at a convenient venue where pregnancy tests are available. Should the patient become pregnant because of the assault, she must be referred for sympathetic counseling. If the pregnancy is terminated, it may be relevant to seek permission from the patient for the products of conception to be retained for DNA analysis.

13.4. Sexually Transmitted Infections

Adult female complainants of sexual assault are at risk of acquiring a sexually transmitted infection (STI) as result of the assault *(199,200)*. Some male complainants have also described STI acquisition after the sexual assault *(170,171)*. In children who may have been sexually abused, there is a low prevalence of infections that are definitely sexually transmitted, although other organisms possibly associated with sexual activity may be identified *(201)*. Therefore, STI testing should be offered when the history and/or physical findings suggest the possibility of oral, genital, or rectal contact.

Some guidelines advocate STI screening for all adults at the time of presentation in recognition of the significant incidence of pre-existing STI amongst women who allege rape and a high default rate for follow-up consultations *(202,203)*. However, disclosure in court of pre-existing STI can be detrimental to the complainant *(40,204)*. Consequently, it may be more appropriate for the first tests to be deferred until 14 d after the assault. When interpreting the results of STI tests in young children, consideration must be given to the possibility that the sexually transmitted organisms could have been acquired perinatally *(201,205,206)*.

Some centers prescribe antibiotic prophylaxis for all complainants of penile penetrative sexual assaults at the time they present *(6,207,208)*. The use of antibiotic prophylaxis reduces the need for repeated examinations, avoids the anxiety incurred in waiting for the results, and is acceptable to the majority of women to whom it is offered *(209)*. Antibiotic prophylaxis should cover the prevalent, treatable organisms in the local population, and advice should be sought from the local center for disease control regarding an appropriate regimen.

Hepatitis B virus (HBV) can be acquired through consensual and nonconsensual sexual activity *(210)*. Therefore, HBV vaccine should be offered to all adult victims of sexual assault *(202)*. In children and young people, a risk/benefit analysis will inform the decision regarding whether the vaccine should be offered.

It is not known how soon after the sexual assault the HBV vaccine needs to be given to have an effect. However, because of the long incubation period an accelerated course of the vaccine (0, 1, and 2 months or 0, 1, and 6 months) may be efficacious if is initiated within 3 weeks of the exposure *(202)*.

Human immunodeficiency virus (HIV) can be acquired through sexual activity *(210)*. Although preventive antiretroviral treatment (postexposure prophylaxis [PEP]) is increasingly being offered to patients who may have had a sexual exposure to HIV infection, there are no studies that prove the efficacy of PEP in these circumstances *(211)*.

There are two approaches to the management of HIV PEP after a sexual assault. The first approach is to offer HIV PEP to all patients whose mucosa has been or is believed to have been exposed to the blood or semen of the assailant, regardless of the geographic location or likelihood of HIV infection in the assailant *(212)*. The second is for a forensic/genitourinary medicine physician to undertake a risk assessment taking account of the prevalence of HIV in the area where the assault occurred, the timing and nature of the assault, and any HIV risk behaviors exhibited by the assailant *(202,212)*. Animal studies suggest that the sooner HIV PEP is given, the greater the chance of preventing seroconversion. Therefore, it is currently recommended that HIV PEP is commenced no more than 72 hours after the assault, although it still may be effective up to 14 days after exposure *(202,213)*. Patients considering HIV PEP should be advised of the unproven efficacy, side effects, and potential toxicity of the treatment *(202,211)*.

Regardless of whether prophylaxis is given, complainants should be counseled and offered baseline serological tests for syphilis, HBV, hepatitis C, and HIV, which will be repeated at the relevant periods after assault.

13.5. Psychological

Complainants of sexual assault must be offered immediate and ongoing counseling to help them cope with the recognized immediate and long-term psychological sequelae of a sexual assault *(214)*. Some examination facilities have 24-h access to trained counselors *(215)*.

REFERENCES

1. Bays, J., Chadwick, D. Medical diagnosis of the sexually abused child. Child Abuse Negl. 17:91–110, 1993.
2. Heger, A., Emans, S. J., Muram, D., eds. Evaluation of the Sexually Abused Child. Oxford University Press, New York, NY, 2000.
3. Royal College of Physicians. Physical Signs of Sexual Abuse in Children. RCP, London, UK, 1997.
4. General Medical Council. Intimate Examinations. GMC, London, UK, 1996.
5. Hicks, D. J. Rape: Sexual assault. Am. J. Obstet. Gynecol. 137:931—935, 1980.
6. Evrard, J. R., Gold, G. M. Epidemiology and management of sexual assault victims. Obstet. Gynecol. 53:381–387, 1979.
7. Keating, S. M., Allard, J. E. What's in a name? Medical samples and scientific evidence in sexual assaults. Med. Sci. Law. 34:187–201, 1994.
8. Keating, S. M. The laboratory's approach to sexual assault cases. Part 1: sources of information and acts of intercourse. J. Forensic. Sci. Soc. 28:35–47, 1988.
9. Clark, M. D. B. Metropolitan Police Laboratory Examination Kit for Sexual Offences. Police Surg. 15:447–452, 1979.
10. Ranson, D. The forensic medical examination. In: Forensic Medicine and the Law. Melbourne University Press, Victoria, Australia, pp. 119–127, 1996.
11. Kafarowski, E., Lyon, A. M., Sloan, M. M. The retention and transfer of spermatozoa in clothing by machine washing. Can. Soc. Forensic Sci. J. 29:7–11, 1996.
12. Benecke, M. DNA typing in forensic medicine and in criminal investigations: a current survey. Naturwissenschaften. 84:181–188, 1997.
13. Mannucci, A., Sullivan, K. M., Ivanov, P. L., Gill, P. Forensic application of a rapid and quantitative DNA sex test by amplification of the X–Y homologous gene amelogenin. Int. J. Leg. Med. 106:190–193, 1994.
14. Foreman, L. A., Evett, I. W. Statistical analyses to support forensic interpretation for a new ten-locus STR profiling system. Int. J. Leg. Med. 114:147–155, 2001.

15. Gill, P. Role of short tandem repeat DNA in forensic casework in the UK—past, present and future perspectives. Biotechniques. 32:366–372, 2002.
16. Werrett, D. J. The national database. Forensic Sci. Int. 88:33–42, 1997.
17. Hoyle, R. The FBI's national database. Biotechnology. 16:987, 1998.
18. Gill, P., Sparkes, B., Fereday, L.,Werrett, D. J. Report of the European Network of Forensic Science Institutes (ENFSI): formulation and testing of principles to evaluate STR multiplexes. Forensic Sci. Int. 108:1–29.
19. Bar, W., Brinkman, B., Budowle, B., et al. DNA recommendations. Further report of the DNA Commission of the ISFH regarding the use of short tandem repeat systems. International Society for Forensic Haemogenetics. Int. J. Leg. Med. 110:175–176, 1997.
20. Olaisen, B., Bar, W., Brinkmann, B., et al. DNA recommendations of the International Society for Forensic Genetics. Vox-Sang. 74:61–63, 1998.
21. Leriche, A., et al. Final report of the Interpol Working Party on DNA profiling. Proceedings from the 2nd Eurpoean Symposium on Human Idenitification. Promege Corporation, 48–54, 1998.
22. The Forensic Science Service. Low copy number DNA profiling. Available at Website: (http://128.1.18.1/html/corpcomm/hotnews/low.copy.htm).
23. Monckton, D. G., Jeffreys, A. J. DNA profiling. Curr. Opin. Biotechnol. 4:660–664, 1993.
24. Rutty, G. An investigation into the transference and survivability of human DNA following simulated manual strangulation with consideration of the problem of third party contamination. Int. J. Leg. Med. 116:170–173, 2001.
25. Sweet, D. J. Human bite marks—examination, recovery and analysis. In: Bowers, C. M. and Bell, G. L., eds., Manual of Forensic Odontology. American Society of Forensic Odontology, Colorado Springs, CO, 1995.
26. Clift, A., Lamont, C. M. Saliva in forensic odontology. J. Forensic Sci. Soc. 14:241–245, 1974.
27. Bowers, C. M., Bell, G. L., eds. Manual of Forensic Odontology. American Society of Forensic Odontology, Colorado Springs, CO, 1995.
28. Sweet, D., Lorente, M., Lorente, J. A., Valenzuela, A., Villanueva, E. An improved method to recover saliva from human skin: the double swab technique. J. Forensic Sci. Soc. 42: 320–322, 1997.
29. Girardin, B. W., Faugno, D. K., Seneski, P. C., Slaughter, L., Whelan, M. Care of the sexually assaulted patient. In: Color Atlas of Sexual Assault.Mosby, St. Louis, MO, 1997, p. 96.
30. Lynnerup, N., Hjalgrim, H. Routine use of ultraviolet light in medicolegal examinations to evaluate stains and skin trauma. Med. Sci. Law. 35:165–168, 1995.
31. Santucci, K., Nelson, D., Kemedy, K., McQuillen, K., Duffy, S., Linakis, J. Wood's lamp utility in the identification of semen. Pediatrics. 104:1342–1344, 1999.
32. Jones, D. N. The task of the Forensic Science Laboratory in the investigation of sexual offences. J. Forensic Sci. Soc. 3:88–93, 1963.
33. Stoilovic, M. Detection of semen and blood stains using Polilight® as a light source. Forensic Sci. Int. 51:289–296, 1991.

34. Marshall, S., Bennett, A., Fravel, H. Locating semen on live skin using visible fluorescence. Paper presented at the Sixth International Conference in Clinical Forensic Medicine of the World Police Medical Officers, March 17–22, Sydney, Australia, 2002.

35. Nelson, D. G., Santucci, K. A. An alternative light source to detect semen. Acad. Emerg. Med. 9:1045–1048, 2002.

36. Sweet, D., Lorente, J. A., Valenzuela A., Lorente, M., Villanueva, E. PCR-based DNA typing of saliva stains recovered from human skin. J. Forensic Sci. Soc. 42:447–451, 1997.

37. Cartwright, P. S. Reported sexual assault in Nashville-Davidson County, Tennessee, 1980–1982. Am. J. Obstet. Gynecol. 154:1064–1068, 1986.

38. Everett, R. B., Jimerson, G. K. The rape victim: a review of 117 consecutive cases. Obstet. Gynecol. 50:88–90, 1977.

39. Soules, M. R., Stewart, S. K., Brown, K. M., Pollard, A. A. The spectrum of alleged rape. J. Reprod. Med. 20:33–39, 1978.

40. Kerr, E., Cottee, C., Chowdhury, R., Jawad, R., Welch, J. The Haven: a pilot referral centre in London for cases of serious sexual assault. Br. J. Obstet. Gynaecol. 110: 267–271, 2003.

41. Riggs, N., Houry, D., Long, G., Markovchick, V., Feldhaus, K. Analysis of 1,076 cases of sexual assault. Ann. Emerg. Med. 35:358–362, 2000.

42. Vale, G. L., Noguchi, T. T. Anatomical distribution of human bite marks in a series of 67 cases. J. Forensic Sci. Soc. 28:61–69, 1983.

43. Wright, R., West, D. J. Rape—a comparison of group offences and lone assaults. Med. Sci. Law. 21:25–30, 1981.

44. Muller, C., Vogt, S., Goerke, R., Kordan, A., Weinmann, W. Identification of selected psychopharmaceuticals and their metabolites in hair by LC/ESI-CID/MS and LC/MS/MS. Forensic Sci. Int. 113:415–421, 2000.

45. Kintz, P., Cirimele, V., Jamey, C., Ludes, B. Testing for GHB in hair by GC/MS/MS after single exposure. Application to document sexual assault. J. Forensic Sci. 48:195–199, 2003.

46. Negrusz, A., Moore, C. M., Hinkel, K. B., et al. Deposition of 7-aminoflunitrazepam and flunitrazepam in hair after a single dose of Rohypnol®. J. Forensic Sci. 46:1–9, 2001.

47. Guterman, L. Nailing the drug rapists. New Scientist. 160:4, 1998.

48. Wicks, J. Managing Director Tricho-Tec Ltd. Paper presented at the Association of Police Surgeons Autumn Symposium, Northamtpon, UK, November 2001.

49. Ledray, L. (1993) Evidence collection: an update. J. Sexual Abuse. 2:113–115.

50. Young, W., Bracken, A. C., Goddard, M. A. A., Matheson, S. The New Hampshire sexual assault medical examination protocol project committee sexual assault: review of a national model protocol for forensic and medical evaluation. Obstet Gynecol. 80:878–883, 1992.

51. Salter, M. T., Cooke, R. The significance of transfer of fibres to head hair, their persistence and retrieval. Forensic Sci. Int. 1981:211–221, 1996.

52. Exline, D. L., Smith, F. P., Drexler, S. G. Frequency of pubic hair transfer during sexual intercourse. J. Forensic Sci. 43:505–508, 1998.

53. Mann, M. J. Hair transfers in sexual assault: a six-year case study. J. Forensic Sci. Soc. 35:951–955, 1990.

54. Stone, I. C. Hair and its probative value as evidence. Texas Bar J. 45:275–279, 1982.

55. Riis, R. Sexual assault combing evidence. Presented at the NWAFS Meeting, Jackson Hole, WY, 1990.

56. Higuchi, R., Von Beroldingen, C. H., Sensabaugh, G. F., Erlich, H. A. DNA typing from single hairs. Nature. 332:543–546, 1988.

57. Prahlow, J. A., Lantz, P. E., Cox-Jones, K., Rao, P.N., Pettenati, M. J. Gender identification of human hair using fluoresence in situ hybridisation. J. Forensic Sci. 41:1035–1037, 1996.

58. Cirimele, V., Kinttz, P., Staub, C., Mangin, P. Testing of human hair of flunitrazepam and 7-amino-flunitrazepam by GC/MS-NCY. Forensic Sci. Int. 84:189–200, 1997.

59. Ropero-Miller, J. D., Goldberger, B. A., Cone, E. J., Joseph, R. E. The deposition of cocaine and opiate analytes in hair and fingernails of humans following cocaine and codeine administration. J. Anal. Toxicol. 24:496–508, 2000.

60. Tsatsakis, A. M., Psillakis, T., Paritsis, N. Phenytoin concentration in head hair sections: a method to evaluate the history of drug use. J. Clin. Psychopharmacol. 20:560–573, 2000.

61. Enos, W. F., Beyer, J. C. The importance of examining skin and hair for semen in sexual assault cases. J. Forensic Sci. Soc. 26:605–607, 1981.

62. Thomas, F., Baert, H. A new means of identification of the human being: the longitudinal striation of the nails. Med Sci Law. 5, 39–40, 1965.

63. Lederer, T., Betz, P. Seidi, S. DNA analysis of fingernail debris using different multiplex systems: a case report. Int J Legal Med. 114, 263–266, 2001.

64. Evans, B. A., Bond, R. A., Macrae, K. D. Sexual behaviour in women attending a genitourinary medicine clinic. Genitourin Med. 64:43–48, 1988.

65. Keating, S. M., Higgs, D. F. Oral sex—further information from sexual assault cases. J Forensic Sci Soc. 32:327–331, 1992.

66. Bradham, G. B. The establishment of a treatment center for victims of rape. JSC Med Assoc. June, 283–286, 1981.

67. Sexual Offences Act. Website: (www.publications.parliament.uk), Home Office, London, UK, 2003.

68. Lind, W., Carlson, D. Recovery of semen from chewing gum in an oral sexual assault. J Forensic Identification. 45, 280–282, 1995.

69. Hampton, H. L. Care of the woman who has been raped. N. Engl. J. Med. 332:234–237, 1995.

70. Willott, G. M., Crosse, M. A. The detection of spermatozoa in the mouth. J. Forensic Sci Soc. 26:125–128, 1986.

71. Allard, J. E. The collection of data from findings in cases of sexual assault and the significance of spermatozoa on vaginal, anal and oral swabs. Sci. Justice. 37:99–108, 1997.

72. Enos, W. F., Beyer, J. C. Spermatozoa in the anal canal and rectum and in the oral cavity of female rape victims. J. Forensic Sci. Soc. 23:231–233, 1978.

73. Schlesinger, S. L., Borbotsina, J., O'Neill, L. Petechial hemorrhages of the soft palate secondary to fellatio. Oral Surg. 40:376–378, 1975.

74. Giansanti, J. S., Cramer, J. R., Weathers, D. R. Palatal erythema, another etiologic factor. Oral Surg. 40:379–381, 1975.
75. Damm, D. D., White, D. K., Brinker, C. M. Variations of palatal erythema secondary to fellatio. Oral Surg. 52:417–421, 1981.
76. Girardin, B. W., Faugno, D. K., Seneski, P. C., Slaughter, L., Whelan, M. Findings in sexual asault and consensual intercourse. In: Color Atlas of Sexual Assault. Mosby, St. Louis, MO, 1997, p. 41.
77. Bellizzi, R., Krakow, A. M., Plack, W. Soft palate trauma associated with fellatio: case report. Mil. Med. 145:787–788, 1980.
78. Girardin, B. W., Faugno, D. K., Seneski, P. C., Slaughter, L., Whelan, M. Findings in sexual asault and consensual intercourse. In: Color Atlas of Sexual Assault. Mosby, St. Louis, MO, 1997, p. 38.
79. Johnson, A. M., Wadsworth, J., Wellings, K., Field, J. Heterosexual practices. In: Sexual Attitudes and Lifestyles. Blackwell Scientific Publications, Oxford, UK, 1994, p. 160.
80. Bolling, D. R. Prevalence, goals and complications of hetcrosexual anal intercourse in a gynecologic population. J. Reprod. Med. 19:121–124, 1977.
81. Keating, S. M. Oral sex—a review of its prevalence and proof. J. Forensic Sci. Soc. 28:341–355, 1988.
82. Keating, S. M., Higgs, D. F. The detection of amylase on swabs from sexual assault cases. J. Forensic Sci. Soc. 34:89–93, 1994.
83. Skerlavy, M., Epstein, J. A., Sobrero, A. J. Cervical mucus amylase levels in normal menstrual cycles. Fertil. Steril. 19:726–730, 1968.
84. Banaschak, S., Moller, K., Pfeiffer, H. Potential DNA mixtures introduced through kissing. Int. J. Leg. Med. 111:284–285, 1998.
85. Mader, C. L. Lingual frenulum ulcer resulting from orogenital sex. J. Am. Dent. Assoc. 103:888–890, 1981.
86. Johnson, A. M., Wadsworth, J., Wellings, K., Field, J. Heterosexual practices. In: Sexual Attitudes and Lifestyles. Blackwell Scientific Publications, Oxford, UK, 1994.
87. Wellings, K., Nanchahai K., Macdowall, W., Sexual behaviour in Britan: early heterosexual experience. Lancet. 358:1843–1850, 2001.
88. Howitt, J., Rogers, D. J. Adult sexual offences and related matters. In: McLay, W. D. S., ed., Clinical Forensic Medicine. Greenwich Medical Media, Hong Kong, 1996, pp. 193–218.
89. Lines 1844 I.C. and K. 393.
90. Slaughter, L., Brown, C. R. V., Crowley, S., Peck, R. Patterns of genital injury in female sexual assault victims. Am. J. Obstet. Gynecol. 176:609–616, 1997.
91. Jenny, C., Kunhs, M. L., Fukiko, A. Presence of hymens in newborn female infants. Pediatrics. 80:399–400, 1987.
92. Chadwick, D. L., Berkowltz, C. D., Kerns, D., McCann, J., Reinhart, M. A., Strickland, S. Color Atlas of Child Sexual Abuse. Year Book Medical Publishers, Chicago, IL, 1989.
93. Berenson, A., Chacko M. R., Wiemann, C. M., Mishaw, C. O., Friedrich, W. N., Grady, J. J. A case control study of anatomic changes resulting from sexual abuse. Am. J. Obstet. Gynecol. 182:820–834, 2000.

94. Berenson, A., Heger, A., Andrews, S. The appearance of the hymen in the newborn. Pediatrics. 87:458–465, 1991.

95. Berenson, A. Appearance of the hymen in prepubertal girls. Pediatrics. 89:387–394, 1992.

96. Emans, S. J., Woods, E., Allred, E., Grace, E. Hymenal findings in adolescent women, impact of tampon use and consensual sexual activity. Pediatrics. 125:153–160, 1994.

97. Muram, D. Anatomic and physiological changes. In: Evaluation of the Sexually Abused Child. Oxford University Press, New York, NY, 1992, p. 72.

98. Emans, S. J. H., Goldstein, D. P. The physiology of puberty. In: Pediatric and Adolescent Gynecology, 3rd Ed., Little, Brown, Boston, MA, pp. 95–97, 1990.

99. Porkorny, S. F. Configuration of the prepubertal hymen. Am. J. Obstet. Gynecol. 157:950–956, 1987.

100. McCann, J., Wells, R., Simon, M., Voris, J. Genital findings in prepubertal girls selected for nonabuse: a descriptive study. Pediatrics. 86:428–439, 1990.

101. Girardin, B. W., Faugno, D. K., Seneski, P. C., Slaughter, L., Whelan, M. Care of the sexually assaulted patient. In: Color Atlas of Sexual Assault. Mosby, St. Louis, MO, pp. 111–118, 1997.

102. Masters, W. H., Johnson, V. E. The vagina. In: The Human Sexual Response. Little Brown, Boston, MA, pp. 69–70, 1966.

103. Robinson, E. G. Management of the rape victim. Can. Med. Assoc. J. 115:520–523, 1976.

104. Reade, D. J. Early scientific investigations of sexual assault. Police Surg. April:42–46, 1986.

105. Eungprabhanth, V. Finding of the spermatozoa in the vagina related to elapsed time of coitus. Z. Rechtamedizin. 74:301–304, 1974.

106. Florence, A. Du sperme et des taches de sperme en medecine legale. Arch. d'Anthropol. Criminelle d' Criminolo Psychol. Normale Pathol. 11:146–165, 1896.

107. Laurell, C. B. Electroimmunoassay. Scand. J. Clin. Lab. Invest. 29:21, 1972.

108. Collins, K. A., Rao, P. N., Hayworth, R., et al. Identification of sperm and non-sperm male cells in cervicovaginal smears using Fluoresecence In Situ Hybrid-isation—applications in alleged sexual assault cases. J. Forensic Sci. 39:1347–1355, 1994.

109. Sibille, I., Duverneuil, C., Lorin de la Grandmaison, G., Y–STR DNA amplification as biological evidence in sexually assaulted female victims with no cytological detection of spermatozoa. Forensic Sci. Int. 125:212–216, 2002.

110. Rao, P. N., Collins, K. A., Geisinger, K. R., et al. Identification of male epithelial cells in routine post-coital cervicovaginal smears using Fluoresecence In Situ Hybridisation—application in sexual assault and molestation. Am. J. Clin. Path. 104:32–35, 1995.

111. Divall, G. B. Methods for the identification and menstrual blood. In: Lee, H.G. and Gaensslen, R.E., eds., Advances in Forensic Science, Biomedical Publications, Foster City, CA, pp. 1–14, 1985.

112. Allard, J. The facts of life. Contact-FSS Internal Publication. 25, 1996.
113. Davis, A., Wilson, E. The persistence of seminal constituents in the human vagina. Forensic Sci. 3:45–55, 1974.
114. Graves, H. C. B., Sensabaugh, G. F., Blake, E. T. Postcoital detection of a male-specific semen protein: application to the investigation of rape. N. Engl. J. Med. 312:338–340, 1985.
115. Wilson, E. M. A comparison of the persistence of seminal constituents in the human vagina and cervix. Police Surg. 22:44–45, 1982.
116. Keating, S. M. The laboratory's approach to sexual assault cases. Part 2. Demonstration of the possible offender. J. Forensic Sci. Soc. 28:99–110, 1988.
117. Dziegelewski, M., Simich, J. P., Rittenhouse-Olson, K. Use of a Y chromosome probe as an aid in the forensic proof of sexual assault. J. Forensic Sci. 47:601–604, 2002.
118. Gaensslen, R. E. Survival of spermatozoa in the vagina. In: Gaensslen, R. E., ed., Sourcebook in Forensic Serology, Immunology and Biochemistry. United States Government Printing Office, Washington, DC, pp. 144–152, 1983,
119. Silverman, E. M., Silverman, A. G. Persistence of spermatozoa in the lower genital tracts of women. JAMA. 240:1875–1877, 1978.
120. Rupp, J. C. Sperm survival and prostatic acid phosphatase activity in victims of sexual assault. J. Forensic Sci. Soc. 14:177–183, 1969.
121. Paul, D. M. Examination of the living. In: Taylor's Principles and Practice of Medical Jurisprudence, 13th Ed. Mant A. K., ed., Churchill Livingstone, Edinburgh, Scotland, pp. 64–105, 1984.
122. Allard, J. E. The collection of data from findings in cases of sexual assault and the significance of spermatozoa on vaginal, anal and oral swabs. Sci. Justice. 37:99–108, 1997.
123. Slaughter, L., Brown, C. R. V. Colposcopy to establish physical findings in rape victims. Am. J. Obstet. Gynecol. 166:83–86, 1992.
124. Cartwright, P. S., Moore, R. A., Anderson, J. R., Brown, D. H. Genital injury and implied consent to alleged rape. J. Reprod. Med. 31:1043–1044, 1986.
125. Ramin, S. M., Satin, A. J., Stone, S. C., Wendel, G. D. Sexual assault in postmenopausal women. Obstet. Gynecol. 80:860–864, 1992.
126. Norvell, M. K., Benrubi, G. I., Thompson, R. J. Investigations of microtrauma after sexual intercourse. J. Reprod. Med. 29:269–271, 1984.
127. Fraser, I. S., Lahteenmaki, P., Elomaa, K., et al. Variations in vaginal epithelial surface appearance determined by colposcopic inspection in healthy sexually active women. Hum. Reprod. 14:1974–1978, 1999.
128. Lauber, A. A., Souma, M. L. Use of toluidine blue for documentation of traumatic intercourse. Obstet. Gynecol. 60:644–648, 1982.
129. McCauley, J., Gorman, R. L., Guzinski, G. Toluidine blue in the detection of perineal lacerations in pediatric and adolescent sexual abuse victims. Pediatrics. 78:1039–1043, 1986.
130. McCauley, J., Guzinski, G., Welch, R., Gorman, R., Osmers, F. Toluidine blue in the corroboration of rape in adult victim. Am. J. Emerg. Med. 5:105–108, 1987.

131. Wilson, K. F. G. Lower genital tract trauma. Aust. N. Z. J. Obstet. Gynaecol. 6:291–293, 1966.
132. Adams, J. A., Girardin, B., Faugno, D. Adolescent sexual assault: documentation of acute injuries using photo-colposcopy. J. Pediatric Adolesc. Gynecol. 14:175–180, 2001.
133. Bowyer, L., Dalton, M. E. Female victims of rape and their genital injuries. Br. J. Obstet. Gynecol. 104:617–620, 1997.
134. Manser, T. Findings in medical examinations of victims and offenders in cases of serious sexual offences—a survey. Police Surg. 38:4–27, 1991.
135. Kellogg, N. D., Parra, J. M. Linea vestibularis: a previously undescribed normal genital structure in female neonates. Pediatrics. 87:926–929, 1991.
136. De San Lazaro, C., Sivaramakrishnan, S. Summer sandal genital injury. J. Clin. Forensic Med. 5:32–33, 1998.
137. Dowd, M. D., Fitzmaurice, L., Knapp, J. F., Mooney, D. The interpretation of urogenital findings in children with straddle injuries. J. Pediatric Surg. 29:7–10, 1994.
138. Ferrell, J. Sexual assault: clinical issues, Foley catheter balloon technique for visualizing the hymen in female adolescent sexual abuse victims. J. Emerg. Nurs. 21: 585–586, 1995.
139. Muram, D. Child sexual abuse: relationship between sexual acts and genital findings. Child Abuse Negl. 13:211–216, 1989.
140. McCann, J., Voris, J., Simon, M. Genital injuries resulting from sexual abuse: a longitudinal study. Pediatrics. 89:307–317, 1993.
141. Berkowitz, C., Evik, S., Logan, M. A simulated 'acquired' imperforate hymen following the genital trauma of sexual abuse. Clin. Pediatr. 26:307–309, 1993.
142. Goodyear-Smith, F. A., Laidlaw, T. M. What is an "intact hymen"? A critique of the literature. Med. Sci. Law. 38:289–301, 1998.
143. Teixera, W. Hymenal colposcopic examination in sexual offences. Am. J. Forensic Med. Pathol. 3:201–214, 1981.
144. Underhill, R., Dewhurst, J. The doctor cannot always tell: medical examination of the 'intact' hymen. Lancet. 1:375–376, 1978.
145. Wilson, F., Swartz, D. P. Coital injuries of the vagina. Obstet Gynecol. 39:182–184, 1972.
146. Fish, S. A. Vaginal injury due to coitus. Am. J. Obstet. Gynecol. 72:544–548, 1956.
147. Metsala, P., Nieminen, U. Traumatic lesions of the vagina. Acta Obstet. Gynecol. Scand. 47:483–488, 1968.
148. Gray, M. J., Norton, P., Treadwell, K. Tampon-induced injuries. Obstet. Gynecol. 58:667–668, 1981.
149. Hakanson, E. Y. Trauma to the female genitalia. Lancet. 86:286–291, 1966.
150. Burgess, A. W., Holmstrom, L. L. The rape victim in the emergency ward. Am. J. Nurs. 73:1741–1745, 1973.
151. Slaughter, L., Brown, C. R. V. Cervical findings in rape victims. Am. J. Obstet. Gynecol. 164:528–529, 1991.

152. Fraser, I. S., Lahteenmaki, P., Elomaa, K., et al. Variations in vaginal epithelial surface appearance determined by colposcopic inspection in healthy, sexually active women. Hum. Reprod. 14:1974–1978, 1999.

153. Masters, W. H., Johnson, V. E. The penis. In: The Human Sexual Response. Little Brown, Boston, MA, pp. 171–203, 1966.

154. Muram, D. Anatomy. In: Hegar, A. and Emans, S. J., eds., Evaluation of the Sexually Abused Child. Oxford University Press, New York, NY, p. 73, 1992.

155. Girardin, B. W., Faugno, D. K., Seneski, P. C., Slaughter, L., Whelan, M. Anatomy and the human sexual response. In: Color Atlas of Sexual Asault. Mosby, St. Louis, MO, p. 11, 1997.

156. Stephen, J. C., Collins, K. A., Pettenati, M. J., Fitts, M. Isolation and identification of female DNA on post-coital penile swabs. Am. J. Forensic Med. Pathol. 21:97–100, 2000.

157. Farah, R., Cerny, J. C. Penis tourniquet syndrome and penile amputation. Urology. 11:310–311, 1973.

158. Garty, B. Z., Mimouni, M., Varsano, I. Penile tourniquet sydrome. Cutis. 31:431–432, 1983.

159. Kerry, R. L., Chapman, D. D. Strangulation of appendages by hair and thread. Pediatric Surg. 8:23–27, 1973.

160. Wheatley, J. K. Genital injury during intercourse. Med. Aspects Hum. Sex. 17:24A–24J, 1983.

161. Ball, T. P., Pickett, J. D. Traumatic lymphangitis of penis. Urology. IV:594–597, 1975.

162. Davies, D. M., Mitchell, I. Fracture of the penis. Br. J. Urol. 50:426, 1978.

163. Pryor, J. P., Hill, J. T., Packham, D. A., Yates-Bell, A. J. Penile injuries with particular reference to injury to the erectile tissue. Br. J. Urol. 53:42–46, 1981.

164. Paul, D. M. The medical examination of the live rape victim and the accused. Leg. Med. Ann. 139–153, 1977.

165. Wells, D. L. Genital trauma amongst young boys. J. Clin. Forensic Med. 3:129–132, 1996.

166. Hobbs, C. J., Wynne. J. M. Physical signs of child abuse. W. B. Saunders, Philadelphia, PA, 1996.

167. Johnson, A. M., Wadsworth, J., Wellings, K., Field, J. Heterosexual practices. In: Sexual Attitudes and Lifestyles. Blackwell Scientific Publications, Oxford, UK, p. 163, 1994.

168. Johnson, A. M., Wadsworth, J., Wellings, K., Field, J. Sexual diversity and homosexual behaviour. In: Sexual Attitudes and Lifestyles. Blackwell Scientific Publications, Oxford, UK, pp. 183–223, 1994.

169. Bang, L. Rape victims—assaults, injuries and treatment at a medical rape trauma service at Oslo Emergency Hospital. Scand. J. Primary Health Care. 11:15–20, 1993.

170. Hillman, R. J., O'Mara, N., Taylor-Robinson, D., Williams Harris, J. R. Medical and social aspects of sexual assault of males: a survey of 100 victims. Br. J. Gen. Pract. 40:502–504, 1990.

171. Hillman, R., O'Mara, N., Tomlinson, D., William Harris, J. R. Adult male victims of sexual assault: an underdiagnosed condition. Int. J. STD AIDS. 2:22–24, 1991.

172. Temkin, J. Rape and the Legal Process. Sweet & Maxwell, London, UK, 1987.

173. Royal College of Physicians. Glossary of terms. In: Physical Signs of Sexual Abuse in Children. RCP, London, UK, pp. 67–68, 1997.

174. Girardin, B. W., Faugno, D. K., Seneski, P. C., Slaughter, L., Whelan, M. Anatomy and the human sexual response. In: Color Atlas of Sexual Assault. Mosby, St. Louis, MO, pp. 14–16, 1997.

175. Fenger, C. Anal canal. In: Sternberg, S. S., ed., Histology for Pathologists, 2nd Ed., Lippincott-Raven, Philadelphia, PA, pp. 551–571, 1997.

176. Nivatovongs, S., Stern, H. S., Fryd, D. S. The length of the anal canal. Dis. Colon Rectum. 24:600–611, 1981.

177. Goligher, J. Surgical anatomy and physiology of the anus, rectum and colon. In: Surgery of the Anus, Rectum and Colon, 5th Ed. Baillière Tindall, London, UK, p. 15, 1984.

178. Parks, A. G., Porter, N. H., Melzak, J. Experimental study of the reflex mechanism controlling the muscles of the pelvic floor. Dis. Colon Rectum. 5:401–414, 1962.

179. Davies, A. Discussion of spermatozoa in the anal canal and rectum and in the oral cavity of female rape victims. J. Forensic Sci. Soc. 24:541–542, 1979.

180. Green, R. J., Sayce, M. D. Problems associated with the typing of semen on anal swabs. J. Forensic Sci. Soc. 25:55–56, 1985.

181. Willott, G. M., Allard, J. E. Spermatozoa—their persistence after sexual intercourse. Forensic Sci. Int. 19:135–154, 1982.

182. Bush, R. A., Owen, W. F. Trauma and other noninfectious problems in homosexual men. Med. Clin. North Am. 70:549–566, 1986.

183. Goligher, J. Anal fissure. In: Surgery of the Anus, Rectum and Colon, 5th ed. Baillière Tindall, London, UK, p. 150, 1984.

184. Keighley, M. R. B., Williams, N. S. Fissure in ano. In: Surgery of the Anus, Rectum and Colon. Saunders, Philadelphia, PA, pp. 364–386, 1993.

185. Girardin, B. W., Faugno, D. K., Seneski, P. C., Slaughter, L., Whelan, M. Findings in sexual assault and consensual intercourse. In: Color Atlas of Sexual Assault. Mosby, St. Louis, MO, p. 50, 1997.

186. Girardin, B. W., Faugno, D. K., Seneski, P. C., Slaughter, L., Whelan, M. Glossary. In: Color Atlas of Sexual Assault. Mosby, St. Louis, MO, p. 192, 1997.

187. Crass, R. A., Tranbaugh, R. F., Kudsk, K. A., Trunkey, D. D. Colorectal foreign bodies and perforation. Am. J. Surg. 142:85–88, 1981.

188. Barone, J. E., Yee, J., Nealon, T. F. Management of foreign bodies and trauma of the rectum. Surg. Gynecol. Obstet. 56:453–457, 1983.

189. Rakotomalala, L., de Parades, V., Parisot, C., Atienza, P. Ruptures multiples du sphincter interne après viol anal: une cause peu connue d'incontinence anale. Gastroenterol. Clin. Biol. 20:1142–1143, 1996.

190. Chun, A. B., Rose, S., Mitrani, C., Silvestre, A. J., Wald, A. Anal sphincter structure and function in homosexual males engaging in anoreceptive intercourse. Am. J. Gastroenterol. 92:465–468, 1997.

191. Miles, A. J. G., Allen-Mersh, T. G., Wastell, C. Effect of anoreceptive intercourse on anorectal function. J. R. Soc. Med. 86:144–147, 1993.

192. Blackledge, R.D., Condom trace evidence: a new factor in sexual assault investigations. FBI Law Enforcement Bull, May 12–16, 1996.

193. Greaves, C. Safe sex? Is it so safe? Contact-FSS Internal Publication. 25:20–21, 1998.

194. McCrane W.C., Delly J.G. (1973) The Particles Atlas. 3:600, 702, 1973.

195. Blackledge, R. D., Vincenti, M. Identification of polydimethylsiloxane lubricant traces from latex condoms in cases of sexual assault. J. Forensic Sci. Soc. 34:245–256, 1994.

196. Jansen, K. Date rape drugs. Bull. Int. Assoc. Forensic Toxicol. 28:18–20, 1998.

197. Ferner, R. E. Ethanol. In: Forensic Pharmacology. Oxford University Press, Oxford, UK, pp. 122–124, 1996.

198. Kubba, A., Wilkinson, C. Recommendations for Clinical Practice: Emergency Contraception. FFP & RHC RCOG, London, UK, 1998.

199. Jenny, C., Hooton, T. M., Bowers, A., et al. Sexually transmitted diseases in victims of rape. N. Engl. J. Med. 322:713–716, 1990.

200. Estreich, S., Forster, G. E., Robinson, A. Sexually transmitted diseases in rape victims. Genitourin Med. 66:433–438, 1990.

201. Robinson, A. J., Watkeys, J. E. M., and Ridgeway, G. L. Sexually transmitted organisms in sexually abused children. Arch. Dis. Child. 79:356–358, 1998.

202. British Association for Sexual Health and HIV. National guidelines on the management of adult victims if sexual assault. Available at Website: (www.mssvd.org). Accessed on November 3, 2002.

203. Ross, J. D. C., Scott, G. R., Busuttil, A. Rape and sexually transmitted diseases: patterns of referral and incidence in a department of genitourinary medicine. J. R. Soc. Med. 84:657–659, 1991.

204. Lacey, H. B. Rape, the law and medical practitioners. Br. J. Sex. Med. Winter:89–92, 1991.

205. Hammerschlag, M. R. Sexually transmitted diseases in sexually abused children: medical and legal implications. Sex. Transm. Inf. 74:167–174, 1998.

206. Thomas, A., Forster, G., Robinson, A. Rogstad K. National guidelines on the management of suspected sexually transmitted infections in children and young people. Available at Website: (www.mssvd.org). Accessed 2003.

207. Girardin, B. W., Faugno, D. K., Seneski, P. C., Slaughter, L., Whelan, M. Care of the sexually assaulted patient. In: Color Atlas of Sexual Assault. Mosby, St. Louis, MO, p. 123, 1997.

208. Hochbaum, S. R. The evaluation and treatment of the sexually assaulted patient. Emerg. Med. Clin North Am. 5:601–622, 1987.

209. Gibb, A. M., McManus, T., Forster, G. E. Should we offer antibiotic prophylaxis post sexual assault? Int. J. STD AIDS. 14:99–102, 2003.

210. Crowe, C., Forster, G. E., Dinsmore, W. W., Maw, R. D. A case of acute hepatitis B occurring four months after multiple rape. Int. J. STD AIDS. 7:133–134, 1996.

211. Limb, S., Kawsar, M., and Forster, G. E. HIV post-exposure prophylaxis after sexual assault: the experience of a sexual assault service in London. 13:602–605, 2002.

212. Weinberg, G. A. Post-exposure prophylaxis against human immunodeficiency virus infection after sexual assault. Pediatr. Infect. Dis. 21:957-960, 2002.
213. National HIV Prevention Information Service. Post-exposure prophylaxis (PEP) against HIV infection following sexual and injection drug use exposure. Edward King of NAM Publications, London, UK, 1998.
214. Burgess, A. W., Holmstrom, L. L. Rape trauma syndrome. Am. J. Psychiatry. 131: 981–986.
215. Duddle, M. Emotional sequelae of sexual assault. J. R. Soc. Med. 84:26–28, 1991.

Chapter 4

Injury Assessment, Documentation, and Interpretation

Jason Payne-James, Jack Crane,
and Judith A. Hinchliffe

1. INTRODUCTION

The ability to appropriately assess, document, and interpret injuries that have been sustained is a key part of the work of any forensic physician or forensic pathologist. Crimes of violence are increasing throughout the world. Nonjudicial assault, such as torture, has also become more widely recognized *(1)*. It has been suggested that the definition of physical injury in the forensic medical context should be "damage to any part of the body due to the deliberate or accidental application of mechanical or other traumatic agent" *(2)*. This chapter specifically addresses the issues of physical assault and the assessment and documentation of wounds or injury.

The purpose of assessment and documentation is to assist in establishing how a wound or injury is caused, which may often be at issue in courts or tribunals of law. These two skills should be within the remit of any doctor, although they are rarely done fully and appropriately. The interpretation of the causes of wounds and injuries is probably best undertaken by those with forensic expertise, because there may be many factors involved in such interpretation. Because interpretation of wounds and injuries may be undertaken by review of documents, for example written descriptions, body chart mapping, or photographs, it is imperative that the descriptions are comprehensible to all. For

From: *Clinical Forensic Medicine: A Physician's Guide, 2nd Edition*
Edited by: M. M. Stark © Humana Press Inc., Totowa, NJ

the term *wound* has specific meaning in certain jurisdictions, for example relating to whether the skin or mucosa is completely breached. It is more appropriate for those who are documenting injuries to ensure that they have documented them in detail and unambiguously so that the courts can then make the decision regarding the most appropriate judicial interpretation of the injury or injuries described and their relevance to the case.

In many cases, the initial examination and assessment may have been undertaken for purely therapeutic purposes, and the forensic significance of the injuries may not become apparent until several weeks or months later. Scrutiny of the doctor's notes at a later stage, possibly in court, may reveal serious deficiencies, which not only bring discredit on the individual practitioner and the profession as a whole but also can seriously prejudice the legal proceedings. Pediatricians and emergency medicine specialists are typical of those nonforensic practitioners who may encounter patients with injuries that may be contentious within court proceedings.

2. ASSESSMENT AND DOCUMENTATION

Assessment and interpretation of injury depends on establishing a good history and undertaking an appropriate physical examination and recording the findings contemporaneously, clearly, and unambiguously. Such documentation (whether notes, body charts, or computer records) may be reviewed by other doctors, legal advisers, and the courts. Consent for the examination and for subsequent production of a medical report should be sought from the individual being examined. It should also be remembered that vexatious or frivolous accusations of assault can be made, and the examiner should be aware that false allegations and counter allegations do occur, which may only become obvious at a later date.

2.1. Key Factors

Table 1 identifies key factors that may be relevant in the examination of anyone with injuries and that, if relevant, should be determined when the history is taken from the injured person.

It is important to document the time at which the injury was said to have occurred. Injuries heal, and thus the appearance of an injury after assault is time dependent. Assaults may not be reported for days or weeks after the incident. There may be several injuries from different incidents. Specific times should be sought for each. If more than one type of assault has occurred, clear records must be made of which injury was accounted for by which implement. Document the handedness (left, right, or both) of both the victim and

Table 1
Potential Relevant Factors to Determine From History

- How was the injury sustained?
- Weapon or weapons used (is it [are they] still available?)
- What time was the injury sustained?
- Has the injury been treated?
- Pre-existing illnesses (e.g., skin disease).
- Regular physical activity (e.g., contact sports).
- Regular medication (e.g., anticoagulants, steroids).
- Handedness of victim and suspect.
- Use of drugs and alcohol.
- Clothing worn.

Table 2
Potential Relevant Information Required When Assessing Injury

• Location (anatomical—measure distance from landmarks)	• Type (e.g., bruise, cut, or abrasion)
	• Size (use metric values)
	• Shape
• Pain	• Color
• Tenderness	• Orientation
• Stiffness	• Age
• Causation	• Time
• Handedness	• Transientness (of injury)

the assailant, if known, because this may affect the interpretation of injury causation. Witnesses may give different accounts of the incident; it is the forensic physician's role to assist the court in determining the true account. These accounts may also be influenced by the effect of drugs and/or alcohol, and it is appropriate to assess the influence that these may have in each case. Knowledge of the type of weapon used can be important when assessing injury because particular implements can give identifiable injuries. The type of clothing worn (e.g., long-sleeved shirts or armless vests) should be noted. When examining any individual for injury, all these features should at least be considered to see whether they may have relevance to the case; others may become relevant as the examination progresses or as other accounts of any assault are given.

Documentation of injuries can be in several formats, including hand-drawn notes, annotated pro forma diagrams, and photographic. Figure 1 illustrates one form of body chart and note system *(3)*. Table 2 lists the characteristics of each injury that may be needed for appropriate documentation.

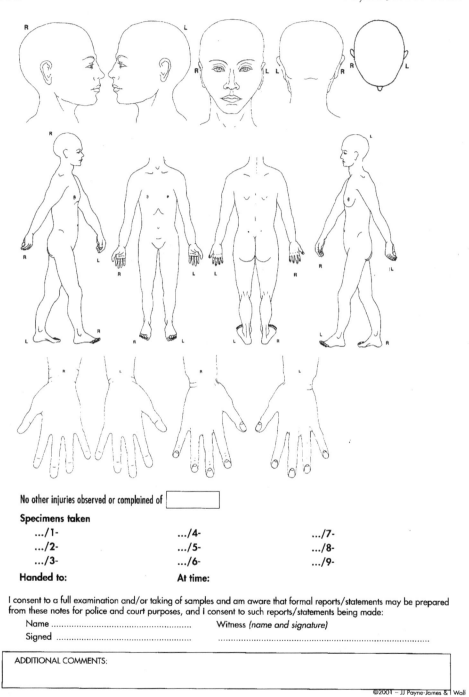

No other injuries observed or complained of [   ]

Specimens taken

...	1-	...	4-	...	7-
...	2-	...	5-	...	8-
...	3-	...	6-	...	9-

Handed to: **At time:**

I consent to a full examination and/or taking of samples and am aware that formal reports/statements may be prepared from these notes for police and court purposes, and I consent to such reports/statements being made:

Name ....   Witness *(name and signature)*

Signed ....

ADDITIONAL COMMENTS:

©2001 – JJ Payne-James & Wall

Fig. 1. Body chart and note system.

Table 3
Classification of Injuries

• Wheals and erythema (reddening)	• Bruises (contusion or ecchymosis)
• Hematoma	• Petechiae
• Abrasions (grazes)	• Scratches
	• Point abrasion
• Scuff/brush abrasions	• Incisions
• Lacerations	• Chop
• Slash	• Firearms
• Stab wounds	• Bites

Digital images have now become an appropriate way of documenting injury, and the digital image evidence should be supported by contemporaneous written and hand-drawn notes. Ensure at the time of examination that each injury is accounted for by the account given. If an injury is not consistent with the account given, question it at the time. In many cases, individuals who have been involved in fights or violent incidents are simply unaware of the causation of many sites of injury. It may be appropriate (particularly with blunt injury) to reexamine injuries 24–48 hours later to see how injuries evolve and whether bruises have appeared or other sites of injury noted. Pretreatment and posttreatment examination and photography may be useful.

2.2. Types of Injury

It is important that anyone who is involved in injury assessment understand the range of terms that can be applied to different injury, and this may depend on certain factors, such as country of origin or medical specialty. Thus, each practitioner should have a system of his or her own that ensures that the nature of each injury is described clearly, reproducibly, and unambiguously in note form, using accepted terms of classification. The most common reason why medical evidence on injuries given in court is contentious is the confusing assortment of terms used by doctors and the inappropriate or inaccurate description of a wound, for example, using the term *laceration* to describe a clean-cut wound caused by a bladed weapon, such as a knife, when the wound was, in fact, an incision *(4)*. It is therefore essential that for medicolegal purposes a standard nomenclature be adopted when describing injuries. The following classification is one that is appropriate and clear, and most visible injuries will fall into one of the groups listed in Table 3. These injuries type are explained in the following paragraphs.

Deliberate injury may be divided into two main types: blunt impact or blunt force injury and sharp implement injury. Blunt force injury describes the cause of injuries not caused by instruments or objects with cutting edges. The injury may be caused by traction, torsion, or shear stresses. The body may move toward the blunt object (e.g., a fall or push against a wall), or the blunt object may move towards the body. Examples of objects that cause blunt impact injuries include fists, feet, baseball bats, and police batons. A blunt force blow can cause a range of symptoms or signs, and the resultant injuries depend on numerous factors, including force, location, and impacting surface, which range from no visible evidence of injury to tenderness or pain at the impact sites, reddening, swelling, bruising, abrasions, cuts (lacerations), and broken bones. Each injury type may be present alone or in combination. Such injuries are seen at the point of contact of the impacting object on the body. Bruises may migrate from the point of contact by gravity after a period of time. Abrasions give a clear indication of the impact site. In some cases, injury patterns may indicate whether a particular impacting object was involved. Blunt impact injuries can be described in terms of force applied as being weak, weak/moderate, moderate, moderate/severe, or severe.

Sharp injuries are those caused by any implement with cutting edges (e.g., knives, scissors, or glass). The injuries may be of varied types, including incised, where the cutting edge runs tangentially to the skin surface cutting through skin and deeper anatomical structures, or stab, where the sharp edge penetrates the skin into deeper structures. An incised wound is generally longer than it is deep, whereas a stab wound is generally deeper than it is wide. Forces required to cause sharp injuries and the effect of such injuries are variable because a sharp pointed object may penetrate vital structures with minimal force. Special types of cutting injuries included slash- or chop-type injuries from weapons such as machetes.

Many impacts may cause initial pain and discomfort, which resolves within a few minutes, and tenderness, which may still be elicited hours or days later, with no visible sign of injury. The lay person must be aware that the absence of visible injury does not imply that no assault or injury has occurred.

Wheals and erythema are also nonpermanent evidence of trauma caused by initial vasodilatation and local release of vasoactive peptides after an injury, such as a slap, scratch, or punch, which will leave no mark after a few hours. The classic features of the triple reaction are present, but no specific damage is done to any tissues. Thus, an initial reddening associated with pain with possible subsequent development of local swelling may be present initially, but after a few hours has completely resolved, unlike bruising, which will still be present after 24 hours or more.

2.3. Size and Shape of the Injury

Even though the size of an injury is perhaps the easiest measurement to ascertain, it is probably the most common omission from medical records. It should be ascertained using a ruler or a pair of calipers and recorded in centimeters or millimeters. Because measurements given in imperial units may be easier for some individuals to understand, it is also acceptable to include the equivalent size of an injury in inches. The shape of the wound should also be noted; simple terms, such as circular, triangular, V-shaped, or crescent-shaped, best express this characteristic, but if the wound shape is irregular or complex, then it is possibly easier to record this feature on a body chart. Wounds may also have depth, but it is often not possible to determine this accurately in the living.

2.4. Position of the Injury

The best method of pinpointing the location of an injury is to use fixed anatomical landmarks. On the head, one can use the eyes, ears, nose, and mouth; on the neck, the prominence of the thyroid cartilage and the sternocleidomastoid muscles can be used; and on the trunk, the nipples, umbilicus, and bony prominences can be used as points of reference. The advantages of using simple anatomical diagrams and body charts for locating the injury are self-evident. It is a simple process to record the position of an injury accurately, yet when medical records are reviewed, it is both surprising and disappointing to find only a vague indication of location.

2.5. Aging Injuries

Allotting a specific time or time frame to the infliction of an injury is one of the most frequently requested and most contentious of issues in forensic medicine. Injuries inflicted shortly before examination (both of the living and the dead) show no sign of healing. The healing process depends on several variables, including the site of injury, the force applied, the severity of tissue damage, infection, treatment, etc., and these all make assessment of the age of a wound extremely difficult and inaccurate. Bruises often become more prominent a few hours or even days after infliction because of diffusion of blood closer to the skin surface; on occasion, a recent deep bruise may be mistaken for an older, more superficial lesion. Bruises resolve over a variable period ranging from days to weeks; the larger the bruise, the longer it will take to disappear. The colors of a bruise can include (dependent on the examiner) blue, mauve, purple, brown, green, and yellow, and all tints and hues associated with these. Many bruises exhibit multiple colors. The only substantial study that looks at bruise evolution by color showed that a bruise with a yellow color was more than 18 hours old and that red, blue, and purple/ black could occur anytime within 1 hour of bruising to resolution (up to 21 days in the study) *(5)*. Thus, coloration of bruises and the progress and change of color patterns cannot, with the exception of a yellow bruise, which may be considered to be more than 18 hours old, be used to time the injury. It should be emphasized that estimation of bruise age from color photographs is also imprecise and should not be relied on because the color values are not accurate *(6)*. This has recently been confirmed in another study *(7)* that identified great interobserver variability in color matching both in vivo and in photographic reproductions. Other specific information (e.g., a witnessed blow) is the only way of reliably timing a bruise.

Abrasions sustained during life are usually red-brown and exude serum and blood, which hardens to form a scab. This scab organizes over a period of days before detaching to leave a pink, usually intact, surface.

In the absence of medical intervention, lacerations tend to heal with scarring, usually over a period of days or weeks, whereas incisions, the edges of which may be apposed, can heal within a few days, although some may scar significantly.

2.6. Transient Lesions

Swelling, redness, and tenderness, although frequently caused by trauma, are not specific signs of injury. Although it is important to record whether these features are present, it must be remembered that there also may be nontraumatic causes for these lesions (e.g., eczema/dermatitis or impetigo).

Red marks outlining an apparent injury, for example, the imprint of a hand on the slapped face or buttock of a child, should be photographed immediately because such images may fade within an hour or so and leave no residual marks.

3. Types of Injury

3.1. Bruises

The terms *contusion* and *ecchymosis* have been used to differentiate between different types of injury that can more simplistically be called bruising. These terms have been used variously to describe different injury sizes but do not enhance understanding of either causation or mechanism of injury and should no longer be used. A hematoma is best used to refer to a collection of blood forming a fluctuant mass under the skin and may be associated with substantial trauma. The difference between that and a standard bruise is that a hematoma may be capable of being aspirated in the same way a collection of

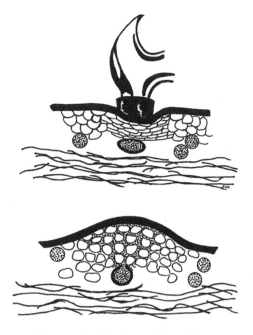

Fig. 2. Production of bruising.

pus is aspirated. Bruising is caused when an impact damages blood vessels so that blood leaks into the perivascular tissues and is evident on the skin surface as discoloration. Such discoloration changes in color, shape, and location as the blood pigment is broken down and resorbed. In some cases, although blood vessels may be damaged, there may be no visible evidence on the skin. In certain cases, it may take hours or days for any bruise to become apparent because the blood diffuses through damaged tissue. The blunt force ruptures small blood vessels beneath the intact skin, and blood then escapes to infiltrate the surrounding subcutaneous tissues under the pumping action of the heart (*see* Fig. 2). Thus, theoretically at least, bruising is not produced after death. In fact, severe blows inflicted after death may cause some degree of bruising, although this is usually only slight. Bruises may be associated with other visible evidence of injury, such as abrasions and lacerations, and these lesions may obscure the underlying bruise.

Bruising may need to be differentiated from purpura, which develop spontaneously in those with a hemorrhagic tendency and in the elderly and tend to be rather blotchy, are less regular in outline, and are usually confined to the forearms and lower legs. Bruises vary in severity according to the site and nature of the tissue struck, even when the force of the impact is the same.

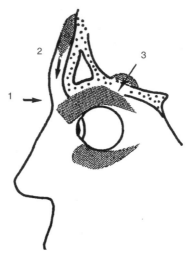

1. Direct blow to the orbit
2. Injury to the front of the scalp
3. Fracture of base of skull

Fig. 3. Production of a black eye. **(1)** Direct blow to the orbit. **(2)** Injury to the front of the scalp. **(3)** Fracture of base of scull.

Where there is an underlying bony surface and the tissues are lax, as in the facial area, a relatively light blow may produce considerable puffy bruising. The orbit is the most vulnerable, giving rise to the common "black eye." However, remember that there are other mechanisms for the production of a black eye, such as an injury to the front of the scalp draining down over the supraorbital ridge or a fracture of the base of the skull allowing blood to escape through the roof of the orbit (*see* Fig. 3).

Bruises can enlarge over a variable period of time, which can be misleading regarding the actual site of injury. Because a bruise is a simple mechanical permeation of the tissues by blood, its extension may be affected by movement and gravity. Thus, bruising of the face can result from an injury to the scalp. Further difficulties arise if a bruise, as it extends, tracks along tissue planes from an invisible to a visible location. Bruising of this kind may not become apparent externally for some time and then some distance from the site of the original impact. This delay in the appearance of bruising is of considerable significance because absence of apparent injury at an initial examination is not necessarily inconsistent with bruising becoming apparent 24–48 hours later. Thus, in cases of serious assault, it is often advisable to conduct a further examination a day or so later.

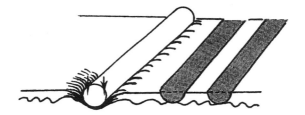

Fig. 4. Tramline bruising caused by a blow from a rod-like implement.

Generally, bruises, unless superficial and intradermal, tend to be nonspecific injuries, and it is usually not possible to offer any detailed opinions on the agent responsible. However, some bruises may have a pattern (a patterned bruise), or because of their shape or size or location, may have particular significance. Common patterning types include petechial bruising reproducing the texture of clothing, the ridge pattern from the sole of a shoe or tire, or the streaky linear purple bruising seen on the neck, wrists, or ankles caused by the application of a ligature. Beating with a rod-like implement often leaves a patterned bruise consisting of an area of central pallor outlined by two narrow parallel bands of bruising, so-called tramline bruising (*see* Fig. 4).

Other bruises of particular medicolegal significance are the small circular or oval bruises, usually approx 1–2 cm in diameter, characteristic of fingertip pressure from either gripping or grasping with the hand, prodding with the fingers, or the firm impact of a knuckle. They may be seen on the limbs in cases of child abuse when the child is forcibly gripped by the arms or legs and shaken or on the abdomen when the victim is poked, prodded, or punched. However, such nonaccidental injuries must be differentiated from bruises seen on toddlers and children associated with normal activities, play, or sports. Bruises may be seen on the neck in cases of manual strangulation and are then usually associated with other signs of asphyxia.

When sexual assault is alleged, the presence of bruising on the victim may help support the victim's account and give an indication of the degree of violence that was used. For example, grip marks or "defense" injuries may be present on the upper arms and forearms, whereas bruising on the thighs and the inner sides of the knees may occur as the victim's legs are forcibly pulled apart. Bruising of the mouth and lips can be caused when an assailant places a hand over the face to keep the victim quiet. Love bites ("hickeys") may be present often in the form of discrete areas of ovoid petechial bruising on the neck and breasts. However, it is important to recognize that the latter may be the sequelae of consensual sexual encounters.

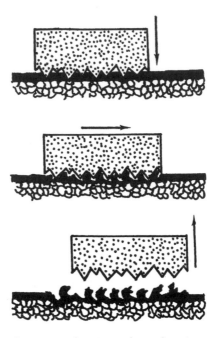

Fig. 5. Production of an abrasion.

3.2. Abrasions

An abrasion (or a graze) is a superficial injury involving only the outer layers of the skin and not penetrating the full thickness of the epidermis. Abrasions exude serum, which progressively hardens to form a scab, but they may also bleed because occasionally they are deep enough to breach the vascular papillae that corrugate the undersurface of the epidermis in which case frank bleeding may be present at an early stage. More superficial abrasions that barely damage the skin with little or no exudation of serum (and thus little or no scab formation) may be termed *brush* or *scuff* abrasions. Scratches are linear abrasions typically caused by fingernails across the surface of the skin. Pointed but noncutting objects may also cause linear abrasions and to differentiate them from fingernail scratches may be termed "point abrasions."

Abrasions often result from movement of the skin surface over a rough surface or vice versa (*see* Fig. 5). Thus they may have a linear appearance, and close examination may show ruffling of the superficial epidermis to one end, indicating the direction of travel of the opposing surface. Thus, a tangential blow could be horizontal or vertical, or it may be possible to infer that the victim had been dragged over a rough surface.

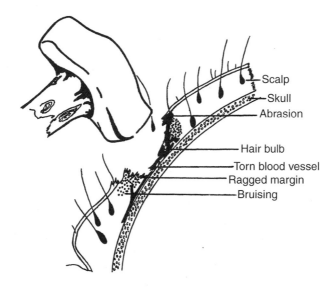

Fig. 6. Laceration of the scalp.

The patterning of abrasions is clearer than that of bruises because abrasions frequently take a fairly detailed impression of the shape of the object causing them and, once inflicted, do not extend or gravitate; therefore, they indicate precisely the area of application of force. In manual strangulation, small, crescent-shaped abrasions caused by the fingernails of the victim or assailant may be the only signs visible on the neck. A victim resisting a sexual or other attack may claw at her assailant and leave linear parallel abrasions on the assailant's face. Some abrasions may be contaminated with foreign material, such as dirt or glass, which may have important medicolegal significance. Such material should be carefully preserved for subsequent forensic analysis. In such cases, consultation with a forensic scientist can ensure the best means of evidence collection and preservation.

3.3. Lacerations

Lacerations are caused by blunt force splitting the full thickness of the skin (*see* Fig. 6) most frequently when the skin and soft tissues are crushed between impacting force and underlying bone. Boxers classically develop lacerations when a boxing glove presses on the orbital rim. As with abrasions, the injury site is indicative of the impact site. Lacerations can bleed profusely, particularly on face and scalp. When inflicted deliberately, the force may cause the assailant and weapon to be contaminated with blood.

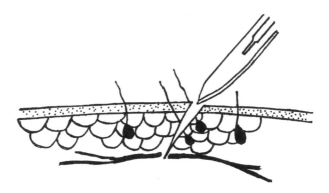

Fig. 7. Cross-section of an incision.

Lacerations have characteristic features but often mimic incised wounds (or vice-versa), particularly where the skin is closely applied to underlying bone, for example, the scalp. Close examination of the margins of the wound, which are usually slightly inverted, normally resolves the issue. Lacerations are ragged wounds caused by crushing and tearing of the skin. They tend to gape open, and their margins are often bruised and abraded. Blood vessels, nerves, and delicate tissue bridges may be exposed in the depth of the wound, which may be soiled by grit, paint fragments, or glass.

The shape of the laceration may give some indication regarding to the agent responsible. For example, blows to the scalp with the circular head of a hammer or the spherical knob of a poker tend to cause crescent-shaped lacerations. A weapon with a square or rectangular face, such as the butt of an axe, may cause a laceration with a Y-shaped split at its corners.

3.4. Incisions

These wounds are caused by sharp cutting implements, usually bladed weapons, such as knives and razors, but sharp slivers of glass, the sharp edges of tin cans, and sharp tools, such as chisels, may also cause clean-cut incised injuries. Axes, choppers, and other similar instruments, although capable of cutting, usually cause lacerations because the injury caused by the size of the instrument (e.g., axe head) overrides the cutting effect of the tool. Mixed wounds are common, with some incised element, some laceration, bruising, and swelling and abrasion also present. Each element of the injury must be documented. Machetes and other large-blade implements are being used, producing large deep cuts known as slash or chop injuries.

The features of an incision contrast with those of a laceration (*see* Fig. 7). The margins tend to be straight, unbruised, unabraded, and not inverted. They gape, and the deeper tissues are all cut cleanly in the same plane. Hemorrhage tends to be greater than from similarly located lacerations. If the blade of the weapon is drawn across the skin while it is lax, it may cause a notched wound if the skin creases. The direction of travel of the blade of the weapon is not always easy to decide, but usually the deeper part of the wound is near the end that was inflicted first, the weapon tending to be drawn away toward the end of the wound.

The head and neck are usual targets when an assailant inflicts incised wounds. In an attempt to ward off the assailant, the arms are often raised in a protective gesture and incisions are then often seen on the ulnar borders of the forearms. If the blade of the weapon is grasped, then incised wounds are apparent on the palmar surfaces of the fingers. Such injuries are known as *defense wounds*.

Incised wounds may be a feature of suicide or attempted suicide (*see* Subheading 3.6.). They are usually located on the wrists, forearms, or neck, although other accessible areas on the front of the body may be chosen. The incisions usually take the form of multiple parallel wounds, most of them being tentative and superficial; some may be little more than simple linear abrasions.

3.5. Stab Wounds

Stab wounds are caused by sharp or pointed implements and wounds with a depth greater than their width or length. They are usually caused by knives but can also be inflicted with screwdrivers, pokers, scissors, etc. Although the external injury may not appear to be particularly serious, damage to vital structures, such as the heart, liver, or major blood vessels, can lead to considerable morbidity and death, usually from hemorrhage. In those individuals who survive, it is common for little information to be present about the forensic description of the wound because the priority of resuscitation may mean that no record is made. If operative intervention is undertaken, the forensic significance of a wound may be obliterated by suturing it or using the wound as the entry for an exploratory operation. In such cases, it is appropriate to attempt to get a forensic physician to assess the wound in theatre or subsequently.

Stab wounds are rarely accidental and occasionally suicidal, but usually their infliction is a result of criminal intent. In the case of suicide, the wounds are usually located on the front of the chest or upper abdomen and, as with self-inflicted incisions, may be associated with several superficial tentative puncture wounds (*see* Subheading 3.6.). When deliberately inflicted by an assailant, stab wounds may be associated with defense injuries to the arms and hands.

The appearance of the skin wound will vary depending on the weapon used and can easily be distorted by movement of the surrounding skin. Typi-

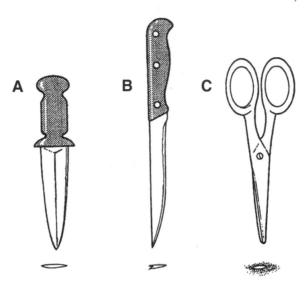

Fig. 8. Elliptical **(A)**, fish-tailed **(B)**, and bruised ovoid **(C)** stab wounds.

cally, when inflicted with a knife, the wound is usually elliptical because the natural elasticity of the skin causes its length to shrink. If the blade is double-edged, such as that of a dagger, the extremities of the wound tend to be equally pointed. A stab wound from a single-edged blade, such as a kitchen knife, will usually have one extremity rounded, squared-off, or fish-tailed (caused by the noncutting back of the blade). When blunt weapons are used—a pair of scissors, for example—the wound tends to be more rounded or oval, with bruising of its margins (*see* Fig. 8). Scissor wounds can sometimes have a cross-shape caused by the blade screws or rivets. Notched wounds are often caused by the blade of the weapon being partially withdrawn and then reintroduced into the wound or twisted during penetration.

It is rarely possible from an inspection of the skin wound alone to comment usefully on the width of the blade because the skin retracts and the knife is unlikely to have been introduced and removed perfectly perpendicularly. Surprisingly, long skin wounds may be caused with quite narrow-width blades.

3.6. Deliberate Self-Harm

Deliberate self-harm refers to any attempt by an individual to harm himself or herself. When assessing injuries, it is important to understand which factors may indicate the possibility that an injury was caused by deliberate

Table 4
Indicators of Possible Deliberate Self-Harm Injuries

- Must be on an area of body accessible to the person to injure themselves.
- Superficial or minor.
- Regular with an equal depth at the beginning and end (for cuts).
- Regular and similar in style or shape (for scratches, burns, etc.).
- Multiple.
- Parallel or grouped together.
- In right-handed persons, the injuries are predominantly on the left side (and the converse for left-handed individuals).
- There may be lesser injuries where initial attempts at self-harm are made (tentative scars).
- There may be old scars of previous self-harm.
- There may be a psychiatric history.

From ref. 2.

self-harm. Individuals injure themselves for numerous reasons, including psychiatric illness and others, such as attempting to imply events took place that did not or for motives of gain. Self-inflicted injuries have several characteristics, which are not diagnostic but that together may give an indication of self-infliction. Table 4 lists features that may assist in the recognition or suspicion that cuts or other injury, such as scratches, are self-inflicted—all or some may be present—their absence does not preclude self-infliction nor does their presence necessarily imply self-infliction *(2)*.

4. FIREARM INJURIES

The examination of fatal firearm injuries should be left to an experienced forensic pathologist; however, it is not unusual in cases of nonfatal injuries for a hospital clinician or forensic physician to be asked to comment on the nature of the wound or wounds *(8)*. As with all injuries within the forensic setting it is essential in these nonfatal cases that the initial appearances of the injuries be accurately described and the wounds photographed. This is particularly important because subsequent surgical treatment may distort or completely obliterate the wound characteristics. Furthermore, any fragments, bullets, or pellets found within the wounds must be carefully removed and handed over to the appropriate authorities.

There are two main types of firearm: smooth bore and rifled. Injuries occurring from both are discussed in the following subheadings.

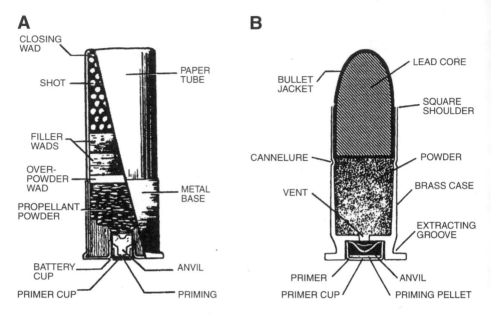

Fig. 9. Components of a shotgun cartridge (**A**) and a rifled bullet (**B**).

4.1. Smooth-Bore Weapons

Shotguns, which fire a large number of small projectiles, such as lead shot, are the most common type of smooth-bore weapons. They are commonly used in sporting and agricultural activities and may be either single or double-barreled. The ammunition for these weapons consists of a plastic or cardboard cartridge case with a brass base containing a percussion cap. Inside the main part of the cartridge is a layer of propellant, plastic, felt, or cardboard wads and a mass of pellets (lead shot of variable size) (*see* Fig. 9A). In addition to the pellets, the wads and/or cards may contribute to the appearance of the wounds and may be important in estimating range and possible direction.

4.2. Rifled Weapons

Rifled weapons are characterized by having parallel spiral projecting ridges (or lands) extending down the interior of the barrel from the breach to the muzzle. This rifling causes the projectile, in this case a bullet (*see* Fig. 9B), to spin as it is ejected from the weapon and thus impart gyroscopic stability along its flight path. The rifling also leaves characteristic scratches and rifling marks that are unique to that weapon on the bullet surface. There are three common types of rifled weapons: the revolver, the pistol, and the rifle. The revolver, which tends to have a low muzzle velocity of 150 m/s, is a short-barreled weapon with its ammunition held in a metal drum, which rotates each time the trigger is released. The spent cartridge case is retained within the cylinder after firing. In the self-loading pistol, often called "semi-automatic" or erroneously "automatic," the ammunition is held in a metal clip-type magazine under the breach. Each time the trigger is pulled, the bullet in the breach is fired, the spent cartridge case is ejected from the weapon, and a spring mechanism pushes up the next live bullet into the breach ready to be fired. The muzzle velocity of pistols varies between 300 and 360 m/s. The rifle is a long-barreled shoulder weapon capable of firing bullets with velocities up to 1500 m/s. Most military rifles are "automatic," allowing the weapon to continue to fire while the trigger is depressed until the magazine is empty; thus, they are capable of discharging multiple rounds within seconds.

4.3. Shotgun Wounds

When a shotgun is discharged, the lead shot emerges from the muzzle as a solid mass and then progressively diverges in a cone shape as the distance from the weapon increases. The pellets are often accompanied by particles of unburned powder, flame, smoke, gases, wads, and cards, which may all affect the appearance of the entrance wound and are dependent on the range of fire. Both the estimated range and the site of the wound are crucial factors in determining whether the wound could have been self-inflicted.

If the wound has been sustained through clothing, then important residues may be found on the clothing if it is submitted for forensic examination. It is absolutely essential that the advice of the forensic science team and crime scene investigator is sought when retrieving such evidence. When clothing is being cut off in the hospital, staff should avoid cutting through any apparent holes.

Contact wounds are caused when the muzzle of the weapon is held against the skin. The entrance wound is usually a fairly neat circular hole, the margins of which may be bruised or abraded resulting from impact with the muzzle. In the case of a double-barreled weapon, the circular abraded imprint of the nonfiring muzzle may be clearly seen adjacent to the contact wound. The wound margins and the tissues within the base of the wound are usually blackened by smoke and may show signs of burning owing to the effect of flame. Because the gases from the discharge are forced into the wound, there may be subsidiary lacerations at the wound margin, giving it a stellate-like shape. This is seen particularly where the muzzle contact against the skin is tight and the skin is closely applied to underlying bone, such as in the scalp. Carbon monoxide contained within the gases may cause the surrounding skin and soft tissues to turn pink resulting from the formation of carboxyhemoglobin. Contact wounds to the head are particularly severe, usually with bursting ruptures of the scalp and face, multiple explosive fractures of the skull, and extrusion or partial extrusion of the underlying brain. Most contact wounds of the head are suicidal in nature, with the temple, mouth, and underchin being the sites of election. In these types of wounds, which are usually rapidly fatal, fragments of scalp, skull, and brain tissue may be dispersed over a wide area.

At close, noncontact range with the muzzle up to about 15 cm (6 in) from the skin, the entrance wound is still usually a single circular or oval hole with possible burning and blackening of its margins from flame, smoke, and unburned powder. Blackening resulting from smoke is rarely seen beyond approx 20 cm; tattooing from powder usually only extends to approx 1 m. The wads and cards rarely travel more than approx 2 m.

As distance increases, the pellets begin to diverge. Up to approx 1 m they are still traveling as a compact mass, but between approx 1–3 m, the pellets start to scatter and cause variable numbers of individual satellite puncture wounds surrounding a larger central hole. At ranges greater than 8–10 m, there is no large central hole, only multiple small puncture wounds, giving the skin a peppered appearance.

Exit wounds are unusual with shotgun injuries because the shot is usually dispersed in the tissues. However, the pellets may penetrate the neck or a limb and, in close-range wounds to the head, the whole cranium may be disrupted.

4.4. Rifled Weapon Wounds

Intact bullets penetrating the skin orthogonally, that is, nose-on, usually cause neat round holes approx 3–10 mm in diameter. Close examination reveals that the wound margin is usually fairly smooth and regular and bordered by an even zone of creamy pink or pinkish red abrasion. A nonorthogonal nose-on strike is associated with an eccentric abrasion collar, widest at the side of the wound from which the bullet was directed (*see* Fig. 10). Atypical entrance wounds are a feature of contact or near contact wounds to the head where the thick bone subjacent to the skin resists the entry of gases, which accumulate beneath the skin and cause subsidiary lacerations to the wound margins, imparting a stellate lacerated appearance. Contact wounds elsewhere may be bordered by the imprint of the muzzle and the abraded margin possibly charred and parchmented by flame. Punctate discharge abrasion and sooty soiling are usually absent from the skin surface, but the subcutaneous tissues within the depth of the wound are usually soiled. The effects of flame are rarely seen beyond 10 cm (4 in), with sooty soiling extending to approx 20 cm (8 in).

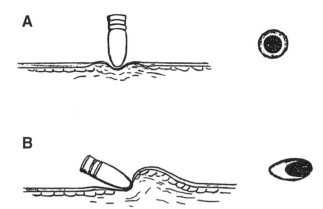

Fig. 10. Entrance wounds caused by perpendicular **(A)** and tangential **(B)** bullet strikes.

Punctate discharge abrasions, which may be particularly heavy with old revolver ammunition, are often present at ranges up to approx 50 cm (20 in). It is important to remember that sooty soiling of the skin surrounding a wound is easily removed by vigorous cleaning carried out by medical or nursing staff. The soiling of contact close-range entrance wounds may be absent if clothing or other material is interposed between the skin surface and the muzzle of the weapon.

Bullet exit wounds tend to be larger than entrance wounds and usually consist of irregular lacerations or lacerated holes with everted, unabraded, and unbruised margins. When the skin at the site of an entrance wound has been supported by tight clothing, eversion of the margins of the wound may be absent and the margins may even be abraded, albeit somewhat irregularly, but nevertheless making differentiation from entrance wounds more difficult.

Entrance wounds caused by damaged or fragmented bullets may be so atypical that it may not be possible to offer a useful opinion as to their nature. It is inappropriate to offer an opinion on the caliber of a bullet based on the size of an entrance wound, and it is not possible to state whether the bullet was fired from a revolver, pistol, or rifle by only the appearance of the wound.

5. DEFENSE INJURIES

Certain types of injuries may be described as defense injuries. These injuries typically are seen when an individual has tried to defend himself or herself against an attack and are the result of instinctive reactions to assault. Some individuals, for example, the very young and the very old, are less capable of offering much defense against the perpetrators of assault. When attacked with blunt objects, most individuals will attempt to protect their eyes, head, and neck by raising their arms, flexing their elbows, and covering their head and neck. As a result, the exposed surfaces of the arms become the impact point for blows. Thus, the extensor surface of the forearms (the ulnar side), the lateral/posterior aspects of the upper arm, and the dorsum of the hands may receive blows. Similarly, the outer and posterior aspects of lower limbs and back may be injured when an individual curls into a ball, with flexion of spine, knees, and hips to protect the anterior part of the body.

In sharp-blade attacks, the natural reaction is to try and disarm the attacker, often by grabbing the knife blade. This results in cuts to the palm and ulnar aspect of the hand. Occasionally, the hands or arms may be raised to protect the body against the stabbing motion, resulting in stab wounds to the defense areas.

In blunt-force attacks, the injuries sustained usually take the form of bruises if the victim is being punched or kicked, but there may also be abrasions and/or lacerations depending on the nature of the weapon used. If the victim is lying on the ground while being assaulted, he or she will tend to curl up into a fetal position to protect the face and the front of the trunk, particularly from kicks. In these circumstances, defensive bruising is likely to be seen on other surfaces of the trunk and limbs.

The absence of defense injuries in persons otherwise apparently capable of defending themselves against an assault may be particularly significant if it is believed that other injuries found on the victim could have been self-inflicted or if it is believed that they were incapacitated through alcohol, drugs, or other injury.

6. TORTURE

The World Medical Association's Declaration of Tokyo in 1975 defined torture as "the deliberate, systematic or wanton infliction of physical or mental suffering by one or more persons acting alone or on the orders of any authority, to force another person to yield information, to make a confession, or for any other reason" *(9)*. The declaration also established guidelines for doctors when faced with cases of suspected torture. Clinicians view torture in two main contexts: first, torture that is perpetrated by criminals and terrorist organizations, and second, torture that is carried out, or allegedly carried out, by the police or other security force personnel during the detention and interrogation of prisoners and suspects. Nonjudicial justice is now meted out worldwide in several ways.

Criminal groups and paramilitary organizations may torture their captives for numerous reasons. It may be to extract information from an opposing gang or faction, to discipline informants and others engaged in unsanctioned criminal activity, or simply to instill fear and division within a community. The methods used are crude and barbaric. The victim is usually bound, blindfolded, and gagged, and the wrists and ankles may bear the pale streaky linear bruises and abrasions caused by ligatures. "Beating up" is typical, with extensive bruises and abrasions scattered on the head, trunk, and limbs. Black eyes, fractures of the nose and jaws, and dislodgment of the teeth are all fairly typical. Cigarette burns, usually seen as discrete circular areas of reddish-yellow, parchmented skin, are also quite common. Patterned injuries resulting from being struck with the butt of a gun or tramline bruising owing to blows with a truncheon or baseball bat may be seen; in Northern Ireland, shooting through the lower limbs ("knee-capping") is a favored method of punishment by paramilitary organizations.

Systematic torture by security personnel, usually during interrogation of suspects, ranges from the subtle use of threats and intimidation to physical violence. Hooding, prolonged standing, and the use of high-pitched sound have all been used, as have attempts to disorientate prisoners by offering food at erratic times, frequent waking up after short intervals of sleep, and burning a light in the cell 24 hours a day. Physical abuse includes beating of the soles of the feet, so-called falanga, which, although extremely painful and debilitating, does not usually cause any significant bruising. Repeated dipping of the victim's head under water, known as *submarining*, may prove fatal if prolonged, as can the induction of partial asphyxia by enveloping the head in a plastic bag.

Electric torture is well documented and carries the risk of local electric shocks and fatal electrocution. *Telefono*, as it is known in Latin America, consists of repeated slapping of the sides of the head by the open palms, resulting in tympanic membrane rupture.

Doctors who have access to prisoners in custody have a heavy responsibility to ensure that they are properly treated during detention and interrogation. In all cases of suspected or alleged ill-treatment of prisoners, it is essential that the doctor carry out a methodical and detailed "head-to-toe" examination. All injuries and marks must be accurately recorded and photographed, and the appropriate authorities must be informed immediately. Increasingly, forensic physicians are involved in assessments of refugees and asylum seekers to establish whether accounts of torture (both physical and psychological) are true. This role is likely to expand in the future, and the principles of independent assessment, documentation, and interpretation are, as with other areas discussed, vital in ensuring that courts and tribunals have the appropriate information to allow fair judgments to be reached (1).

7. BITE MARK INJURIES

7.1. Introduction

The term *bite mark* has been described as "a mark caused by the teeth alone, or teeth in combination with other mouth parts" (10).

Biting is a dynamic process, and bite marks are complex injuries. Recognition, recording, analysis, and interpretation of these injuries are the most intriguing challenges in forensic dentistry. Biting can establish that there has been contact between two people—the teeth being used for offense or defense. When individual tooth characteristics and traits are present in the dentition of the biter and are recorded in the biting injury, the forensic significance of the bite mark is greatly increased. Early involvement of the forensically trained dentist, with experience in biting injuries, is essential to ensure that all dental evidence from both the victim and any potential suspect(s) is appropriately collected, preserved, and evaluated. There may be insufficient evidence to enable comparisons to be made with the biting edges of the teeth of any particular person, but, if the injury can be identified as a human bite mark, it may still be significant to the investigation. It is important that the forensic dentist discusses with investigators the evidential value of the bite mark to enable resources to be wisely used. Clearly, conclusions and opinions expressed by the forensic dentist often lead him or her into the role of the expert witness subject to rigorous examination in court.

The forensic physician will mostly be involved with biting injuries to human skin and any secondary consequences, including infection and disease transmission, but should be aware that bites in foodstuffs and other materials may be present at a crime scene and be easily overlooked. It is essential that a human bite can be distinguished from an animal bite, thus exonerating (or incriminating) the dog or cat next door. The following sections will consider issues surrounding bites to human skin caused by another human. Early recognition of a patterned injury (suspected of being caused by biting) by medical personnel, social services, and other investigating agencies is extremely important; the injury may be the only physical evidence and must not be lost. Ideally, the forensic dentist should be contacted sooner rather than later when a possible biting injury is discovered to ensure that all evidence is collected appropriately. All too often the dentist is brought in at a later date, when there has been incorrect recording of the bite mark and the injury is partly healed and distorted or fully healed and no longer visible. Reliance may then have to be placed on ultraviolet photography to demonstrate the "lost" injury (11).

Bites can be found on the victim or the assailant (living, deceased, child, or adult). It is well known that biting is often a feature in nonaccidental injury to children (*see* Chapter 5). We must all beware of the so-called "amorous" bite and self-inflicted bite. If a bite mark is found on an anatomical site that is accessible to the victim, it becomes necessary to exclude him or her from the investigation.

7.2. Bite Mark Information

7.2.1. Initial Considerations

1. Is it a biting injury?
2. Is it human?
3. What should I do?

If the answer to the first question is "don't know," "possibly," or "yes," then request the assistance of the forensic dentist. Ensure that swabs are taken from the injured site (with controls) and photographs should be taken. Make sure that you know which forensic dentists are available in your area; this will prevent delays and frustration. You will need to know whether your local forensic dentist has experience and training in bite mark analysis or whether he or she focuses mainly on identifications.

The forensic dentist will examine the suspected biting injury and consider the following:

- Whether the injury is oval or round.
- Whether the injury has central sparing or discoloration from suction or nipping between teeth.
- Whether the mark is made by two dental arches. However, note that a mark from only one arch does not mean that it is not a biting injury.
- Are marks made by individual teeth within the dental arch clearly visible?
- If so, is detail of that individual tooth visible? Characteristics, such as tooth size, shape, displacement, rotations, wear facets, etc. will be considered. Individual tooth absences from the arch will be noted.
- Is there sufficient detail for comparisons to be made with the biting edges of the teeth of any particular person or persons?
- Does the appearance of the injury fit the alleged time frame of the incident?

7.2.2. Differential Diagnosis

It is important to remember that other injuries can mimic bite marks. The following have all been queried as biting injuries:

- Dermatological conditions.
- Marks made by electroencephalogram electrodes.
- Heel marks.

- Patterned door knobs.
- Burns.

7.2.3. Range of Bite Mark Appearance

- Erythema.
- Laceration.
- Bruising.
- Avulsion of tissue.
- Abrasion.

In a single bite mark, one or any combination of several or all of these components may be present, and they may be discrete or superimposed. Furthermore, scrape marks made by tooth movement over the skin may be present. However, the complex situation may become even more complicated when there are multiple bite marks at a single location where they may overlap as a result of the biter trying to get a better "grip;" all this leads to interpretation difficulties.

7.2.4. Helpful Information From Bitten Person (When Possible)

- When were they bitten?
- How many bites were there?
- What was the victim's position?
- What was the assailant's position?
- Has the injury been washed?
- Was the victim clothed over the bitten area?
- Did the victim bite the assailant?

In attempting to get answers to these questions, a clearer picture of the incident may develop.

7.2.5. Anatomical Distribution of Bitten Sites

It can be seen from the anatomical distribution of the bite marks studied by the author (*see* Fig. 11) that no part of the body is spared. This graph does not distinguish between male and female, child or adult, or whether there were multiple bites to one person, but serves purely to illustrate that it is essential for medical personnel to thoroughly examine the body for biting injuries and carefully document the findings. Record the anatomical location and nature of the injury and its size, shape, and color. However, photographic documentation is essential for bite mark analysis. In many cases, there are multiple bite marks on the body, some that the victim may not be aware of or recall. Multiple bite marks on the body, produced by the same perpetrator, may vary

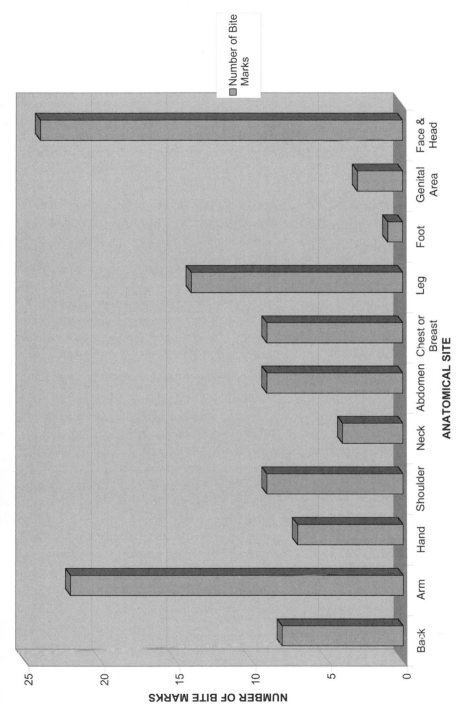

Fig. 11. Anatomical distribution of last 110 bite marks studied by the author (Hinchliffe).

153

considerably in appearance depending on several factors; these include the site bitten, number of teeth involved, thickness of the skin, elasticity of the skin, force involved, relative movement between biter and victim, etc.. In short, do not jump to the conclusion that there are multiple biters or vice-versa. Nor should it be assumed that a small biting injury has been caused by a child; it may be an incomplete adult bite. Where bruising is diffuse or confluent, size is not always easy to determine. If the marks on the skin can be identified as being made by the smaller deciduous (baby) teeth, it would suggest the mark has been inflicted by a young child. It is widely appreciated that it is easy to miss bruising on dark skins.

7.3. Evidence Collection

As soon as it has been established that the injury has been caused by biting, the injury should be photographed and swabbed for saliva. In addition, it may be necessary to take an impression of the injured site to preserve any possible indentations. Clearly, the taking of forensic samples is not always possible when the injured party needs urgent medical attention. Often, the forensic dentist is provided with photographs taken some time after the incident date and after medical intervention (*see* Fig. 12); by this time dental evidence has been lost, but it may still be possible to identify the injury as a possible biting injury.

7.3.1. Saliva

Saliva is deposited on the skin (and clothing, if present) during biting and sucking. The quantity and quality of this may enable DNA analysis after swabbing of the unwashed injury site. The double-swab technique is effective for this procedure (*12*). Please note that salivary DNA has been reported as having been recovered from the bitten breast of a young deceased woman found submerged in water (*13*). The saliva swabs (with controls) must be clearly and correctly labeled and stored appropriately (*see* Chapter 3).

Oral saliva samples will be needed from any potential suspect, and the victim of an assault if there is a possibility that the victim bit the assailant (or self-infliction is suspected).

7.3.2. Photography

Photographs should be taken when the bite mark is first discovered. It is essential for correct photographic procedures to be followed to minimize distortions. Police photographers experienced in crime scene and other injury photography may still find the assistance of the forensic dentist useful, because

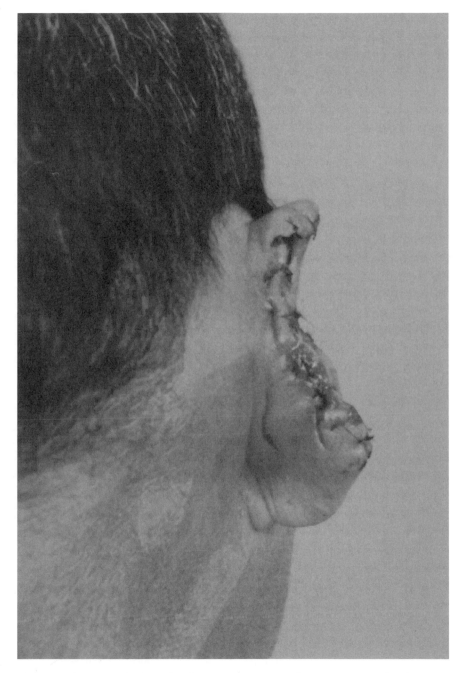

Fig. 12. Photograph showing biting injury to right ear after medical intervention. © Northumbria Police. Used with permission.

complications arise from curved surfaces and the correct positioning of the camera and scales. The American Board of Forensic Odontology no. 2 scale, being small and "L" shaped, is very effective *(14)* and is now used by many police forces.

Skin is not the best impression material, and various papers and reports have shown the importance of photographing the victim in the same position as when bitten in an attempt to minimize distortion *(15,16)*. However, this is not always possible. Changes in the injury with time (in both the living and the deceased) may mean that the injury pattern appears clearer after a day or two. There is no reliable way of knowing when an injury will reveal the most detail, and, therefore, repeat photography (e.g., every 24 hours for 3–5 days) can prove useful.

7.3.3. Photograph Protocol

- Anatomical location of bite mark (and identification of bitten person).
- Victim in same position as when bitten (when possible).
- Close up of bite mark without scales (nothing is being hidden) in color and black and white (in addition, black and white with a green filter may be useful).
- Close up of bite mark with scales in color and black and white (in addition, black and white with a green filter may be useful). Scales should be close to injury but not so close as to obscure the injury.
  Note: scales should be in the same plane as the bite mark.
- Photograph with the scales and injury parallel to the film plane (right angles to injury).
- Each dental arch may need to be photographed separately when on a curved surface.
- Repeat at intervals.
- Consider ultraviolet photography for older injuries that may no longer be visible.

Ultimately, the forensic dentist will select the best photographs and have them reproduced to life-size (1:1) for analysis and comparison work. At the time of writing, conventional film photography is still widely used, but the use of digital photography is progressing rapidly. Whatever the future brings, it is essential that standards, protocols, and appropriate training are in place.

7.3.4. Dental Impressions

Dental impressions taken from the potential biter by the dentist (or appropriately qualified person) after a thorough dental examination will be cast into hard dental models. Dental impressions taken of an individual in custody are intimate samples and require the appropriate authority and consent for your jurisdiction. Transparent overlays of the biting edges of the

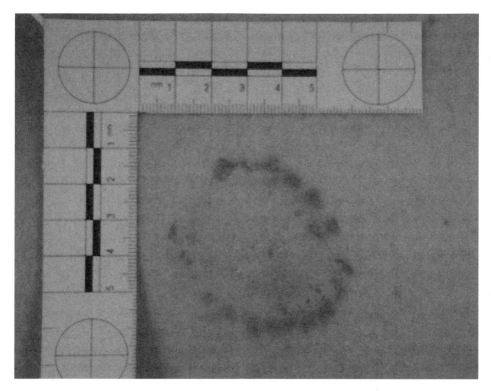

Fig. 13. Photograph showing bite mark on back, with scales. Individual tooth detail is visible. © Northumbria Police. Used with permission.

teeth from the dental models will be produced to facilitate physical comparisons. Currently, the best method for overlay production to achieve accuracy and reproducibility is the computer-generated method *(17)*.

The importance of following the correct procedures for evidence documentation, collection, preservation, and storage with continuity of evidence cannot be overstressed.

7.4. Summary

The biting injury demonstrating plenty of detail (*see* Fig. 13) that has been carefully examined, recorded, analyzed, and interpreted can be useful to the justice system. It can establish contact between two people or, of equal importance, exclude an innocent party. *Early suspicion and recognition by personnel involved with the investigation, followed by prompt and appropri-*

ate action, will help maximize the opportunity to collect evidence. Awareness by all concerned and early referral to the forensically trained dentist with experience in this field promote teamwork and best practice.

REFERENCES

1. Peel, M., Iacopino, V. The Medical Documentation of Torture. Greenwich Medical Media, London, UK, 2002.
2. Payne-James, J. J. Assault and injury. In: Payne-James J. J., Busuttil A., Smock W., eds. Forensic Medicine: Clinical & Pathological Aspects. Greenwich Medical Media, London, UK, 2003, pp. 543–563.
3. Payne-James, J. J., Wall, I. Forensic Medical Notebook. Greenwich Medical Media, London, UK, 2001.
4. Irvine, A. J. Incisions are not lacerations. Br. Med. J. 325:1113–1114, 2002.
5. Langlois, N. E. I., Gresham, G. A. The ageing of bruises: a review and study of the color changes with time. Forensic Sci. Int. 50:227–238, 1991.
6. Stephenson, T., Bialas, Y. Estimation of the age of bruising. Arch. Dis. Child. 74:5–55, 1996.
7. Munang, L. A., Leonard, P. A., Mok, J. Y. Q. Lack of agreement on color description between clinicians examining childhood bruising. J. Clin. Forensic Med. 9:171–174, 2002.
8. Dana, S., DiMaio, V. J. M. Gunshot trauma. In: Payne-James J. J., Busuttil A., Smock W., eds. Forensic Medicine: Clinical & Pathological Aspects. Greenwich Medical Media, London, UK, 2003, pp. 149–168.
9. British Medical Association. Report of a Working Party. Medicine Betrayed. British Medical Association, London, UK, 1992.
10. MacDonald, D. G. Bite mark recognition and interpretation. J. Forensic Sci. Soc. 14:229–233, 1974.
11. David, T. J., Sobel, M. N. Recapturing a five-month-old bite mark by means of reflective ultraviolet photography. J. Forensic Sci. 39:1560–1567, 1994.
12. Sweet, D., Lorente, J. A., Lorente, M., Valenzuela, A., Villanueva, E. An improved method to recover saliva from human skin: the double swab technique. J. Forensic Sci. 42:320–322, 1997.
13. Sweet, D., Shutler, G. Analysis of salivary DNA evidence from a bite mark on a body submerged in water. J. Forensic Sci. 44:1069–1072, 1999.
14. Hyzer, W. G., Krauss, T. C. The bite mark standard reference scale—ABFO No. 2. J. Forensic Sci. 33:498–506, 1988.
15. DeVore, D. T. Bite marks for identification? A preliminary report. Med. Sci. Law. 11:144–145, 1971.
16. Barbenel, J. C., Evans, J. H. Bite marks in skin—mechanical factors. J. Forensic Sci. Soc. 14:235–238, 1974.
17. Sweet, D., Bowers, C. M. Accuracy of bite mark overlays: a comparison of five common methods to produce exemplars from a suspect's dentition. J. Forensic Sci. 43:362–367, 1998.

Chapter 5

Nonaccidental Injury in Children

Amanda Thomas

1. INTRODUCTION

Nonaccidental injury (NAI) is a common condition in children and carries a significant morbidity and mortality. Doctors have an important role in recognizing, assessing, and managing children with suspected NAI.

1.1. Definition

Child abuse is difficult to define, and although many definitions exist in the legal and scientific literature, there is no consensus on an absolute definition. Issues that arise in the debate include the influence and attitudes of societies, cultural differences in child rearing, politics, and religious beliefs. In addition, there is a need to examine the factors involved in particular episodes, the context in which the episodes occurred, the opinion of the professionals who are describing or judging these episodes, the current knowledge of the long-term outcomes of particular behaviors to children, and the effectiveness of current interventions. However, definitions are important because they provide a general framework for policy setting, statutory and legal interventions, gathering statistical information, and an understanding of current and future research.

The UK Children Act (1) and the Federal Child Abuse Prevention and Treatment Act *(2)* (CAPTA) define a child as: "a person under the age of eighteen years." (In cases of sexual abuse, CAPTA refers to the age specified by the child protection law of the state in which the child resides.)

From: *Clinical Forensic Medicine: A Physician's Guide, 2nd Edition*
Edited by: M. M. Stark © Humana Press Inc., Totowa, NJ

Working Together to Safeguard Children 1999 *(3)* describes the abuse and neglect of a child as: "Somebody inflicting harm or failing to act to prevent harm" and physical abuse as: "Hitting, shaking, throwing, poisoning, burning or scalding, drowning, suffocating or otherwise causing physical harm to a child including when a parent or carer feigns the symptoms of, or deliberately causes ill-health to a child whom they are looking after, termed Fabricated or Induced Illness (FII)."

In the United States, each state is responsible for providing its own definitions of child abuse and neglect within the civil and criminal codes, but the operational definition of physical abuse (CAPTA) *(2)* is as follows:

"Physical abuse is characterized by the infliction of physical injury as a result of punching, beating, kicking, biting, burning, shaking or otherwise harming a child. The parent or caretaker may not have intended to hurt the child; rather, the injury may have resulted from over-discipline or physical punishment."

1.2. Effects of Child Abuse

There is extensive literature on the effects of child abuse. It is generally accepted that child abuse carries a significant mortality and morbidity with consequences that include the following:

- Death or disability in severe cases.
- Affective and behavior disorders.
- Developmental delay and learning difficulties.
- Failure to thrive and growth retardation.
- Predisposition to adult psychiatric disorders.
- An increased risk of the abused becoming an abuser.

In Gibbons et al.'s study *(4)* of 170 children, an attempt was made to disentangle the effect of the abuse from the contributing circumstances and the results of intervention. The authors found that 10 years after diagnosis, abused children were more likely to show behavior problems at home and at school, had greater difficulties with friendships, and scored lower on certain cognitive tests. There was evidence that persistent abuse, a combination of different kinds of abuse, or abuse and neglect together had a poorer prognosis. Isolated incidents of physical abuse in the context of a nonviolent family and in the absence of sexual abuse or neglect did not necessarily lead to poor long-term outcomes for children. What has emerged from this research has been the importance of the style of parenting in families: children exposed to a harshly punitive, less reliable, and less warm environments are the children with the poorest outcomes.

1.3. Risk Factors for Abuse

The picture of child abuse is complex, with social, psychological, economic, and environmental factors all playing a part. Often there is evidence of family stress followed by a triggering event leading to abuse. Newberger *(5)* pinpointed the following three categories of predisposing family stress:

1. Child factors—disability, learning difficulties, behavior problems, adoption.
2. Parental factors—mental health problems, alcohol or drug abuse, domestic violence, previous abuse as a child.
3. Sociosituational factors—single parent, young parent, new partner, poverty, unemployment.

Gibbons et al. *(6)* studied children on the child protection registers in England and Wales (that is, children identified by agencies as at risk for significant harm and for whom a child protection plan had been developed) and found that domestic violence was recorded in more than one-fourth of cases. A substantial minority of parents had histories of mental illness, criminal behavior, or substance abuse. Substance abuse is more common worldwide and is associated with an elevated risk of neglect in the children of substance-abusing parents. Children with disabilities are at greater risk of becoming victims of abuse and neglect than children without disabilities, estimated at 1.7 times greater, with physical abuse 1.6 times more likely *(7)*.

The harmful effect of socioeconomic deprivation on children is well established. Poverty is associated with postnatal and infant mortality, malnutrition and ill health, low educational attainment, delinquency, teenage pregnancy, and family tension and breakdown. Parental stress leads to greater vulnerability of the children, and common stress factors include unemployment and debt, which are linked to poverty. Abuse occurs throughout all social classes, but children from the most disadvantaged sectors of society are brought to the attention of child protection agencies more frequently *(8)* than those from nondisadvantaged sectors.

1.4. Extent of Abuse

The true prevalence of child abuse is difficult to determine in all countries. Official estimates will only represent a fraction of the total number of cases, because many go unreported or unrecognized, and information systems are incomplete or track just one limited part of the picture. In the United States, the referral rate for child abuse investigations is three times higher than in the United Kingdom, and twice as many children are in state care, with four times as many child abuse deaths *(9)*.

In the United Kingdom, child protection registers hold statistical information on children identified by agencies as at risk of significant harm and for whom a child protection plan has been developed. However, these figures record professional activity and the numbers of children registered, not the numbers of children who have been abused. They exclude cases where abuse has occurred but the child is otherwise protected or no longer at risk, cases where abuse has not been recognized, or cases where the child has not been registered but may still be subject to abuse. In 2002, there were 23 children per 10,000 aged less than 18 years on the child protection register, and 19% were registered under the category of physical injury, the second most frequent type of maltreatment *(10)*.

The 2001 annual statistics on child maltreatment from state child protective services (CPS) agencies in the United States revealed a victimization rate of 12.4 per 1000 children in the population (19% suffered physical abuse) and a child fatality rate of 1.81 children per 100,000 children in the population *(11)*. Neglect is the most common category of registration or type of maltreatment in both the United Kingdom and the United States.

2. NONACCIDENTAL INJURY IN CHILDREN

NAI in children (physical abuse or battering) includes injuries that result from deliberate actions against the child or failure to prevent injury occurring to the child. The spectrum of injury includes the following:

- Soft tissue injury.
- Thermal injury.
- Skeletal injury.
- Internal injuries (brain, abdomen, or eye).
- Fabricated or induced illness (Munchausen syndrome by proxy, factitious illness).

The range of NAI extends from minor (e.g., bruising) to fatal, and younger infants are at risk of more serious injuries.

Different types of abuse overlap. Physical abuse will often coexist with emotional abuse. Injury may occur in the context of neglect, such as leaving a child unsupervised and exposed to dangerous situations. Physically abused children are at increased risk of sexual abuse. Hobbs and Wynne *(12)* found that 1 in 6 of 769 physically abused children and 1 in 7 of 949 sexually abused children had suffered both forms of abuse.

2.1. Role of the Physician

Physicians have a duty (a legal duty in countries, such as the United States and Australia) to recognize and report suspected abuse to the statutory investigative agencies. Physicians need to work together with statutory agencies and have an awareness and understanding of other agencies' roles and responsibilities. Physicians should be aware of current guidance on accountability and confidentiality produced by their professional bodies.

Physicians may be involved in a range of child protection activities, including the following:

- Recognition, diagnosis, and treatment of injury.
- Joint interagency activity.
- Court attendance.
- Ongoing care and monitoring of children following suspected abuse.
- Support for families and children.
- Prevention.
- Teaching, training, supervision, and raising awareness.

2.2. Assessing the Nonaccidentally Injured Child

For the physician faced with the assessment of a child for suspected physical injury, the following points should be remembered:

- Physical abuse often overlaps with other forms of abuse.
- Abuse may involve other siblings and family members.
- Abuse may recur and escalate.
- Younger children and infants are more at risk of physical injury and death than older children.
- The aim of recognition and early intervention is to protect the child, prevent mortality and morbidity, and diagnose and improve disordered parenting.
- Early intervention in families may prevent more serious abuse and subsequent removal of children into care.
- The medical examination is important, but it is only one part of the wider assessment of the child and family.

A recommended approach to the pediatric assessment is as follows:

1. Obtaining background information from professionals, e.g., social worker or police officer, if accompanying the family, or by telephone before the assessment.
2. Full pediatric history from the parent/caregiver and child. Remember to document the responses and the questions asked and any spontaneous disclosures.
3. Assessment of the "whole child," including:
   - Growth plotted on a percentile chart.
   - Development: is this child developmentally capable of what has been described? Is this child's developmental delay part of a wider picture of abuse or neglect?
   - A description of the child's demeanor and behavior: is the child's behavior normal for age?

- Full physical examination, including genitalia and anus.
- Description of injuries: types of lesions, sites, sizes, shapes and patterns, colors, and estimate of ages.

4. Legible, signed, dated, hand-written, contemporaneous record of the assessment with drawings of injuries detailing measurements.
5. Photographs of injuries.
6. Appropriate investigations (discussed in Subheading 3.1.1.4.).
7. Ask to assess siblings.
8. Initial information gathering from other professionals (e.g., family doctor, health visitor, or teachers from nursery or school) already involved with the family. This does not replace the formal investigation procedures but may be helpful for the examining physician, who must consider the wider picture to formulate an opinion and guide the child protection agencies.
9. Provision of a clear, factual report detailing the findings, summarizing the assessment, and providing a medical opinion for child protection agencies and any criminal proceedings.
10. Maintenance of written records of contacts with families and professionals.

2.3. Pointers to the Diagnosis

Suspicion of NAI may arise in the following scenarios (13):

- Delay in presentation of the injury.
- Discrepant or absent history.
- History incompatible with the injury.
- Pattern of injury more suggestive of abuse.
- Repetitive injuries.
- Unusual parental behavior or mood.
- Child's demeanor, behavior, or interaction with the parent/caregiver unusual.
- Disclosure by child or witness.

3. TYPES OF INJURIES (See CHAPTER 4)
3.1. Soft Tissue Injuries
3.1.1. Bruising

A bruise is an escape of blood into the skin, subcutaneous tissue, or both, after the rupture of blood vessels by the application of blunt force (14). The initial color of the bruise is the product of the child's natural skin pigmentation, the color of the pigments in the extravasated blood, and any color added by the inflammatory reaction. The color of the bruise changes as the extracellular hemoglobin breaks down into various pigments (15).

Factors affecting the appearance of a bruise include (16):

- The severity of the force applied to the area.
- The connective tissue support at the site of injury—increased extravasation of blood occurs around lax, loose areas of skin, such as the eye.

- Skin color—bruising is more visible in pale skin.
- Diseases affecting coagulation, blood vessels, or connective tissues.
- Drugs (e.g., steroids and salicylates).
- Continued extravasation of blood and tracking between tissue planes, which may delay the appearance of the bruise or lead to a different site of bruising from the site of injury.
- Bruising is reduced if pressure is maintained over the area until death has occurred or when death has occurred rapidly.
- The use of an implement. The pattern or shape of the bruise can reflect the implement used.

3.1.1.1. Clues to Distinguish NAI From Accidental Bruising

For further information, *see* ref. *17.*

1. Patterns
   - Hand marks.
     - Fingertip bruises consisting of circular or oval bruises from squeezing, poking, gripping, or grabbing injuries.
     - Linear petechial bruises in the shape of a hand caused by capillaries rupturing at the edge of the injury from the high-velocity impact of the hand slap.
     - Pinch marks consisting of paired, crescent-shaped bruises separated by a white line.
   - Implement marks.
     - High-velocity impact causing a rim of petechiae outlining the pattern of the inflicting instrument, e.g., parallel sided marks from sticks—"tramline bruising"
     - Higher velocity impacts causing bruising underlying the injury in the shape of the object used, (e.g., wedge-shaped bruises from kicks with shoes).
     - Pressure necrosis of the skin from ligatures, causing well-demarcated bands partially or fully encircling limbs or the neck.
     - Coarse speckled bruising from impact injuries through clothing.
   - Petechial bruises.
     - Pinprick bruises from ruptured capillaries (e.g., suction bruises, squeezing, slapping, strangulation, or suffocation).
2. Sites more commonly associated with NAI:
   - Facial—soft tissues of the cheek, eye, mouth, ear, mastoid, lower jaw, frenulum, and neck.
   - Chest wall.
   - Abdomen.
   - Inner thighs and genitalia (strongly associated with sexual abuse).
   - Buttock and outer thighs (commonly associated with punishment injuries).
   - Multiple sites.
3. More commonly associated with accidental injury:
   - Bony prominences.
   - On the front of the body.

4. Numbers:
  - The number of accidental bruises increases with increased mobility of a child.
  - More than 10 bruises in an actively mobile child should raise concern.

3.1.1.2. Dating Bruising

For further information, *see* refs. *14–16.*

- Bruises cannot be reliably aged.
- The development of a yellow color in a bruise is the most significant color change, occurring, at the earliest, 18 hours from the time of injury *(16)*.
- Bruises can change color at different rates, and several different colors can be present at the same time in the same bruise.
- Bruises of identical age and etiology may not show the same colors.
- Possible indicators of more recent injury include:
  - Fresh cuts and abrasions overlying a bruise.
  - Swelling underlying the bruising.
  - Pain or tenderness at the site of injury.

3.1.1.3. Differential Diagnosis of Bruising

- Accidental injury—commonly on bony surfaces, appropriate history.
- Artifact—dirt, paint, felt tip, or dye from clothing or footwear.
- Benign tumors—halo nevus, blue nevus, or hemangiomas.
- Vascular and bleeding disorders—thrombocytopenic purpura, Henoch–Schoenlein purpura, hemophilia, or purpura in association with infection (e.g., meningococcal septicemia).
- Disturbances of pigmentation—café-au-lait patches or Mongolian blue spots.
- Erythematous lesions—erythema nodosum.
- Hereditary collagen disorders—osteogenesis imperfecta or Ehlers–Danlos syndrome.

3.1.1.4. Investigations

In the presence of excessive or reported spontaneous bruising, it is reasonable to exclude an underlying bleeding disorder. However, O'Hare and Eden *(18)* found abnormal tests in 16% of 50 children with suspected NAI and concluded that the two conditions can coexist.

Suggested tests include full blood count, platelet count, prothrombin time, thrombin time, partial thromboplastin time, fibrinogen level, and bleeding time (after discussion with a hematologist).

3.1.2. Bite Marks

A bite mark is a mark made by teeth alone or in combination with other mouth parts and may be considered a mirror image of the arrangement and characteristics of the dentition. Human bite marks rarely occur accidentally and are good indicators of inflicted injury. Children can be bitten in the context of punishment, as part of a physical assault, or in association with sexual abuse. Children can also be bitten by other children. (For further information, *see* refs. *19* and *20*.)

Human bite marks have a broad U-shaped arch and broad, shallow, blunt indentation marks on the skin, compared with animal bites, which have a narrower arch size and deeper, smaller skin indentations from sharper teeth.

Factors influencing the appearance of a bite mark include the following:

- The status of the skin (ante- or postmortem) and the skin condition.
- The time period between the bite and the examination.
- The clarity of the marks and the reaction of the surrounding tissue.
- The strength of the bite pressure (stronger bite pressures cause deeper skin depressions).
- The strength of the sucking pressure (stronger sucking pressures lead to reduced markings by the incisors).

3.1.2.1. Good Practice Tips

- When defined bite marks are found, advice should be sought from a forensic odontologist. Impressions and dental casts of suspects can be made that may be able to establish the identity of the perpetrator.
- Bite marks can be found on any site of the human anatomy, and when a single bite mark is found, particular care should be taken to search for other bites. Vale et al. *(21)* found that 40% of their victims had more than one bite and 22% had bite marks in more than one anatomic site.
- Documentation of the bite should include the location, contour of the skin surface, size and number of teeth marks, diameter of the mark, and intercanine distance.
- An intercanine distance of 3 cm or more indicates that the bite was inflicted by a person with a permanent dentition (an adult or a child older than 8 years) *(22)*.
- Plain sterile swabs (moistened, if necessary) can be used to obtain residual saliva from the bite area for forensic purposes. The swabs should be air dried and managed according to standard procedures for the collection of forensic evidence (*see* Chapter 3).
- Good-quality photographs, both black and white and color, should be taken. These should include a scale (rigid L-shaped measuring rule) and, when appropriate, a color standard. Serial daily photographs are useful to record the bite mark's evolution and optimum definition.

3.1.3. Other Soft Tissue Injuries

- Subgaleal hematoma—diffuse, boggy swelling on the scalp can occur following hair pulling (often associated with broken hairs and petechial hemorrhages).
- Periorbital injury—from a direct blow (e.g., a punch).

- Ocular injury
  - Subconjunctival hemorrhage from direct trauma, suffocation, strangulation, chest, or abdominal trauma.
  - Direct trauma can also lead to corneal or scleral laceration or scarring, ruptured globe, vitreous or retinal hemorrhage, acute hyphema, dislocated lens, traumatic cataract, and detached retina.
- Perioral injuries—bruising or laceration to the lips from a direct blow to the mouth.
- Intraoral injuries.
  - Ulceration to the inner lips or cheeks from a blow to the face causing impaction of the tissues against teeth, torn frenulum from a blow to the upper lip, or penetrating injury from a feeding utensil.
  - Abrasions or lacerations to the palate, vestibule, or floor of the mouth from penetrating injuries (e.g., from a feeding utensil).
  - Petechial injury to the palate from direct trauma to the palate or oral abuse.
  - Tooth injury (e.g., breaks, fractures, or avulsions caused by blunt trauma).
- Abrasions—superficial areas of skin loss caused by friction injuries, scratches from fingernails, or sharp-edged objects.
- Cuts or incised wounds—a superficial injury that is longer than it is deep, produced by a sharp-edged object.
- Lacerations producing rugged wounds from crushing or tearing of the skin resulting from blunt force.

3.2. Thermal Injury

Burns and scalds to children can be inflicted, occur accidentally, or follow neglect. The injury can be superficial or partial or full-skin thickness, depending on the temperature and duration of exposure.

3.2.1. Types of Thermal Injury

For further information, *see* ref. *23*.

- Scalds—immersion, pouring or throwing a hot liquid onto a child. The affected skin is soggy, blanched, and blistered. The shape of the injury is contoured. The depth of the burn is variable.
- Contact burns—direct contact of a hot object with the child. Characteristically, the burn is shaped like the hot object, with sharply defined edges and usually of uniform depth. The burn may blister.
- Fire burns—flames from fires, matches, or lighters in close or direct contact with the skin, causing charring and skin loss with singeing of hairs.
- Cigarette burns—inflicted direct contact leaves a characteristically well-demarcated circular or oval mark with rolled edges and a cratered center, which may blister and tends to scar. Accidental contact with a cigarette tends to leave a more superficial, irregular area of erythema with a tail.

- Electrical burns—small, deeply penetrating burns with an entry and exit wound with possible necrosis of underlying tissues.
- Friction burns—dragging or rubbing injury causing superficial skin loss, with broken blisters, usually on bony prominences.
- Chemical burns—the chemical in liquid form is drunk, poured, or splashed onto the skin, or in solid form is rubbed on the skin. The skin may stain, may have the appearance of a scald, and may scar.
- Radiant burns—more extensive areas of erythema and blistering on exposed body parts.

3.2.2. Features of Thermal Injuries Suggestive of NAI

For further information, *see* ref. *24.*

- Those features discussed in Subheading 2.3.
- Repeated burns.
- Sites—backs of hands, buttocks, feet, and legs.
- Types—clearly demarcated burns shaped like a particular object, immersion burns with a tide mark (clear edge) and no splash marks.
- The presence of other NAIs.

3.2.3. Differential Diagnosis of Thermal Injuries

- Accidental burns—appropriate history and presentation.
- Infection—staphylococcal or streptococcal (impetigo or scalded skin syndrome).
- Allergy—urticaria or contact dermatitis.
- Insect bites.
- Bullous diseases—porphyria or erythema multiforme.

3.2.4. Good Practice Tips

- Identify the type, depth, and extent of the burn.
- Accurately measure the injury and document with photographs.
- Manipulate the child's posture to reflect the position at the time of the injury.
- Assess the child's developmental skills. Can the child climb? Turn on a tap?
- Assess for other signs of abuse.
- Assessment of the home or place of injury with reenactment of the episode to include the events leading up to the injury, the child's position at the time of the incident, the length of time the child was exposed to the heat or liquid, the temperature of the appliance or liquid, and measurements of suspected appliances (e.g., the height/depth of the bath, height of the work surface, and position of appliance).
- Remember that burns and infection can coexist.

3.3. Skeletal Injury

Historically, skeletal injury played a major role in the recognition of child abuse *(25,26).* In 1946, Caffey *(27)* described six patients presenting with chronic subdural hematoma in which 23 unexplained fractures of the long bones were found. Caffey concluded that the fractures were traumatic in origin and introduced the concept of inflicted injury.

Most skeletal injuries of NAI occur in children under the age of 2 years, and some may be occult, particularly in the infant younger than 1 yr who has other signs of physical injury. Merten et al. *(28)* found fractures in 47% of abused children under the age of 1 year who had skeletal surveys, in which 67% were occult and 60% were multiple. Fractures in infants and children resulting from falls of under 3 ft are relatively uncommon. Research evidence suggests that 1% of children falling less than 3 ft may sustain a simple linear skull fracture *(29)*.

Accidental fractures in infants and toddlers do occur, usually as a result of falls, often from a height, but they can occasionally occur in long bones of ambulant children from twisting, running, and falling. There is usually a consistent history and a prompt presentation. Fractures cause pain and distress and are often accompanied by nonuse of the affected body part and local swelling.

Any fracture can occur as a result of NAI, but some have a high specificity for abuse, such as:

- Metaphyseal—a shaking, pulling, or twisting force applied at or about a joint, resulting in a fracture through the growing part of the bone.
- Epiphyseal separation—resulting from torsion of a limb, particularly in children younger than 2 years old.
- Rib—resulting from severe squeezing or direct trauma; posterior rib fractures virtually pathognomonic of NAI and commonly associated with shaking injury.
- Scapular—resulting from direct impact.
- Lateral clavicle—resulting from excessive traction or shaking of an arm.
- Humerus or femur—in nonambulant children (under 1 year); transverse fractures from angulation, including a direct blow; spiral fractures from axial twists with or without axial loading; oblique fractures from angulation, axial twisting with axial loading.
- Vertebral—resulting from hyperflexion injuries, impact injuries, or direct trauma.
- Digital—resulting from forced hyperextension or direct blows.
- Skull—resulting from blunt-impact injuries, particularly occipital fractures and fractures that are depressed, wide (or growing), bilateral, complex, crossing suture lines multiply, or associated with intracranial injury *(30)*.
- Periosteal injury—resulting from pulling or twisting of a limb separating the periosteum from the surface of the bone, leading to hemorrhage between the periosteum and the bone and subsequent calcification.

Other features of skeletal injury suggestive of abuse include the following:

- Absence of an appropriate history.
- Multiple fractures.
- Fractures of differing ages.

- Fracture in association with other features of NAI (e.g., bruising at other sites).
- Unsuspected fractures (recent or old) found when X-rays taken for other reasons.

Precise dating of fractures cannot be achieved, although ranges of fracture ages are available. Advice from an experienced pediatric radiologist should be sought to assist with dating injuries, to obtain further radiological or other imaging views, and to exclude other causes of skeletal abnormality.

3.3.1. Dating Fractures

- Resolution of soft tissues — 2 to 10 days.
- Early periosteal new bone — 4 to 21 days.
- Loss of fracture line definition — 10 to 21 days.
- Soft callus — 10 to 21 days.
- Hard callus — 14 to 90 days.
- Remodeling — 3 months to 2 years.

For further information, *see* ref. *31*.

Detecting occult injury is particularly important in the younger child and infant and recommended indications for a skeletal survey include the following *(17,25,28,32)*:

- Any child younger than 2 years when there is a suspicion of physical abuse.
- Any child younger than 2 years presenting with a fracture suggestive of abuse.
- Consider in children aged 2–4 years with severe bruising.
- Older children with severe injuries.
- Children dying in unusual or suspicious circumstances.
- Physical abuse in an infant twin (or multiple birth sets) younger than 1 year— consider skeletal survey of the other infant(s) *(33)*.
- Repeat views, particularly of ribs, may be useful 2 weeks after the initial survey, because periosteal reaction may not have formed around acute injuries.

3.3.2. Differential Diagnosis of Skeletal Injury

- Accidental injury—appropriate, consistent history, and prompt presentation.
- Normal variation—skull suture, physiological periosteal reaction (symmetric and smooth around the long bones of children from 6 weeks to 6 months).
- Birth trauma—commonly clavicle or humerus.
- Infection—osteomyelitis or congenital syphilis.
- Rickets—nutritional, renal, chronic illness, and prematurity.
- Cancers—neuroblastoma or leukemia.
- Osteogenisis imperfecta—a rare condition, incidence of 1 in 20,000, usually accompanied by a family history of fractures, fractures with minimal trauma, easy bruising, joint laxity, early-onset deafness, blue sclerae, and dentinogenesis.
- Copper deficiency—low-birth-weight preterm infants, malnutrition, or malabsorption.

3.4. Internal Injuries

3.4.1. Intracranial Injury

There is a high incidence of mortality and morbidity after inflicted head injury, and it is the most common cause of traumatic death in infancy *(34)*. It has been generally accepted from research evidence that serious or fatal injury from accidental injury, other than that sustained in road traffic accidents or falls from major heights, is rare in children under 2 years and that simple skull fractures in accidental trauma have a low risk of intracranial sequelae *(26)*.

The major acute intracranial lesions of NAI are subdural hematoma, cerebral edema with hypoxic ischemic encephalopathy, and, more rarely, brain lacerations, intracerebral and intraventricular hemorrhage, and extradural hematomas *(26)*.

The mechanism of brain injury is considered to be a whiplash motion of acceleration and deceleration, coupled with a rotational force, during a shaking episode of an infant, where the head is unsupported. Shaking alone may lead to brain injury, although in many instances there may be other forms of head trauma, including impact injuries *(35,36)*. Impact may be against a hard surface, leading to external injury and an associated skull fracture, or against a soft surface, with no associated external injury. Hypoxia may also lead to brain injury from impairment of ventilation during chest squeezing, suffocation, or strangulation *(26)*.

Retinal hemorrhages are strongly suggestive of abuse when accompanied by intracranial injuries and in the absence of a confirmed history of severe accidental injury. Unilateral or bilateral retinal hemorrhages are present in 75–90% of cases of shaken baby syndrome *(36)*. Retinal hemorrhages can also be found after severe closed chest injury, asphyxia, coagulation disorders, carbon monoxide poisoning, acute hypertension, sepsis, meningitis, and normal birth (usually disappearing by 2 weeks, rarely persisting to 6 weeks). When shaking injuries are suspected, retinal examination is essential and should include direct and indirect ophthalmoscopy preferably by an ophthalmologist. Subhyaloid hemorrhages and local retinal detachment occur earliest, are often peripheral, and are found only by indirect ophthalmology. When intraocular injury is present, subdural hemorrhage is likely, and the presence of retinal detachment and multiple hemorrhages may indicate additional cerebral lacerations or intracerebral hemorrhages *(35)*.

Children with acute intracranial injury may present with fits, lethargy, irritability, apnea, unconsciousness and signs of shock, a tense fontanelle, increasing head circumference, and low hemoglobin. Children with chronic subdural hematomas may present with poor feeding, failure to thrive, vomiting, increasing head circumference, and fits. The presentation may suggest sepsis, meningitis, encephalitis, or toxic or metabolic bone disease. The findings of retinal hemorrhages, other signs of abuse, and blood-stained cerebrospinal fluid may assist with the differential diagnosis. Milder forms of shaking may go undetected or present with nonspecific signs that may be minimized by physicians or attributed to a viral illness *(36)*.

When brain injury of abuse is suspected, a full blood count, platelet count and coagulation studies, skull X-ray, skeletal survey, and brain computed tomography (CT) are recommended. Magnetic resonance imaging (MRI) should be undertaken when CT is equivocal or normal and there are neurological signs or symptoms *(26)*. The American Academy of Pediatrics considers MRI as complimentary to CT and recommends MRI 2–3 days1 later, if possible *(36)*.

3.4.2. Abdominal Injuries

Visceral manifestations of NAI are uncommon and considered to contribute 2–4% of injuries in NAI *(37,38)*. However, visceral injuries carry a high morbidity and mortality (estimated mortality of 40–50%) and are the second most common cause of fatal child abuse because of the shear force of trauma, delay in recognition of injury because of frequent lack of signs and symptoms, and delay in recognition of NAI *(38,39)*.

Injuries arise mainly from blunt trauma (punching, kicking, trampling, or stamping) or sudden acceleration/deceleration injuries (swinging or throwing a child into a solid object) and include contusion, laceration, and rupture of solid or hollow viscera. The duodenum, jejunum, pancreas, and liver are common sites of injury in abdominal NAI. Colonic or rectal injuries are associated with sexual abuse *(38)*.

Vomiting, abdominal distension, pain, and shock may be presenting features. Other features of NAI and skeletal injury may provide clues to the underlying etiology. Immediate surgery may be necessary.

Suggested investigations include full blood count, blood biochemistry, pancreatic and liver enzymes, plain, abdominal, and chest X-ray (free air or free fluid), ultrasound, CT, and gastrointestinal contrast studies, where indicated.

3.5. Fabricated or Induced Illness

The fabrication or induction of illness in children by a caregiver is referred to by several different terms, most commonly Munchausen syndrome by proxy, factitious illness by proxy or illness induction syndrome. In the United States, the term *pediatric condition falsification* is being adopted by the American

Professional Society on the Abuse of Children. This terminology is also used by some as if it were a psychiatric diagnosis. The American Psychiatric Association's *Diagnostic and Statistical Manual* has proposed using the term *factitious disorder by proxy* for a psychiatric diagnosis applicable to the fabricator *(40)*.

Fabricated or induced illness is a persistent fabrication of a child's illness either simulated or produced by the child's parent or caretaker. There are three main ways of the caregiver fabricating or inducing illness in a child:

- Fabrication of signs and symptoms. This may include fabrication of past medical history.
- Fabrication of signs and symptoms and falsification of hospital charts and records and specimens of bodily fluids. This may include also falsification of letters and documents;.
- Induction of illness by numerous means.

This form of child abuse is uncommon but severe and carries a high mortality and morbidity. International research findings suggest that up to 10% of children die and approx 50% experience long-term morbidity. There is a high incidence of reabuse and harm to siblings, commonly requiring separation of the child from the abusing parent *(41)*.

The perpetrator is more commonly the mother. The range of fabricated illness is wide and can be complicated further by multiple medical investigations. Among the most common presentations are fits, apnea, bleeding, diarrhea, vomiting, fever, and rash *(42)*. Suffocation, poisoning, drug administration, and lying are mechanisms of fabricating illness. Emotional abuse is associated in almost all cases with considerable overlap with other forms of abuse. Diagnosis is difficult and often delayed. Management should follow the usual child protection procedures. Covert video surveillance can play an important role in detection, offering definitive evidence, but this approach must be a carefully coordinated, multiagency and multidisciplinary approach, with the surveillance undertaken by the police *(40,43)*.

4. SUMMARY

NAI in children is a common condition and carries with it a significant morbidity and mortality. Physicians must be able to recognize NAI and take appropriate action to protect children. Young children and infants are at particular risk, and there is often an overlap with other forms of abuse. A multidisciplinary approach aimed at early intervention, support for families, improvements in parenting styles, and prevention of mortality and morbidity in the child is essential to safeguard the welfare of children.

REFERENCES

1. Department of Health. Children Act 1989—Guidance and Regulations. Her Majesty's Stationery Office, London, UK, 1991.
2. The Child Abuse and Treatment Act Amendments of 1996. PL 104-235. March 10, 1996.
3. Department of Health, Home Office, Department for Education and Employment. Working Together to Safeguard Children. A Guide to Inter-agency Working to Safeguard and Promote the Welfare of Children. The Stationery Office, London, UK, 1999.
4. Gibbons, J., Gallagher, B., Bell, C., Gordon, D. Development After Physical Abuse in Early Childhood: a follow-up study of children on the child protection registers. Her Majesty's Stationery Office, London, UK, 1995.
5. Newberger, E. H. Child physical abuse. Primary Care. 20:317–327, 1993.
6. Gibbons, J., Conroy, S., Bell, C. Operating the child protection system: a study of child protection practices in English local authorities. Her Majesty's Stationery Office, London, UK, 1995.
7. American Academy of Pediatrics. Assessment of maltreatment of children with disabilities. Pediatrics. 108:508–512, 2001.
8. National Commission of Inquiry into the Prevention of Child Abuse. Childhood matters. Report of the National Commission of Inquiry into the Prevention of Child Abuse. Her Majesty's Stationery Office,London, UK, 1996.
9. Child Protection Messages from Research. Studies in Child Protection. Her Majesty's Stationery Office, London, UK, 1995.
10. Department of Health. Referrals, assessments and children and young people on child protection registers year ending 31 March 2002. Department of Health, UK, 2003.
11. Department of Health and Human Services. Child Maltreatment 2001. Reports from the states to the National Child Abuse and Neglect Data System (NCANDS). Administration for Children and Families. US Department of Health and Human Services, Washington, DC, April 2003.
12. Hobbs, C. J., Wynne, J. M. The sexually abused battered child. Arch. Dis. Child. 65: 423–427, 1990.
13. Speight, N. Nonaccidental injury. In: Meadow, R., ed., ABC of Child Abuse, 3rd Ed. British Medical Journal Publishing Group, London, UK, 1997.
14. Stephenson, T., Balias, Y. Estimation of the age of bruising. Arch. Dis. Child. 74: 53–55, 1996.
15. Stephenson, T. Ageing of bruising in children. J. R. Soc. Med. 90:312–314, 1997.
16. Langlois, N., Gresham, G. The ageing of bruises: a review of the study of the color changes with time. Forensic Sci. Int. 50:227–238, 1991.
17. Hobbs, C. J., Hanks, H., Wynne, J. M. Physical Abuse. In: Child Abuse and Neglect. A Clinician's Handbook, 2nd Ed. Churchill Livingstone,London, UK, 1999.
18. O'Hare, A., Eden, O. Bleeding disorders and nonaccidental injury. Arch. Dis. Child. 59:860–864, 1984.
19. McDonald, D., McFarland, T. Forensic odontology—report of a case involving bite marks. Glasgow Dent. J. 3:16–19, 1972.

20. Glass, R., Andrews, E., Jones, K. Bite mark evidence: a case report using accepted and new techniques. J. Forensic Sci. 25:638–645, 1980.
21. Vale, G., Noguchi, T. Anatomical distribution of human bite marks in a series of 67 cases. J. Forensic Sci. 28:61–69, 1983.
22. Scmitt, B. D. The child with non-accidental trauma. In: Helfer, R. E. and Kempe, R. S., eds., The Battered Child, 4th Ed. University of Chicago Press, Chicago, IL, pp. 178–196, 1987.
23. Hobbs, C. Burns and scalds. In: Meadow, R., ed., ABC of Child Abuse, 3rd Ed., British Medical Journal Publishing Group, London, UK, pp. 20–23, 1997.
24. Hobbs, C. When are burns not accidental? Arch. Dis. Child. 61:357–361, 1986.
25. Feldman, K. W. Evaluation of physical abuse. In: Helfer, R. E., Kempe, R. S., and Krugman, R. D., eds., The Battered Child, 5th Ed., University of Chicago Press, Chicago, IL, pp. 175–220, 1997.
26. Carty, H. Non-accidental injury: a review of the radiology. Eur. Radiol. 7:1365–1376, 1997.
27. Caffey, J. Multiple fractures of the long bones of infants suffering from chronic subdural hematoma. Am J Roentgeneol. 56:163–173, 1946.
28. Merten, D., Radkowski, M., Leonidis, J. The abused child: a radiological reappraisal. Radiology. 146:377–381, 1983.
29. Helfer, R., Slovis, T., Black, M. Injuries resulting when small children fall out of bed. Pediatrics. 60:533–555, 1977.
30. Hobbs, C. J. Skull fracture and the diagnosis of child abuse. Arch. Dis. Child. 59:246–252, 1984.
31. O'Connor, J. F., Cohen, J. Dating factures. In: Kleinman, P. K., ed., Diagnostic Imaging of Child Abuse. Williams & Wilkins, Baltimore, MD, p. 112, 1987.
32. American Academy of Pediatrics. Diagnostic imaging of child abuse. Pediatrics. 105:6:1345–1348, 2000.
33. Hansen, K. K. Twins and child abuse. Arch. Pediatr. Adolesc. Med. 148:1345–1346, 1994.
34. Duhaime, A. C., Christain, C. W., Rorke, L. B., Zimmerman, R. Nonaccidental head injury in infants—"the shaken baby syndrome." N. Engl. J. Med. 338:1828–1829, 1988.
35. Green, M. A., Lieberman, G., Milroy, C. M., Parsons, M. A. Ocular and cerebral trauma in non-accidental injury in infancy; underlying mechanisms and implications for paediatric practice. Br. J. Ophthalmol. 80:282–287, 1996.
36. American Academy of Pediatrics. Shaken baby syndrome: rotational cranial injuries—technical report (T0039). Pediatrics. 108:206–210, 2001.
37. Merten, D. F., Carpenter, B. L. M. Radiologic imaging of inflicted injury in the child abuse syndrome. Pediatr. Clin. North Am. 37:815–837, 1990.
38. Ng, C. S., Hall, C. M., Shaw, D. G. The range of visceral manifestations of non-accidental injury. Arch. Dis. Child. 77:167–174, 1997.
39. Cooper, A., Floyd, T., Barlow, B., et al. Major blunt abdominal trauma due to child abuse. J.Trauma. 28:1483–1487, 1988.
40. Department of Health. Safeguarding children in whom illness is fabricated or induced. Department of Health, Washington, DC, 2002.

41. Davis, P., McClure, R. J., Rolfe, K., et al. Procedures, placement, and risks of further abuse after Munchausen syndrome by proxy, non-accidental poisoning, and non-accidental suffocation. Arch. Dis. Child. 78:217–221, 1998.
42. Rosenberg, D. A. Web of deceit: a literature review of Munchausen syndrome by proxy. Child Abuse Negl. Int. J. 11:547–563, 1987.
43. Southall, D. P., Plunkett, M. C., Bank, M., et al. Covert video recordings of life-threatening child abuse: lessons in child protection. Pediatrics. 100:735–760, 1997.

Chapter 6

Crowd-Control Agents

Kari Blaho-Owens

1. INTRODUCTION

Chemical restraint can be used for a variety of reasons: for control of a violent individual or the agitated patient, to disperse crowds (crowd-control agents), or to limit access to specific areas. This type of control has also been used by criminals to subdue the individual in acts such as rape, robbery, and murder. The possibilities are vast, and detection of their use can be obvious, such as that with traditional tear gas or pepper spray, or may take forensic testing in cases where the person was sedated or otherwise drugged.

Forms of chemical restraint were used as early as 423 BC in the Peloponnesian war. Modern chemical crowd-control agents were first employed in the early months of World War I, when the French launched tear gas grenades against the German army. In addition to chlorobenzylidene (tear gas). World War I also saw the introduction of chlorine gas and mustard gas. The Germans first used chlorine gas in the spring of 1915 against the French Army at Ypres. The chlorine gas formed a cloud that was mistaken as a smoke screen behind which the German Army would advance. Instead of evacuating the area, the French army entrenched itself, readying for an attack. Mustard gas was used in 1917 by the German army against the French army. Unlike chlorine, which wafted in a cloud described as a greenish-yellow smoke, mustard gas was nearly odorless, and its effects took much longer to manifest. Although chlorine was an immediate choking agent, rendering severe respiratory distress and death, the full effects of mustard gas take 12–24 hours. Because mustard is an oily substance, it persists in the environment in which it is released, extending its

From: *Clinical Forensic Medicine: A Physician's Guide, 2nd Edition*
Edited by: M. M. Stark © Humana Press Inc., Totowa, NJ

exposure. Any surface exposed to mustard gas is affected. Mucosal membranes, such as the eye, respiratory tract, and skin, develop blisters, slough, and can fully incapacitate the individual for long time periods. It should be noted that the term *gas* may not be completely correct because many of these agents are not true gases but rather are solid particles that can be dispersed. The effectiveness of the crowd-control agent depends on the delivery of adequate amounts and sufficient contact with susceptible surfaces so that the desired effect is achieved. Therefore, temperature, wind conditions, method of delivery, formulation and potential barriers (such as clothing, masks, and eye protection), and ability to decontaminate interject variability into the response.

World War I was the first modern forum that tested chemical weapons to control large numbers of individuals. Since then, agents with wider safety margins have been developed that promote dispersal of large numbers of individuals without significant morbidity and mortality. Modern crowd-control agents, such as chlorobenzylidene ([CS]; also known as tear gas), were first used by the military as training agents, then by law enforcement as alternatives to lethal force, and most recently, some have become available to civilians for personal self-defense. Chemical crowd-control agents can also be used by terrorists to incite fear or panic in crowds, and there is always the potential for accidental dispersal in a public forum or, rarely, the potential for self-abuse.

There is considerable debate concerning the use of chemical agents for crowd control. Three agents have been used as less lethal alternatives to firearms and batons. They are capsaicin oleum (OC) (also known as pepper spray [PS]), chloracetothenon ([CN]; also known as mace), and CS.

There are five major concerns about the use of these agents by law enforcement:

1. Their possible toxicity to the offender.
2. Potential for exposure to the person administering the agent.
3. The potential for any ancillary exposure to health care providers, and to bystanders *(1–4)*.
4. The expansion of their use to nonviolent offenders, such as peaceful protesters.
5. Concern about the long-term effects from repeated exposure and from occupational exposure *(5)*.

Some of these issues become more complicated because chemical control agents are increasingly popular with civilians as readily available, often legal, self-defense weapons.

There have been several incidents in the United States and in other countries that question the appropriateness of use of chemical crowd-control agents *(5,6)*. In one reported incident in the United States, law enforcement officers applied OC liquid via a cotton-tipped applicator directly to the periorbital area

Table 1
Examples of Chemical Restraint Products Available

Brand name	Ingredients	Delivery system
Cap–Stun	5% OC	Spray
Alan's Pepper Spray	10% OC	Spray
Pepper Foam	10% OC	Foam spray
Pepper Gard, Triple Action Spray	10% OC and 10% CS	Spray
Mark III	5% OC and 5% CS	Spray

OC, capsaicin oleum; CS, chlorobenzylidene.

of protesters who were sitting and refused to disperse *(7)*. The use of OC against these nonviolent offenders when other methods of control failed generated negative publicity and resulted in legal action against the law enforcement officials.

When used appropriately, crowd-control agents have a good safety margin and generally do no permanent harm. In addition to the furious debate over the agents, there has been some concern over the safety of the delivery vehicles, particularly methyl-isobutyl ketone (MIBK). Although chronic exposure to MIBK has been associated with neurological and respiratory effects, there are no data to support the theory that acute exposure to the low concentrations that occur with CS spray poses these same problems *(8–10)*. Despite all of the controversy surrounding chemical control agents, they offer a less hazardous method of restraint than other potentially lethal alternatives, such as firearms.

2. CLINICAL FEATURES AND TREATMENT

As mentioned, the three main chemical restraint compounds used by law enforcement for individual or crowd control are OC, CN, and CS. These agents are available in varying concentrations, with several vehicles, in aerosols or foams and in particulate form with dispersal devices. Some of these are listed in Table 1.

Essentially a means of less lethal chemical warfare, chemical crowd-control products are used as defensive agents to temporarily incapacitate individuals or disperse groups without requiring more forceful means. The clinical effects are short-lived once exposure has ended. These agents share common effects that include lacrimation, ocular irritation and pain, dermal irritation, blepharospasm, conjunctivitis, transient impairment of vision, and mild to moderate respiratory distress *(11–13)*. Some corneal defects after exposure have been noted, but whether this is a direct tissue effect of the agent, the vehicle, or dispersant or a result of rubbing the ocular surface is unknown

(14). Contact dermatitis and periocular edema can also result. Other more severe effects, such as pulmonary edema, have been documented when concentrations are several hundred-fold above what produces intolerable symptoms or with trauma associated with the explosive device used to deliver the chemical agent *(6,15)*.

All of these clinical effects produced by chemical crowd-control agents render the recipient temporarily unable to continue violent action or resist arrest. Because they all share a high safety ratio, are effective at low concentrations, and can be used without direct forceful contact by the law enforcement officer, they are ideal agents for control of either the individual offender or riot control. Because of their relative safety, these agents are generally excluded from international treaty provisions that address chemical weapons. The United States, England, Ireland, France, China, Korea, Israel, and Russia are just some examples of countries that use these compounds as riot control agents. The legal availability to law enforcement and the general public differs between countries; however, most can be easily obtained through international markets or ordered through the Internet.

Chemical restraint compounds differ from most agents because some, such as CS, are solid particles with low vapor pressures. They are usually dispersed as fine particles or in a solution. For large crowds, "bombs" have been developed that can be dropped from aerial positions producing wide dispersal of the compound. They are also formulated in grenades or canisters, which can be propelled by either throwing or with a projectile device. The most common method of dispersal is by individual spray cans that deliver a stream, spray, or foam containing the agent. These individual dispersal units were designed to render immediate incapacitation to an offender without the use of more forceful methods, thereby providing an extra means of control in the ladder of force used by law enforcement. Canisters containing a lower concentration of the active ingredient have been marketed to civilians for personal protection. There is no formal training for civilians on securing the devices, laws governing their use, deployment, or decontamination after exposure. This lack of training significantly increases the risk for exposure and adverse events to the users, the intended target, and bystanders.

2.1. Oleum Capsicum

OC selectively stimulates nociceptors in exposed mucous membranes, releasing substance P, bradykinin, histamine, and prostaglandins. The physiological effects of these mediators' results in vasodilation, increased vascular permeability, pain, and altered neurotrophic chemotaxis. Other common symptoms are listed in Table 2.

Table 2
Common Clinical Findings
With Exposure to Crowd-Control Agents

Finding	CS	CN	OC
Ocular			
▪ Lacrimation	✓	✓	✓
▪ Blepharospasm	✓	✓	
▪ Pain and/or burning at exposure site	✓	✓	✓
▪ Conjunctival injection	✓	✓	✓
▪ Conjunctival edema	✓	✓	
▪ Photophobia	✓	✓	
▪ Corneal abrasion	✓	✓	✓
▪ Impaired vision	✓	✓	✓
Upper airway			
▪ Pain and/or burning	✓	✓	
▪ Shortness of breath	✓	✓	✓
▪ Increased secretion	✓	✓	
▪ Congestion	✓		
▪ Coughing	✓	✓	✓
▪ Throat irritation	✓	✓	✓
▪ Wheezing	✓	✓	✓
▪ Irregular respiration[a]	✓	✓	
Dermal			
▪ Pain	✓	✓	✓
▪ Contact dermatitis		✓	✓
▪ Blistering	✓	✓	✓
Miscellaneous			
▪ Nausea/vomiting	✓		
▪ Bad taste	✓		
▪ Headache	✓		
▪ Increased blood pressure	✓ [a]		

[a] Initial response believed to be associated with pain.
CS, chlorobenzylidene; CN, chloracetothenon; OC, capsaicin oleum.

Capsicum in its pure form is a crystalline material. The oleoresin extract of capsicum contains more than 100 volatile compounds that act similarly to capsicum *(16)*. Because of the variability in the individual components of OC, the relative pungency of the pepper type and geographical origin of the pepper, and variation in quality control, products containing this extract have differences in efficacy *(16,17)*. Commercially available OC products lack

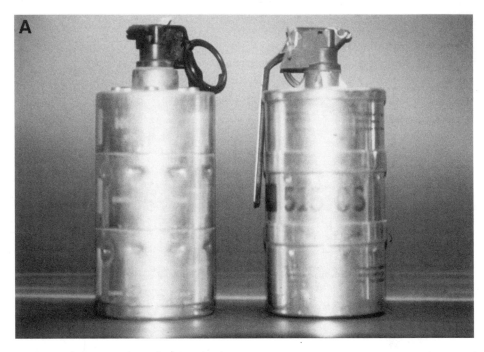

Fig. 1(A). Examples of individual spray containers containing crowd-control agents.

standardization for capsaicinoid content, which may alter potency, ultimately lead to variability in its efficacy, and jeopardize the safety of the user because of lack of effect *(18)*. Most OC preparations are formulated in a propylene vehicle to enhance adherence to the skin surface. PS is the most common spray marketed to civilians for a less lethal, noncontact, self-defense method. It can be purchased in numerous sprays or foams, in various concentrations, or combined with other crowd-control agents, such as CS *(see* Fig. 1).

In a retrospective study by Watson et al. *(8)*, patients presenting to an emergency department (ED) after PS exposure during a law enforcement action were evaluated. Most patients complained of ocular irritation and irritation and pain at the exposure site. The symptoms were transient, and few required treatment. The most significant adverse effects were corneal abrasions, which were treated with topical anesthetics and topical antibiotics. Five of 94 patients complained of wheezing or shortness of breath. No patient required treatment for wheezing, and two of the five had a history of reactive airway disease. No patient in this study had significant morbidity or mortality,

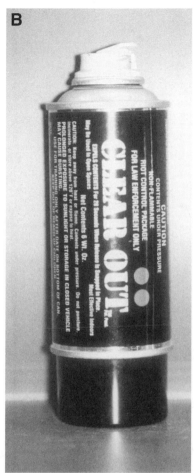
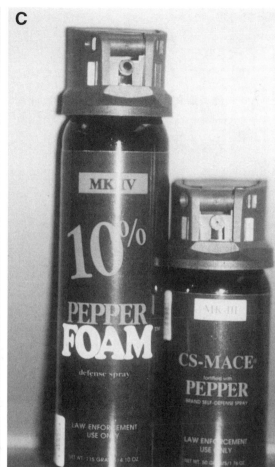

Fig. 1 (B,C).

and all were discharged from the ED. There are no data to support that PS exacerbates pulmonary disease or that patients with reactive airway disease are more sensitive to the effects *(8,19–21)*.

There have been a few reports of severe reactions to PS. One case report summarized respiratory distress that necessitated extracorporeal membrane oxygenation in a 4-wk-old infant after a 5% PS was accidentally discharged in his face *(22)*. The infant had a rocky clinical course but recovered. Another case report summarized the clinical course of an 11-yr-old child who intentionally sprayed and inhaled PS from an individual canister and developed reversible wheezing *(23)*. These case reports are anecdotal in that they report symptoms temporally related to PS exposure and demonstrate that when used improperly these compounds can cause severe symptoms. Thus far, these adverse events have been rare.

Of concern were reports of violent prisoners who died after being sprayed with PS and being physically restrained *(24)*. It was assumed that the police used excessive force and that the prisoners died from "positional asphyxia" from the restraints and that PS played a role in their deaths *(24)*.

The cause of in-custody deaths can be difficult to determine because many times these deaths have other confounding factors besides restraint and chemical control agents. Risk factors for sudden death, such as mental illness, drug abuse, and seizure disorders, may not be readily visible, and autopsy reports can often be inconclusive or incomplete. There is no evidence that PS causes any type of respiratory effects sufficient to cause death, nor is there evidence to conclude that positional asphyxia caused the deaths of those in question. All of the prisoners who died exhibited characteristics consistent with excited delirium from substance abuse. Most were obese, had hyperthermia, were violent, and had measurable cocaine on postmortem analysis. The lesson learned from these cases is that all violent prisoners, regardless of whether a chemical restraint has been used, should be closely monitored and evaluated by appropriate health care professionals. A small population of acutely intoxicated individuals is at risk of sudden death, independent of their treatment.

To refute the association between restraint and OC exposure, Chan et al. performed a randomized, crossover, controlled trial to assess the effect of OC spray inhalation with OC exposure plus restraint in a prone position *(25)*. Results from 35 subjects exposed to OC or placebo showed that inhalation of OC did not result in abnormal spirometry, hypoxemia, or hypoventilation when compared to placebo in either sitting position or in a maximal restraint position.

Treatment of exposure to PS is based on severity of symptoms. The first order of treatment should always be decontamination, which includes actions to limit exposure, such as the removal of contaminated clothing. Copious irrigation of affected areas will attenuate the burning sensation *(26,27)*. However, one must use caution not to contaminate other sites with the irrigant (e.g., washing PS from the hair into the eyes or oral pharyngeal mucosa). In a study, topical proparacaine was helpful in alleviating ocular pain associated with OC exposure (approx 50% of those treated experienced an improvement in their symptons) when compared to a topical nonsteroidal antiinflammatory agent (0.03% topical flurbiprofen) or placebo *(28)*. It is important to note that there were no corneal abrasions in any of the 11 subjects in this study and that 21% of the eyes had slit lamp evidence of punctuate epithelial erosions. In this

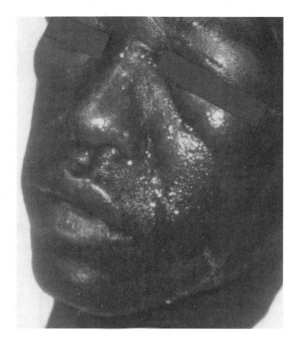

Fig. 2. Periocular swelling and facial contact dermatitis from pepper spray exposure during an arrest by law enforcement.

study, as well as an additional exposure trial, the focal epithelial damage healed within 1 d, independent of treatment *(29)*.

For those with ocular exposure to OC, a slit lamp examination of the anterior chamber is warranted to rule out corneal abrasion in patients who remain symptomatic for more than 30 min. If present, the abrasion should be treated appropriately with topical local anesthetics, topical antibiotics, cycloplegics, analgesics, and follow-up care. Dermatitis associated with PS has been reported *(30,31)*. Topical corticosteroids, systemic antihistamines, and analgesics have been employed in reducing symptoms. An example of rather severe PS dermatitis and ocular swelling is shown in Fig. 2. This particular patient was sprayed during arrest by police officers and brought to an ED for evaluation. He was treated with irrigation, systemic antihistamines, and steroids, with resolution of his symptoms within 4 d.

2.2. CS Malononitrile and CN

CS, or tear gas, is used frequently by the military and law enforcement as a method of controlling both individuals and crowds. The military also uses it during exercises to train personnel in the use of protective equipment. CN, known by its common name, Mace®, is the oldest of the crowd-control agents. CS was developed in the 1950s, and it has largely replaced the use of CN.

CS and CN are both lacrimating agents. CS is usually mixed with a pyrotechnic compound for dispersal in grenades or canisters as a fine particulate, which forms the characteristic smoke. CN is usually prepared for aerosol dispersal by individual canisters. Both agents are available in individual containers or large bombs, or they can be dispersed through a hand-held aerosolizer. They are formulated with several solvents, such as alcohol, ether, carbon sulfide, and methylchloroform (32), or can be dispersed as solid particles. In the United States, a combination of CS (10%) and PS (10%) is used by some law enforcement for chemical restraint.

CS and CN are highly soluble in numerous agents. When contact with mucous membranes is made, the symptoms described in Table 2 occur. Even though there is the perception of shortness of breath, pulmonary function tests performed shortly after exposure to either agent have shown minimal alterations (33). Its mechanism of irritation is not fully understood. The effects of CS are believed to be related to the formation of highly irritating chlorine atoms and hydrochloric acid when it comes in contact with water in mucous membranes (1,34). CS and CN have also been described as alkylating agents that target sulfhydryl groups (33). In addition, there is some controversy surrounding the production of cyanide molecules at the tissue level with exposure to high CS concentrations (35,36). Regardless, the effects of CS and CN are usually manifested without permanent tissue injury. Exposure is most often limited because exposed individuals will voluntarily flee the scene to avoid further exposure. Exposure can be significant if the affected person is forced into a confined space for extended periods of time.

A cluster of adverse events associated with CS exposure during a training exercise in the US Marines has been reported. Nine Marines were exposed to CS without the benefit of personal protective equipment. All participated in rigorous physical exercise within 3–4 d after exposure to CS and were subsequently hospitalized with various pulmonary symptoms, including cough, shortness of breath, hemoptysis ($n = 5$) and hypoxia ($n = 4$). Four required hospitalization in an intensive care setting, five in a non-monitored setting. All symptoms of respiratory distress abated within 72 hours of onset, and all nine Marines had normal lung function 1 week after CS exposure (37).

Most of the dispersal methods for CS and CN achieve concentrations far below what is considered to be lethal (38). However, there is some question regarding concentrations achieved near grenades or other delivery devices or for those who cannot or will not leave the exposure area (6,38). Based on animal studies, it is generally believed that a concentration of 25,000–150,000 mg/m^3/min or 200 mg/kg body mass represents the LD50 for CS. A grenade can generate a concentration of 2000–5000 mg/m^3 at the center, with concentrations becoming significantly less within a few yards from the center of the explosion *(38)*. Regardless of the amount of exposure, all exposures that occur without the use of personal protective equipment where respiratory symptoms do not improve should be evaluated.

Treatment of CS exposure is based largely on the severity of clinical findings. The majority of patients will fully recover within minutes of removal from the agent and will not require medical attention *(39)*. The most common lasting complaints are facial and ocular irritation. In contrast to other forms of chemical exposure, irrigating the affected area will only intensify and prolong the effects of CS gas or particles. For patients who require medical evaluation, the first order of treatment should always be removal of contaminated clothing with special attention to eliminating secondary exposure by using protective equipment and not placing a contaminated patient in a confined space. Clothing should be removed outside and placed inside a plastic bag, then bagged again. Blowing dry air directly onto the eye assists in vaporizing the dissolved CS gas *(40)*. Some clinicians have recommended copious ocular irrigation with sterile saline, although this has been believed to cause an initial acute increase in ocular irritation *(40,41)* in some cases. A careful slit lamp examination of the anterior segment of the eye, including under the lids, should be done for persistent ocular irritation. If particles have become imbedded in the cornea or under the lids, they should be removed. If corneal abrasions are present, a few days of topical broad-spectrum antibiotics, cycloplegics, and appropriate analgesics in addition to close follow-up should be prescribed.

Dermal irritation in the form of burning and blistering can be treated with irrigation, preferably with an alkaline solution other than sodium hypochlorite *(30)*. Erythema can be common in skin that has been freshly abraded but resolves 45–60 minutes after exposure. Contact dermatitis can be effectively treated with topical corticosteroids and/or antihistamines, such as diphenhydramine. Typically, dermatitis associated with CS exposure resolves within a few days *(30)*.

Home remedies, such as application of cooking oils, are contraindicated and pose an increase risk for irritation and infection *(41)*. Sodium hypochlorite solutions will exacerbate any dermal irritation and should not be used. Plain soap and water is effective, but in most cases, removal of clothing in a well-ventilated area is all that is needed.

There are conflicting reports about the long-term effects of CS exposure. With an exposure to high concentrations, usually for prolonged periods in a

Table 3
Options for Treatment for Exposure to Chemical Crowd-Control Agents

Treatment	PS	CS	CN
Removal of contaminated clothing	✓	✓	✓
Ocular irrigation	✓		✓
Dermal irrigation	✓	✓	✓
Alkaline solution irrigation of skin		✓	✓
Soap and water decontamination	✓	✓	✓
Topical steroids for dermatitis	✓	✓	✓
Systemic antihistamines for dermatitis	✓	✓	✓
Systemic steroids for dermatitis	✓	✓	✓
Topical antibiotics for corneal abrasion	✓	✓	✓
Cycloplegics	✓	✓	✓
Analgesics for pain	✓	✓	✓

PS, pepper spray; CS, chlorobenzylidene; CN, chloracetothenon.

confined space, pulmonary edema, pneumonitis, heart failure, hepatocellular damage, and death have been reported *(12,42)*. There are no data to support any claims of teratogenicity, or toxicity to the pregnant woman *(12,43)*. These agents do not exacerbate chronic diseases, such as seizure disorders, respiratory disease, or psychiatric illnesses. Contact allergies in those previously exposed have also been reported *(44–46)*.

The possibility of secondary exposure to health care and law enforcement providers exists with the use of chemical crowd-control agents. Although published reports are few, effects can be minimized with common sense practices, such as decontamination before the patient is placed in a confined area (e.g., police car, ambulance, or a confined room in the emergency department). The use of protective personal equipment, such as gloves and careful washing of exposed areas, avoids cross-contamination.

3. CONCLUSIONS

The most important considerations in using chemical crowd-control agents is that they be used judiciously, correctly, and in place of more forceful means of controlling violent or potentially violent prisoners or crowds. Law enforcement officers should be educated on the common clinical effects and the appropriateness of seeking medical care. Medical care should never be withheld from those who request it or in those prisoners who have lingering effects. Treatment of exposure is summarized in Table 3. To limit injury or potential liability, many police forces regulate the use of chemical crowd-control agents by establishing policies to guide their use. One example is the "ladder of force" employed by some police departments. Words are used first, followed by more defensive actions (such as chemical agents), then batons, and finally firearms. Use of these agents is monitored, and formal reports are filed when they are used. These agents afford control of violent offenders with much less risk to life and limb than do firearms, explosives, and battering.

REFERENCES

1. Bhattacharya, S. T., Hayward, A. W. CS gas-implications for the anesthetist. Anaesthesia. 48:896–897, 1993.
2. "Safety" of chemical batons [editorial]. Lancet. 352:159, 1998.
3. Stark, M. M., Knight, M. "Safety" of chemical batons. Lancet. 352:1633, 1998.
4. Blaho, K., Winbery, S. "Safety" of chemical batons. Lancet. 352:1633, 1998.
5. Gray, P. J. CS gas is not a chemical means of restraining a person. Br. Med. J. 314:1353, 1997.
6. Hu, H., Fine, J., Epstein, P., Kelsey, K., Reynolds, P., Walker, B. Tear gas—harassing agent or toxic chemical weapon. JAMA. 262:660–663, 1989.
7. Van Derbeken, J. Pepper spray in the eyes—protesters sue police. San Francisco Chronicle 1A, 1997.
8. Spencer, P. S., Schaumburg, H. H., Raleigh, R. L., Terhaar, C. J. Nervous system degeneration produced by the industrial solvent methyl n-butyl ketone. Arch. Neurol. 32:219–222, 1975.
9. Iregren, A., Tesarz, M., Wigaeus-Hjelm, E. Human experimental MIBK exposure: effects on heart rate, performance, and symptoms. Environ. Res. 63:101–108, 1993.
10. Dick, R. B., Krieg, E. F., Setzer, J., Taylor, B. Neurobehavioral effects from acute exposures to methyl isobutyl ketone and methyl ethyl ketone. Fund. Appl. Toxicol. 19:453–473, 1992.
11. Watson, W. A., Stremel, K. R., Westdorp, E. J. Oleoresin capsicum (Cap-Stun) toxicity from aerosol exposure. Ann. Pharmacother. 30:733–735, 1996.
12. Tominack, R. L., Spyker, D. A. Capsicum and capsaicin—a review: case report of the use of hot peppers in child abuse. Clin. Toxicol. 25:591–601, 1987.
13. Weaver, W., Jett, M. B. Oleoresin Capsicum Training and Use. FBI Academy Firearms Training Unit, Quantico, VA, 1987.
14. Lee, R. J., Yolton, R. L., Yolton, D. P., Schnider, C., Janin, M. L. Personal defense sprays: effects and management of exposure. J. Am. Optomol. Assoc. 67:548–560, 1996.
15. Himsworth, H. Report of the inquiry into the medical and toxicological aspects of CS (Ortho-Chlorobenzylidene Malonitrile), II: inquiry into toxicological aspects of CS and its use for civil purposes. Her Majesty's Stationery Office, London, UK, 1971.
16. Cordell, G. A., Araujo, O. E. Capsaicin: identification, nomenclature, and pharmacotherapy. Ann. Pharmacother. 27:330–336, 1993.
17. Haas, J. S., Whipple, R. E., Grant, P. M., Andresen, B. D., Volpe, A. M., Pelkey, G. E. Chemical and elemental comparison of two formulations of oleoresin capsicum. Sci. Justice. 37:15–24, 1997.

18. Reilly, C. A., Crouch, D. J., Yost, G. S. Quantitative analysis of capsaicinoids in fresh peppers, oleoresin capsicum and pepper spray products. J. Forensic Sci. 46: 502–509, 2001.

19. Fuller, R. W. Pharmacology of inhaled capsaicin in human. Respir. Med. 85:31–34, 1991.

20. Maxwell, D. L., Fuller, R. W., Dixon, C. M. S. Ventilatory effects of inhaled capsaicin in man. Eur. J. Clin. Pharmacol. 31:715–717, 1987.

21. Collier, J. G., Fuller, R. W. Capsicum inhalation in man and the effects of sodium cromoglycolate. Br. J. Pharmacol. 81:113–117, 1984.

22. Billmire, D. F., Vinocur, C., Ginda, M., et al. Pepper-spray induced respiratory failure treated with extracorporeal membrane oxygenation. Pediatrics. 98:961–963, 1996.

23. Winograd, H. L. Acute croup in an older child: an unusual toxin orgin. Clin. Pediatr. 16:884–887, 1977.

24. Karch, S. B., Stephens, B. G. Drug abusers who die in custody. J. Royal Soc. Med. 92:110–113, 1999.

25. Chan, T. C., Vilke, G. M., Clausen, J., et al. The effect of oleoresin capsicum "pepper" spray inhalation on respiratory function. J. Forensic Sci. 47:299–304, 2002.

26. Burnet, J. Capsicum pepper dermatitis. Cutis. 43:534, 1989.

27. Jones, L. A., Tandberg, D., Troutman, W. G. Household treatment of chili burns of the hands. Clin. Toxicol. 25:483–491, 1987.

28. Zollman, T. M., Bragg, R. M., Harrison, D. A. Clinical effects of oleoresin capsicum (pepper spray) on the human cornea and conjunctiva. Ophthalmology. 107:2186–2189, 2000.

29. Vesaluoma, M., Muller, L., Gallar, J., et al. Effects of oleoresin capsicum pepper spray on human corneal morphology and sensitivity. Invest Ophthalmol. Vis. Sci. 41:2183–2147, 2000.

30. Holland, P., White, R. G. The cutaneous reactions produced by CS and CN when applied directly to the skin of human subjects. Br. J. Dermatol. 86:150–155, 1972.

31. Penneys, N. S., Israel, R. M., Indgin, S. M. Contact dermatitis due to 1-chloroacetophenone and chemical mace. N. Engl. J. Med. 281:413–415, 1969.

32. Schmutz, J. L., Rigon, J. L., Mougeolle, J. M., Weber, M., Beurey, J. Cutaneous accidents caused by self-defense sprays. Ann. Dermatol. Venerol. 114:1211–1216, 1987.

33. Chemical Casualty Care Office. Medical Management of Chemical Casualties Handbook, 2nd Ed., US Army Medical Research Institute of Chemical Defense, Aberdeen Proving Ground, MD, 1995.

34. Ballantyne, B. Riot control agents: biomedical and health aspects of the use of chemicals in civilian disturbances. Med. Annu. 7–14, 1977.

35. Jones, G. R. N. Verdict on CS. Br. Med. J. 170, 1971.

36. Jones, G. R. N., Israel, M. S. Mechanism of toxicity of injected CS gas. Nature. 228: 1315–1316, 1979.

37. Thomas, R. J., Smith, P. A., Rascona, D. A., Louthan, J. D., Gumpert, B. Acute pulmonary effects from O-chlorobenzylidemalonitrile "tear gas": a unique exposure outcome unmasked by strenuous exercise after a military training event. Mil. Med. 167:136–139, 2002.

38. Weigand, D. A. Cutaneous reactions to the riot control agent CS. Mil. Med. 134:437–440, 1969.
39. Punte, C. L., Owens, E., Gutentag, P. J. Exposures to ortho-chlorobenzylidene malonitrile. Arch. Environ. Health. 67:366–374, 1963.
40. Yih, J. P. CS gas injury to the eye. Br. Med. J. 311:276, 1995.
41. Folb, P. I., Talmud, J. Tear gas—its toxicology and suggestions for management of its acute effects in man. S. Afr. Med. J. 76:295, 1989.
42. Krapf, R., Thalmann, H. Akute Exposition durch CS-Rauchgas und linische Beobachtungen. Schweiz Med Wockenachr. 11:2056–2060, 1981.
43. Upshall, D. G. Effects of o-chlorobenzylidene malononitrile (CS) and the stress of aerosol inhalation upon rat and rabbit embryonic development. Toxicol. Appl. Pharmacol. 24:45–59, 1973.
44. Maucher, O. M., Stengel, R., Schopf, E. Chloroacetophenone allergy. Hautarzt. 37:397–401, 1986.
45. Fuchs, T., Ippen, H. Contact allergy to CN and CS tear gas. Derm Beruf umwelt. 34:12–14, 1986.
46. Fuchs, T., in der Wiesche, M. Contact allergies to CN and CS (tear gas) in participants in demonstrations. Z Hautkr. 65:288–292, 1990.

Chapter 7

Medical Issues Relevant to Restraint

Nicholas Page

1. INTRODUCTION

In 2000–2001, there were 1.25 million people arrested for notifiable offenses in the United Kingdom by 130,000 officers, with each detention involving the potential for several restraint techniques, so it is inevitable that forensic physicians will have involvement with restraint issues *(1)*. Although this topic is common, doctors ignore it at their potential peril. Forensic physicians' involvement with these issues involves many of the core attributes needed in the practice of high-quality forensic medicine, including the need for good history taking from as many involved parties as is practical to clearly establish events, and a precise examination recorded clearly and contemporaneously. Objectivity must be maintained in the light of differing histories, and there is a need to keep abreast of developing restraint techniques that may bring new clinical problems. However, regardless of how careful police officers may be, there is the potential for serious injury requiring further medical intervention, and the real possibility of being a witness in a legal process, such as police disciplinary procedures.

During restraint, any force used must be proportionate to the threat faced, lawful, and necessary. The restraint process is particularly challenging where the potential detainee has a mental health problem or is intoxicated. In addition, the officer, in retrospect and under close scrutiny, must be able to demonstrate that his or her actions were entirely appropriate. It must be recognized

From: *Clinical Forensic Medicine: A Physician's Guide, 2nd Edition*
Edited by: M. M. Stark © Humana Press Inc., Totowa, NJ

that at the time of restraint, officers may not have the luxury of time for a full analysis using prior information or the knowledge that experience, combined with extensive training and retraining, brings. As an independent doctor, excellent clinical management by the forensic physician throughout the case enables the doctor to act as a high-quality witness if needed. The doctor also has a duty to report any instance where excessive restraint appears to have been used, and such concerns should be communicated to the senior police officer on duty immediately. The forensic physician needs to be aware that equipment may be misused; for example, a long-barreled metal torch could be used as a striking weapon in some circumstances, and, indeed such lights were withdrawn in the United States to prevent this from happening.

Although the basic principles of restraint are similar throughout the world, there are many variations both throughout countries and within individual states where there are no national police forces. It is also an evolving subject involving research by organizations, such as the Police Scientific Development Branch in the United Kingdom, as well as the practical outcome of restraint techniques when used by officers.

2. RIGID HANDCUFFS

Until the early 1990s, handcuffs linked both wrists by a short metal chain, but apart from restricting arm movements, they offered little else in terms of restraint, and if only one wrist were attached to them, the handcuffs could quickly become a flail-like weapon. Rigid handcuffs, such as Kwik Cuffs, were first trialed in 1993 and have since become standard issue in the United Kingdom and the United States. In Australia, there is a mixed use of chain-link and fixed-link handcuffs.

Although the ratchet mechanism is the same as with the older cuffs, the fixed joint between the cuffs gives several distinct advantages. Holding the fixed joint allows easy application because simple pressure against the wrist enables the single bar to release over the wrist and engage the ratchet. The ratchet can be locked to prevent further tightening but can also only be released with the key, which requires the detainee to cooperate by keeping still. If the cuffs are not locked, then progressive tightening can occur. Correctly tightened cuffs should just have enough space for an additional finger between the applied cuff and wrist. The hands are usually cuffed behind the back one above the other, because handcuffing to the front may provide opportunities to resist detention.

Even with only one wrist in the cuffs, control by the officer can be gained by essentially using the free cuff and rigid link as a lever to apply local painful pressure to the restrained wrist. Techniques allow a detainee to be brought to the ground in a controlled manner or the other wrist to be put within the cuffs.

A gentle application, such as may be experienced by the forensic physician in a personal trial, will demonstrate that it is clearly an effective way of gaining control of most individuals. This may not be the case in those who are intoxicated, have mental health issues, or are violent. Cuffs should fit firmly but not tightly at the narrowest part of the wrist just distal to the radial and ulna styloid processes.

2.1. Injuries From Handcuffs

Injuries from handcuffs either reflect relative movement between the cuff and wrist or are the result of direct pressure from the cuff to the tissues of the wrist. It is important to remember that injuries may be unilateral, especially where there has been resistance to their application.

The most common injuries found are erythema, abrasions, and bruising, particularly to the radial and ulna borders of the wrist *(2)*. The erythema is often linear and orientated circumferentially around the wrist following the line of the handcuffs, reflecting direct pressure from the edge of the cuffs. Bruising is commonly seen on the radial and ulna borders, with tender swelling often associated with abrasions or superficial linear lacerations from the edge of the cuff. Abrasions reflect relative movement between the cuff and skin surface. However, it is not possible to determine whether this movement is from the cuff moving over the wrist or the wrist moving within the cuff, because either can produce the same skin abrasions. All of these soft tissue injuries will resolve uneventfully during the course of several days, and only symptomatic treatment with simple analgesia and possibly a cold compress is required. Although rare, it is possible to have wrist fractures from restraint using handcuffs. The styloid processes are the most vulnerable, but scaphoid fractures have been reported *(3)*. Tenderness beyond that expected for minor injuries and especially tenderness in the anatomical snuffbox will need an X-ray assessment as soon as possible.

The earliest reports of sensory damage to the nerves of the wrist first appear in the 1920s, with sensory disturbance often restricted to a small patch of hyperesthesia and hyperalgesia on the extensor aspect of the hand between the thumb and index finger metacarpals *(4)*. This area reflects damage to the superficial branch of the radial nerve and subsequent studies confirm that this nerve is most commonly affected by compression between handcuffs and the dorsal radius *(5)*. However, injuries to the median and ulna nerves can also occur, and these may be isolated or in any combination. The superficial branch of the radial nerve may be spared with others being damaged *(6)*. Resultant symptoms are reported as lasting up to 3 years in one case; pain may be severe and prolonged, although the most disturbing symptom to patients is paresthesia *(5)*. Nerve conduction studies may be used to distinguish between a compressive mononeuropathy and a radiculopathy. The majority of cases with significant nerve damage either involve detainees who are intoxicated or have a clear history of excessive pressure being applied by the officers *(5)*. Intoxication may cause problems through a decreased awareness of local pain, marked uncooperativeness, or poor memory for the restraining episode when a significant struggle occurred. It is possible to have nerve damage with no skin breakage, reflecting undue pressure. Although some of the quoted studies predate the introduction of rigid handcuffs, because of the similar ratchet mechanism, direct pressure problems are still possible.

Sensory nerve damage causes loss of pain, touch, and temperature sensation over an area of skin that is smaller than the nerve's sensory supply because of the considerable overlap between the sensory territories of adjacent peripheral nerves. Lesser degrees of damage lead to tingling, pain, and numbness in the appropriate sensory distribution. In acute compression of the nerve, symptoms appear more or less abruptly, and relief of this acute compression should lead to resolution in the course of some weeks. Associated motor weakness can be demonstrated by the correct clinical test within the hand. It should be noted that compression of the radial nerve at the wrist does not result in weakness.

3. BATONS

Until the early 1990s, UK police officers were equipped with a short wooden truncheon approx 40 cm long and weighing just under 300 g. There was little formal training with these, but actual use was not that common, either because they were not terribly effective or the situations faced at that time could be dealt with differently. In 1993, trials of both side-handled and numerous straight batons were introduced, because there was a rise in the number of officers injured on duty and the adequacy of their equipment was called into question.

Within the United Kingdom, there are the following three types of batons:

1. The Monadnock PR24 side-handled baton can be either a rigid one-piece baton or extendable from a shorter form for easier transport. Weighing approx 600 g with a shaft of polycarbonate plastic or aluminium, it has a fixed grip at right angles to the shaft toward one end. It is approx 60 cm long. The addition of the handle to the shaft makes it versatile, with more than 30 blocking and striking techniques available to the officer. Correct use in stressful and challenging situations requires extensive and ongoing training. In some restraint situations, a baton strike from the PR24 type is ineffective at producing the desired effect because not enough energy can be imparted from the strike.

2. The straight friction lock baton (e.g., the Asp) weighs less at 560 g and extends from 13 to 39 cm when racked (extended) with a flick of the wrist. It is carried unobtrusively on the belt and does not impede the general movement of the officer. It is made of hollow gun metal, with a small metal knob at the far end. This gives more weight distally, but it is prone to becoming flattened and rough over time because the baton is closed by striking this end against the ground. This change in shape may increase the chance of injury in a forceful strike.

3. The acrylic patrol baton has a solid or hollow nylon shaft with a ring of rubber separating the shaft and handle. It has fixed lengths of 56, 61, and 66 cm. It is broader than the friction lock type and, therefore, less likely to cause injury because the imparted energy is spread over a larger area. This is even though its weight is slightly less at 500–580 g. The heavier weights of these types of batons are used in public order disturbances.

In the United States, a 26-in hickory (wooden) straight baton is used (similar to group 3 in the previous list). The situation throughout the Australian states is variable, with intrastate differences relating to specific police staff; for example, plain clothes staff may use an Asp-type baton, whereas uniformed officers are equipped with straight or side-handled batons.

Batons are used in offensive and defensive strikes, blocks, or jabs. Strikes are made from an officer's strong (dominant) or weak (nondominant) side, and clearly the potential for injury varies with the baton mass and velocity at impact, the target area, and to how much of the surface area the force is applied. Although no body area is absolutely forbidden to strike, an officer must use a proportionate response to the situation he or she faces knowing the potential to injure. Although target areas are divided into low-, medium-, and high-risk areas, maintaining a distinction between them can be difficult because strikes are made in dynamic situations where an initial target area may change as the potential detainee moves.

Target areas with a low injury potential are the areas of the common peroneal, femoral, and tibial nerves on the legs and those of the radial and median nerves on the arms. There is a low probability of permanent injury, with the main effects being seen as short-lived motor nerve dysfunction, as in a "dead leg" and bruising. The medium injury potential areas involve bones and joints, including the knees and ankles, wrist, elbow, hands, upper arms, and clavicle. In these cases fractures, dislocations, and more extensive soft tissue injuries would be expected. Finally, those areas with the highest risk of injury include the head, neck and throat, spine, kidneys, and solar plexus.

The most common injury is bruising, and this is often in the pattern of so-called "tramline bruising," where two parallel lines of bruising are separated by a paler area. This is not unique to a baton injury but reflects an injury caused by any cylindrical hard object. The absence of bruising or other findings does not mean that a baton was not used because, for example, a degree of cushioning can occur from clothing. If the baton end is used to jab, then circular bruises may be seen. It is possible for a detainee to have signs but minimal symptoms or even be unaware of being struck. However, a move toward the friction lock batons makes this less likely.

An impact over a bony surface may produce a laceration. Abrasions are possible from the surface of a damaged baton. Fractures need to be considered where there are the traditional clinical signs of local pain, swelling, and loss of function. X-ray confirmation is needed as soon as possible.

Considering the forces that can be applied when necessary, there is the potential for significant injury with bruising and rupture of internal organs, including the heart, liver, spleen, or kidneys or a head injury. The forensic physician should refer suspected cases for hospital review without delay, especially if a confirmatory history for events is unavailable. Particular care is needed in those who are intoxicated because they are difficult to assess.

4. PLASTIC WRIST CONSTRAINTS

These are thin plastic ties that self-lock when the end is threaded through the catch at the other end of the strap. Because they cannot be released themselves, snips to cut them are always available at the same time. Although quick and easy to apply, they have no way of being locked in position, so they can tighten in an uncontrolled manner, resulting in direct compression injuries. At least two ties are used on each detainee; one is placed on each wrist and then interlocked with the other. These plastic constraints are used in preplanned operations, where numerous arrests are expected or in specialized operations.

5. UNARMED COMBAT

Numerous arm locks and holds, pressure-point control, and knee and elbow strikes may be used. Excessive force, either directly applied by the officer or from a detainee continuing to move, can result in strains to joints, such as the wrist, elbow, and shoulder. Other soft-tissue injuries may occur. Officers in the United Kingdom are not trained in any neck holds because of the high risk of serious injury or death as a result of large blood vessel or airway compression. Fatalities can occur quickly, and if a detainee complains of such holds being used, the neck should be examined carefully. Petechial bruising should be looked for in the face, particularly in and around the eyes, on the cheeks, and behind the ears. It is common for clothing to be held in a struggle to restrain, which may tighten it around the neck. Linear bruising may be seen at the site of tightening, as well as petechial bruising on the neck and above on the face.

6. RESTRAINT AT A DISTANCE

One of the major problems facing police officers is how to restrain a violent or potentially violent individual, who may be carrying an offensive weapon, using the minimum appropriate force. Clearly, the tactical firearms units are often required in these situations, but there is an increasing trend to look for other "nonlethal" options, which will incapacitate with a lower risk of serious injury. In the United Kingdom, the investigation of firearm incidents under the auspices of the Police Complaints Authority with its attendant recommendations is a major influence when looking at developments in this area *(7)*. Different countries use different restraint equipment, such as water cannon or the firing of different projectiles (e.g., bean bags), and these are subject to consideration for police use at certain times. In 2003, trails of the use of the Taser were commenced in the United Kingdom.

6.1. Baton Rounds

In the United Kingdom, baton rounds, previously known as plastic bullets, are solid PVC cylinders measuring 10×3.7 cm fired from a shoulder held gun-like device (Cooper G, personal communication, 2003). They were first introduced in Northern Ireland in 1970; 125,000 rounds have been fired, and 17 fatalities have resulted, the last one occurring in 1989. Deaths have usually been associated with direct hits to the head. With time, the delivery systems have improved, and this is reflected in the mortality figures. In June 2001, the L21A1 baton round was introduced to replace the "plastic bullet" in combination with a new baton gun and optical sight (L104 baton gun). This gives much better accuracy, both decreasing the chances of dangerous inaccurate direct impacts and avoiding hitting unintended persons.

When used in situations of public order, they are fired at ranges between 20 and 40 m, with the target being the belt buckle area. The aim is to hit the individual directly and not bounce the baton around before this, because this will both cause the projectile to tumble around its axes, making injury more likely, and decrease the accuracy of the shot. Injuries are mainly bruises and abrasions, with fewer lacerations, depending on how and where the body is hit. More serious injuries are possible, with occasional fractures and contusions to internal organs. Although intra-abdominal injury is unusual, impacts to the chest can give rib fractures and pulmonary contusions. As an alternative to using armed response against those who may use firearms or where there is major risk to life, the baton round can be used within a 1-m range.

A similar system is used in the United States and is based on the Anti-Riot Weapon Enfield system, the Sage SL-6, and this is the preferred less lethal option of restraint. This system has a projectile with a tail and is smaller and faster than the baton round. The injury pattern will be similar, but if the projectile becomes unstable in flight so that the surface area striking the target is smaller (because of altered orientation), then the potential for injury is increased.

6.2. Taser

First developed in 1970 by John Cover, the "Thomas A. Swift's Electrical Rifle," or Taser (8–10), is a small hand-held, battery-powered device allowing the transmission of pulsed high-voltage shocks to a person along fine wires fired from the front of the unit. This shock incapacitates the victim, allowing further restraint. Onset is almost instant, providing the circuit is completed from Taser to target with an accurate weapon discharge. Either compressed nitrogen or a rifle primer acts as a propellant to fire two barbs from the front of the unit to the skin or clothing of the individual requiring restraint. The barbs remain attached to the unit by lengths of wire to a maximum range in some units of 6.4 m. As the range increases, so does the separation between the barbs at impact. This increased separation gives more effect from the 50,000-V shocks as more muscle groups are affected. The barbs are not barbed like a fish hook but only have small projections on them.

The generalized involuntary muscular contractions produced by the Taser result in victims falling in a semicontrolled fashion. There is a potential for injuries depending on the exact nature of the fall, but normally, recovery is prompt and uneventful. The barbs penetrate bare skin to a depth of just more than 0.5 cm, giving some punctate wounds and surrounding erythema after electrical discharge. In the target areas of the torso and legs, there are few complications, but a direct hit on the eye could cause a penetrating injury, requiring urgent specialist assessment, and superficial blood vessels elsewhere could be punctured. The barbs themselves are easily withdrawn from the tissues.

Taser usage has been associated with fatalities, although the exact cause is not known. Nearly all who died in one study either had taken drugs (phencyclidine, amphetamine, or cocaine), had heart disease (that may only be found postmortem) or had other contributing injuries. Death was delayed for up to 30 min after Taser use, but it should be noted that the Tasers used in this study were using lower energy levels than those in current usage.

Just as those suffering from extreme agitation need careful consideration when in custody, individuals who have been agitated or unwell at the time of

Taser use should have their acid–base balance checked. Taser use could exacerbate an already disturbed acid–base balance by increasing skeletal muscle activity and predispose to the development of ventricular arrhythmias. This would be especially true in the presence of stimulants.

Taser is being tested in a few United Kingdom police forces to be used by firearms-trained officers, and it seems likely to be issued nationally. In the United States, it has decreased in use since mace oleoresin capsicum sprays became widely issued because the latter appeared more effective. Tasers are available in parts of Australia to specialist officers and also subject to review of their effectiveness. More research on the medical effects of Taser usage will no doubt be forthcoming over time.

6.3. Bean Bag Rounds

Available widely in the United States and some Australian states but not the United Kingdom, bean bag rounds consist of rectangular, square, or circular synthetic cloth bags filled with lead pellets and fired from a shotgun. For example, the "Flexible Baton" fires a bag containing 40 g of number 9 lead shot with a projectile velocity of approx 90 m/s. At impact, projectiles are designed to have separated from the shotgun shell and wadding, opened out to strike the target with its largest surface area before collapsing as they lose energy. The effect is to provide sufficient blunt force from an ideal range of 10–30 m to stop an adult's progress.

In one study *(11)*, the most common injuries were bruising and abrasions, followed by lacerations without having retention of the actual bean bag. However, significant other serious injuries have been documented, including closed fractures, penetrating wounds with retention of the bean bag projectile (and at times parts of the shell and/or wadding), and internal organ damage. Serious penetrating injuries involved the thorax, eye, abdomen, and limbs. Thoracic penetration resulted in one fatality from a massive hemothorax. Blunt injuries included splenic rupture, pneumothorax, compartment syndrome, testicular rupture, subcapsular liver hematoma, and cardiac contusions. It was noted that retention of the bag was not always suspected on an initial clinical examination, being detected on subsequent scans. The distance between gun and target was not formally examined in this study.

Clearly, this device has potential for significant trauma to anywhere on the body. Just as with other nonlethal alternatives for restraint, the forensic physician should always consider why such techniques needed to be deployed; use of drugs or alcohol and psychiatric illness are all common concurrent problems in these situations.

ACKNOWLEDGMENTS

The author thanks Dr. G. Cooper, Biomedical Sciences, Defence Science and Technology Laboratory, Porton, England, for information regarding baton rounds, and Sgt. Ross Proctor of the Memphis Police Department and Dr. John Gall and colleagues from Australia for providing information relevant to their jurisdiction.

REFERENCES

1. Conference of the Police Complaints Authority at the Synod. Police Complaints Authority, London, UK, 2002.
2. Rogers, D. J., Stark, M.M., Davie, M. Medical complications associated with the use of rigid handcuffs: a pilot study. J. Clin. Forensic Med. 5:34–37, 1998.
3. Haddad, F. S., Goddard, N.J., Kanvinde, R. N., et al. Complaints after handcuffs should not be dismissed [letter]. Br. Med. J. 318:55, 1999.
4. Stopford, J. S. B. Neuritis produced by a wristlet watch. Lancet. 1:993, 1922.
5. Stone, D.A., Lauren, O. R. Handcuff neuropathies. Neurology. 41:145–147, 1991.
6. Richmond, P., Fligelstone, L., Lewis, E. Injuries cause by handcuffs. Br. Med. J. 297:111–112, 1988.
7. Police Complaints Authority. Review of shootings by police in England and Wales from 1998 to 2001. PCA. The Stationery Office, London, UK, 2003.
8. Kornblum, R. N., Reddy, S. K. Effects of the Taser in fatalities involving police confrontation. J. Forensic Sci. 36: 434–448, 1991.
9. Allen, T. B. Discussion of "Effects of the Taser in fatalities involving police confrontation." J. Forensic Sci. 37:956–958, 1992.
10. Fish, R. M., Geddes, L. A. Effects of stun guns and tasers. Lancet. 358:687–688, 2001.
11. de Brito, D., Challoner, K.R., Sehgal, A., Mallon, W. The injury pattern of a new law enforcement weapon: the police bean bag. Ann. Emerg. Med. 38: 383–390, 2001.

Chapter 8

Care of Detainees

Guy Norfolk and Margaret M. Stark

1. INTRODUCTION

Doctors may be asked by the police to assess the fitness of adults and juveniles who are arrested in connection with an offense, are detained by immigration, require a place of safety (children and the mentally ill), or are remanded or sentenced (convicted) prisoners. A person in police custody is referred to as a detainee in this chapter. Detainees may have to be interviewed regarding their involvement in an offense and possibly further detained overnight for court; guidance may therefore have to be given to the custodians regarding their care.

Although various laws govern the powers of the police in different jurisdictions *(1)*, the basic principles remain the same *(2,3)*. If an individual who is detained in police custody appears to be suffering from a mental or physical illness and needs medical attention or has sustained any injuries whether at arrest or before arrest, such attention should be sought as soon as possible. Increasingly, the police have to deal with individuals who misuse alcohol and drugs or are mentally disordered; if the detainee's behavior raises concern, medical advice should be sought.

Custody staff should also seek medical advice if an individual requests a doctor or requires medication or if the custody staff members suspect that the detainee is suffering from an infectious disease and need advice. In some areas, when a person under arrest is discharged from the hospital and taken to a police station, a doctor is called to review the detainee and assess whether he or she is fit to be detained and fit for interview *(4)*.

From: *Clinical Forensic Medicine: A Physician's Guide, 2nd Edition*
Edited by: M. M. Stark © Humana Press Inc., Totowa, NJ

Table 1
Briefing on Arrival

- Discuss reason called (physical or mental illness/medication/injuries).
- Obtain details from the custody record and any risk assessment performed by police personnel or other health care professional, including reason for arrest (may be related to drugs).
- Ask the arresting officer for information regarding the circumstances of arrest (concerns regarding behavior/use of force).
- Other information may be obtained from relatives/friends/family doctor/hospital/ police computer.
- Is request to assess fitness for detention only?
- The anticipated length of detention, if known.
- Is the detainee to be interviewed?
- Are any samples required?
- Whether the detainee will be in custody overnight.

Medical assessments of detainees may be performed by either a doctor or a nurse retained to attend the police station *(5,6)* or by staff in the local hospital accident and emergency department *(7)*. The basic principles on which doctors should base their conduct have already been outlined in Chapter 2. The health and welfare of detainees should be paramount, with any forensic considerations of secondary importance. The role of any physician in this field should be independent, professional, courteous, and nonjudgmental.

If the police bring a detainee to the accident and emergency department or if the health professional is contacted by the police to attend the police station, it is important to find out why a medical assessment is required. It is essential that the doctor or nurse be properly briefed by the custody staff or investigating officer (Table 1).

Fully informed consent from the detainee should be obtained after explaining the reason for the examination. Detainees should understand that they are under no obligation to give consent and that there is no right to absolute confidentiality. Notwithstanding the latter, custody staff should be given only that information necessary for them to care for detainees while they are in police detention. Such information will include details of any medical concerns, required observations, medication, and dietary requirements.

Although those detained in police custody are usually young, there remains the potential for considerable morbidity and mortality among this group. Therefore, it is essential that a full medical assessment be performed and detailed contemporaneous notes made. Obtaining an accurate account of a detainee's drug

Table 2
The DRUGS Mnemonic

D octor	Any medication prescribed by a registered medical or dental practitioner
R ecreational	Tobacco, alcohol, illicit drugs, anabolic steroids, etc
U ser	Over-the-counter purchases/alternative medicine/homeopathy
G ynecological	Contraceptive or hormone replacement treatment
S ensitivities	Including the exact nature of the response

From: ref. *8.*

history, including prescribed and illicit drugs, can be difficult. A useful aid to obtaining a better drug history has been described (Table 2) *(8)*.

2. MEDICATION ADMINISTRATION

The doctor should ensure that clear and detailed instructions regarding any medication to be administered while the detainee is in police custody (including the dose, times of administration, and special instructions) are given to custodians, with confirmation that these instructions are understood *(9)*. A sufficient quantity of medication should be prescribed to cover the time in detention. The medication should be given to the police in appropriately labeled individual containers or sachets; alternatively, medication may be prescribed and collected from the local pharmacist.

It is most important that there is a safe regimen for medication administration to detainees. Records should be kept showing that the prescribed medication is given at the correct time and that any unused medicines are accounted for. Medication should be stored in a locked cupboard. Ideally, police personnel should ensure that when administering medication they are accompanied by another person as a witness, and the detainee should be observed taking the medication to prevent hoarding.

If detainees are arrested with medications on their persons, medical advice should be sought regarding whether they should be allowed to self-administer them. It may be prudent for a physical assessment to be performed either in the custody suite or in the local hospital before self-administration of medications.

Medication brought with the prisoner or collected from the home address should be checked to ensure that it has the correct name and dosage and that the quantity left is consistent with the date of issue. If there is doubt, police personnel should verify with the pharmacist, family doctor, or hospital. If the medicine is unlabeled, it is preferable to issue a new prescription, especially with liquid preparations, such as methadone.

Table 3
Common Medical Problems

• Epilepsy	• Asthma
• Diabetes	• Heart disease
• Sickle cell disease	• Injuries
• Infectious diseases	• Mental health
• Self-harm	• Claustrophobia
• Alcohol	• Drugs

3. Conditions of Detention

The doctor should ensure that the conditions of detention are satisfactory regarding the temperature and ventilation of the detention cells, cleanliness of the cell, bedding, personal hygiene, dietary needs, and fluids (10). The detainee should have access to food and fluids as appropriate and should also have a period of rest of 8 hours during each 24 hours.

4. Medical Problems

Several common medical problems are encountered when the doctor is assessing fitness to be detained in police custody. These are now considered in more detail (Table 3). Alcohol and drugs are fully discussed in Chapter 10.

4.1. Epilepsy

Many detainees state that they have "fits" and there is a need to differentiate, if possible, between epilepsy and seizures related to withdrawal from alcohol or benzodiazepines; it is also important to consider hypoglycemia.

The type of seizure should be ascertained, together with the frequency and date of the most recent one. Medication details should be, obtained including time of the last dose. Treatment may be given if the detainee is in possession of legitimate medication; however, if he or she is intoxicated with alcohol or other central nervous system-depressant drugs, treatment should generally be deferred until the detainee is no longer intoxicated.

The custody staff should have basic first aid skills to enable them to deal with medical emergencies, such as what to do when someone has a fit. If a detainee with known epilepsy has a seizure while in custody, a medical assessment is advisable, although there is probably no need for hospitalization. However, if a detainee with known epilepsy has more than one fit or a detainee has a "first-ever" fit while in custody, then transfer to a hospital is recommended.

Table 4
Signs of Acute Asthma

Parameter	Severe	Life-threatening
Pulse rate	>110/min	Bradycardia
Respiratory rate	>25/min	
PEFR	33–50%	<33% predicted
Blood pressure	Pulsus paradoxus	Hypotension
Speech	Inability to complete sentences	
Chest auscultation		Silent
Mental State	Agitation Restlessness	Exhaustion Confusion Coma

From ref. *12*.

Diazepam intravenously or rectally is the treatment of choice for status epilepticus *(11)*. Any detainee requiring parenteral medication to control fits should be observed for a period in the hospital.

4.2. Asthma

Asthma is a common condition; a careful history and objective recording of simple severity markers, such as pulse and respiratory rate, blood pressure, speech, chest auscultation, mental state, and peak expiratory flow rate, should identify patients who require hospitalization or urgent treatment (Table 4) *(12)*. Detainees with asthma should be allowed to retain bronchodilators for the acute relief of bronchospasm (e.g., salbutamol or the equivalent), with instructions left with the custody sergeant on other treatment if required.

4.3. Diabetes

It is often desirable to obtain a baseline blood glucose measurement when detainees with diabetes are initially assessed and for this to be repeated if necessary throughout the detention period. All doctors should have the means to test blood glucose, using either a strip for visual estimation or a quantitative meter. Several small portable meters are now available.

Oral hypoglycemics and insulin should be continued and consideration given to supervision of insulin injections. Regular meals and snacks should be provided, and all patients with diabetes should have access to rapidly absorbed, carbohydrate-rich food.

Hypoglycemia is easily treated. If the blood glucose is less than 4 mmol/L in a conscious person, oral carbohydrates should be given. In a detainee who is unconscious or restless, an intravenous bolus of 50 mL of 50% dextrose solution may be difficult to administer and may result in skin necrosis if extravasation occurs; therefore, 1 mg of glucagon can be given intramuscularly, followed by 40% glucose gel orally or applied to the inside of the mouth. Glucagon can give an initial glycemic response even in a patient with alcoholic liver disease *(13)*; however, it should be remembered that in severe alcoholics with depleted glycogen stores, the response to glucagon may be reduced or ineffective.

4.4. Heart Disease

The main problems encountered include a history of hypertension, angina, cardiac failure, and stable dysrhythmias. Basic cardiovascular assessment may be required, including examination of the pulse and blood pressure, together with auscultation of the heart and lungs for evidence of murmurs or cardiac failure.

Prescribed medication should be continued, and detainees should be allowed to keep their glyceryl trinitrate spray or tablet with them in the cell. Chest pain that does not settle with glyceryl trinitrate will obviously require further assessment in the hospital.

4.5. Sickle Cell Disease

Most detainees with sickle cell disease are aware of their illness and the symptoms to expect during an acute sickle cell crisis. Medical management in custody should not pose a problem unless there is an acute crisis, when hospital transfer may be required. Conditions of detention should be suitable, with adequate heating and access to fluids and analgesics as appropriate.

4.6. General Injuries

Detailed documentation of injuries is an important and common request. The injuries may have occurred before or during the arrest, and documentation of such injuries may form part of the investigation to refute counter allegations of assault.

A record of each injury, as outlined in Chapter 4, should be made and basic first aid provided. Certain wounds may be treated with Steri-Strips or Histoacryl glue in the police station *(14)*, although occasionally transfer to a hospital will be required for further medical assessment (e.g., suturing or X-rays).

4.7. Head Injuries

Any suspected head injury should receive a detailed assessment *(15)*. The time, place, and nature of the injury should be ascertained from the detainee or from any witnesses who were present. The duration of any loss of conscious-

Table 5
Head Injuries Indications for Hospital Assessment

A patient with a head injury should be referred to the hospital if *any* of the following are present (a head injury is defined as any trauma to the head, other than superficial injuries to the face):

- Impaired consciousness (GCS <15/15) at any time since injury
- Any focal neurological symptoms or signs (e.g., problems understanding, speaking, reading or writing; decreased sensation; loss of balance; general weakness; visual changes; abnormal reflexes; and problems walking)
- Any suspicion of a skull fracture or penetrating injury (e.g., cerebrospinal fluid leak; black eye with no associated damage around the eyes; bleeding from or new deafness in one or both ears; mastoid hematoma; signs of penetrating injury; visible trauma to the scalp or skull of concern to the FP)
- Amnesia for events before or after the injury
- Persistent headache since the injury
- Any vomiting since the injury
- Any seizures since the injury
- Medical comorbidity (e.g., previous cranial surgery; anticoagulant therapy; bleeding or clotting disorder)
- A high-energy head injury (e.g., RTA, fall from a height of >1 m or more than five stairs)
- Current drug or alcohol intoxication
- Significant extracranial injuries
- Continuing uncertainty about the diagnosis after first assessment
- Age greater than or equal to 65 yr

From ref. *19*.

ness and the behavior since the injury should be noted. Examination should include measurement of pulse and blood pressure, Glasgow Coma Scale *(16)*, and neurological assessment. The indications for hospital assessment include situations in which there are problems with the assessment of the patient or an increased risk of skull fracture or an intracranial bleed (Table 5) *(17)*.

Ingestion of alcohol or drugs and relevant past medical history should be ascertained. Although deaths in police custody are rare, head injuries accounted for 10% and substance abuse, including alcohol and drugs, accounted for 25% in a survey of such deaths between 1990 and 1997 in England and Wales *(18)*. There should be a low threshold for referral to hospitals, especially if a detainee with a head injury is also under the influence of alcohol or drugs.

If the detainee is to remain in custody, then instructions regarding the management of patients with head injuries should be left verbally and in writing with the custody staff and given to the patient on release *(19)*. Police

Table 6
Brief Mental State Examination

• Appearance	Self-care, behavior
• Speech	Rate, volume
• Thought	Association, content (delusions)
• Perception	Hallucinations, illusions
• Obsessive/compulsive	Behaviors
• Mood	Biological symptoms
	(sleep, appetite, energy, concentration, memory)
• Cognitive function	Short-term memory, concentration, long-term memory
• Risk behaviors	Self harm, harm to others

should be advised that when checking a detainee's conscious level they are required to rouse and speak with the detainee, obtaining a sensible response. Appendix 3 outlines the Glasgow Coma Scale, a head injury warning card for adults, and an observation checklist for custody staff responsible for the health care of detainees.

4.8. Infectious Diseases

The doctor may be called to advise the police regarding infectious diseases. This subject is now fully covered in Chapter 11. Because the population in police custody is at high risk for blood-borne viruses, such as hepatitis and the human immunodeficiency virus (20), all individuals should be considered a potential risk, and observation of good clinical practice relating to body fluids to avoid contamination risks is essential (21).

5. Mental Health

5.1. General Psychiatric Problems

When a psychiatric disorder is suspected, an assessment involving background information, full psychiatric history (if known), observation of the detainee, and mental state examination (Table 6) should be performed by the doctor to assess whether there is any evidence of mental illness.

The doctor should then consider whether diversion from the criminal justice system is appropriate. If the detainee has committed a minor offense and there is only evidence of minor to moderate mental illness, treatment may be arranged in the community, in outpatients, or in the day hospital. However, if the detainee has an acute major mental illness but has only committed a minor or moderate offense, then admission to the hospital for further assessment and treatment is required either informally or if necessary formally. When the offense is more serious and there is evidence of probable mental illness needing further assessment, then the detainee may need to go before the court for such an assessment to be ordered.

Chronic stable mental health problems usually pose no specific problems for police detention but may require specific safeguards when the detainee is to be interviewed by the police (*see* Subheading 9). Long-term medication should be continued.

5.2. Substance Misuse and Mental Illness

Concurrent substance misuse and mental illness —"dual diagnosis" or "comorbidity"—is an important consideration. In the Epidemiologic Catchment Area study, 29% of individuals with a lifetime history of any mental disorder (other than substance use) had a history of substance use (22% alcohol disorder and 15% a drug disorder) *(22)*.

Comorbidity can be classified on the basis of the primary diagnosis *(23,24)*. There are those with a primary diagnosis of a major mental illness who have a secondary diagnosis of substance misuse that further affects their mental health. Such individuals may use drugs to relieve the adverse symptoms of their mental illness. Conversely, substance misuse may be the primary diagnosis leading to psychiatric complications and mental illness—for example, depression with suicidal ideation may occur among substance abusers. On occasions, mental illness and substance misuse may coexist, such as when an underlying traumatic experience results in both substance misuse and posttraumatic stress disorder.

5.3. Deliberate Self-Harm

Research has shown that episodes of deliberate self-harm (DSH) typically occur soon after arrest. Particular risk factors include a history of DSH and a psychiatric history *(25,26)*. Medical assessments should be requested for those detainees who give a clear intention of DSH, with attention given to any visible evidence of previous DSH acts.

If a detainee commits a DSH act, a medical assessment should be conducted irrespective of whether there has been any physical injury, and an attempt should be made to assess the risk of suicide. When the risk is believed to be high, then referral to a hospital is required, and the detainee should be kept under constant supervision until such transfer is arranged. When the risk is deemed to be low, clear instructions must be given to the police regarding care and supervision. The police may consider removal of the detainee's clothing and personal effects to prevent self-harm. Cells should be checked with respect to their structural integrity to prevent any defects being used for DSH, and bedding should be of an appropriate standard.

Liaison between agencies is essential, and when the detainee is transferred to prison, another police station, or hospital, details regarding the DSH incident should be passed to the custody or hospital staff concerned so they can take appropriate precautions.

5.4. Claustrophobia

Claustrophobia is a common complaint, and a detailed history and examination with an emphasis on the presence or absence of anxiety when faced with the problem in everyday life should be sought. Inquiry regarding behavior at home, such as leaving doors and windows open, avoidance of elevators and underground trains, and a history of the original precipitant for such behavior, should be noted.

Often, reassurance is enough, and it is rarely necessary to give any medication. The custody staff should be advised if genuine claustrophobia is suspected as this may affect the detainee's fitness to be interviewed.

6. Personal Safety Issues

Certain health care groups are at increased risk of violence in the workplace, for example, those working in the custodial environment *(27)* or accident and emergency services *(28)*.

There are numerous strategies for interviewing a difficult patient *(29)*, which include being fully aware of the person's history (be prepared) and considering how the person sees you (as uninterested or hostile), being polite and respectful, avoiding confrontation, using appropriate eye contact, keeping calm, and showing interest. Look for signs of tension and find out why tension may be increasing. Finally, be ready to leave if necessary and consider the need to have a chaperone (appropriately trained in restraint techniques) of the same sex as the patient.

Accurate assessment regarding the possibility of violence will reduce the danger, but it should never be assumed that there is no risk, and every clinical situation should be categorized as high risk owing to an obvious risk or unknown risk resulting from undiscovered factors *(30)*.

7. Drug Searches

Persons unlawfully in possession of illicit drugs for personal use or involved in drug supply or trafficking may ingest drugs or pack them into certain body cavities ("body packers" or "mules"). Third parties may be employed to act as mules, and a case of body packing using children, two boys aged 6 and 12 years, who had concealed heroin has been reported *(31)*. A person who is about to be arrested by the police may swallow drugs ("body swallower" or "stuffer").

Doctors may then be called by the police to conduct intimate searches of those arrested *(see* Chapter 2) *(32)*. Any health care professional who agrees to perform an intimate search should have the required skills and a comprehensive understanding of the risks involved and their management. The doctor should discuss the possible implications of the ingestion of certain drugs and obtain fully informed consent from the detainee before conducting any search that may involve examination of the mouth, nostrils, ears, umbilicus, foreskin, rectum, or vagina.

Variable quantities of drugs, such as heroin, cocaine, cannabis, and amphetamine, may be packaged in layers of cellophane or in condoms. All searches for such drugs should be carried out in premises where there are full facilities for resuscitation *(32a)* in case significant quantities of the drugs leak into the bloodstream, resulting in acute intoxication and death from overdose *(33)*. Other medical problems such as bowel obstruction may also occur.

The aim of medical management is to prevent these complications, but for ethical reasons, the retrieval of packages for legal purposes alone is no indication for intervention without the patient's permission. Therefore, without such permission, the doctor can do nothing except advise the police authorities that the detainee should be observed. In most patients who are asymptomatic, a trial of conservative treatment, provided bowel obstruction or package perforation is not suspected, will result in the uncomplicated elimination of all ingested packages *(34,35)*.

In a genuine emergency when there is no possibility of obtaining consent, the doctor has a duty to perform treatment to safeguard the life and health of a patient in accordance with what would be accepted as appropriate treatment in the patient's best interests *(36)*.

8. FORENSIC SAMPLES

Samples from a detainee, such as dental impressions, blood, saliva, urine, hair, fingernail scrapings and cuttings, and swabs (e.g., mouth or penile), may be requested by police authorities in connection with the investigation of an offense. These samples should only be taken by a doctor or nurse for evidential purposes with the detainee's fully informed consent and should be packaged in accordance with local procedures to ensure the chain of evidence. For further details regarding samples, *see* Chapter 3.

9. FITNESS TO BE INTERVIEWED
9.1. Introduction

The custodial interrogation of suspects is an essential component of all criminal investigation systems. The confessions and other incriminating statements that are obtained during these interrogations have always played an important role in prosecutions and continue to be relied on as evidence of guilt in a substantial number of trials. For example, in England and Wales, confessions provide the single most important piece of evidence against defendants in the Crown Court, being crucial in approx 30% of cases *(37)*. Similarly, an influential American observational study found that interrogation was necessary for solving the crime in approx 17% of cases *(38)*. The quest to obtain confessions from suspects' mouths has seen a slow and uneven move away from the inquisitions aided by torture and oppression of the Middle Ages toward the doctrine that:

> *A free and voluntary confession is deserving of the highest credit, because it is presumed to flow from the strongest sense of guilt and therefore it is admitted as proof of the crime to which it refers; but a confession forced from the mind by the flattery of hope or by the torture of fear comes in so questionable a shape when it is to be considered as the evidence of guilt, that no credit ought to be given to it; and therefore it is rejected (39).*

In the years since this judgment, considerable effort has been expended attempting to regulate the custodial interview to minimize the risk of false confessions while preserving the value of interrogation as a means of solving crime. In this section, the important psychological aspects of interrogation and confession are considered and the role the forensic physician can play in ensuring that suspects are fit to be interviewed is discussed.

9.2. Police Interview Techniques

Numerous American manuals detail the way in which coercive and manipulative interrogation techniques can be employed by police officers to obtain a confession *(40,41)*, with similar techniques being advocated by Walkley *(42)* in the first such manual written for British officers. The authors of these manuals propound various highly effective methods for breaking down a suspect's resistance while justifying a certain amount of pressure, deception, persuasion, and manipulation as necessary for the "truth" to be revealed. Walkley acknowledges that "if an interviewer wrongly assesses the truth-teller as a lie-teller he may subject that suspect to questioning of a type which induces a false confession." Generally, however, the manuals pay scant attention to certain circumstances in which the techniques they recommend may make a suspect confess to a crime he or she did not commit. Although studies in the United Kingdom have suggested that coercive interview techniques are employed less frequently than in the past, manipulative and persuasive tactics continue to be used, particularly in relation to more serious crimes *(43,44)*.

Interrogators are encouraged to look for nonverbal signs of anxiety, which are often assumed to indicate deception. However, the innocent, as well as the guilty, may exhibit signs of nervousness. Innocent suspects may be anxious because they are erroneously being accused of being guilty, because of worries about what is going to happen to them while in custody, and possibly because of concerns that the police may discover some previous transgression. Furthermore, there are three aspects of a police interview that are likely to be as stressful to the innocent as to the guilty: the stress caused by the physical environment in the police station, the stress of being isolated from family and friends, and the stress caused by the suspect's submission to authority. All these factors can markedly impair the performance of a suspect during an interview. Indeed, American research has suggested that for most suspects, interrogations are likely to be so stressful that they may impair their judgment on such crucial matters as the exercise of legal rights *(45)*.

Given the interview techniques employed by the police and the stresses interrogation places on the accused, there is little wonder that false confessions are occasionally made to the police.

9.3. False Confessions

During the last two decades, the United Kingdom has witnessed several well-publicized miscarriages of justice in which the convictions depended heavily on admissions and confessions made to the police that were subsequently shown to be untrue *(46–48)*. In reviewing 70 wrongful imprisonments that occurred between 1950 and 1970, Brandon and Davies *(49)* found that false confessions were second only to incorrect identification evidence as the most common cause of wrongful conviction. More recently, in 1994, Justice *(50)* identified 89 cases in which an alleged miscarriage of justice rested on a disputed confession. Thus, it is clear that people can and do make false and misleading admissions against their own interest. We must turn to modern psychology to obtain insights into why this may happen.

9.3.1. Why Make a False Confession?

There is no single reason why people falsely confess to crimes they have not committed. Indeed, such confessions usually result from a combination of factors unique to the individual case. Nonetheless Kassin and Wrightsman et al. *(51)* identified three distinct types of false confession, which have been developed by Gudjonsson *(52)* and expanded in two respects by Shepherd *(53)*. These categories are voluntary, accommodating-compliant, coerced-compliant, and coerced-internalized.

9.3.2. Voluntary False Confessions

Voluntary false confessions are offered by individuals without any external pressure from the police. Commonly, the individuals go voluntarily to the police to confess to a crime they may have read about in the press or seen reported on television. Often, they do so out of a morbid desire for notoriety because the individual seemingly has a pathological desire to become infamous, even at the risk of facing possible imprisonment.

Alternatively, a voluntary false confession may result from the individual's unconscious need to expiate guilty feelings through receiving punishment. The guilt may concern real or imagined past transgressions or, occasionally, may be part of the constant feeling of guilt felt by some individuals with a poor self-image and high levels of trait anxiety.

By contrast, some people making this type of confession do so because they are unable to distinguish between fact and fantasy. Such individuals are unable to differentiate between real events and events that originate in their thinking, imagination, or planning. Such a breakdown in reality monitoring is normally associated with major psychiatric illness, such as schizophrenia.

Occasionally, people may volunteer a false confession to assist or protect the real culprit. Gudjonsson (52) highlights some evidence that confessing to crimes to protect others may be particularly common in juvenile delinquents.

Finally, Shepherd (53) identifies a subset of individuals who falsely confess to crimes to preempt further investigation of a more serious crime.

9.3.3. Accommodating-Compliant False Confessions

Expanding on the original three distinct categories of false confession, Shepherd recognizes a group of people for whom acquiescing with the police is more important than contradicting police assertions about what happened. In such circumstances, a false confession arises from a strong need for approval and to be liked. Police conduct is noncoercive, although it does involve the use of leading questions sufficiently obvious to suggest to the suspect what answers the police want to hear. People at all intellectual levels are at risk of behaving in this manner, with those who are excessively compliant being at greatest risk.

9.3.4. Coerced-Compliant False Confessions

Coerced-compliant false confessions are typically elicited during persuasive interrogation: the person perceives that there is some immediate instrumental gain from confessing. The suspect does not confess voluntarily but comes to give into the demands and pressures of the interrogators. He or she is fully aware of not having committed the crime of which he or she is accused, and the confession is usually retracted once the immediate threat is gone.

Gudjonsson *(52)* suggests that the four main types of perceived immediate gain are: being allowed home after confessing, bringing the interview to an end, a means of coping with the demand characteristics (including the perceived pressure) of the situation, and avoidance of being detained in police custody.

In these circumstances, the suspect may be vaguely or fully aware of the consequences of making a false self-incriminating statement, but the perceived immediate gain outweighs, in his or her mind, the potential long-term consequences. These suspects may naïvely believe that the truth will come out later in court, perpetuating the belief shared by many police officers and legal advisers that what happens in the police station is not really that important.

9.3.5. Coerced-Internalized False Confessions

Coerced-internalized false confessions occur when suspects are gradually persuaded that they have committed a crime of which they have no recollection or when they have become so confused that they begin to mistrust their own memory and accept a false scenario suggested by the police. This type of confession can happen under the following two distinct conditions:

1. The suspects have no memory of the alleged offense, even whether or not they committed it. This can be a result of amnesia or alcohol-induced memory loss. In essence, the suspects have no clear recollection of what they were doing at the time the offense was committed and believe they must have committed the crime.
2. At the outset of the interview, the suspects have a clear recollection that they were not involved in the alleged offense. However, as a result of subtle manipulative techniques employed by the interrogator, they begin to distrust their own memory and beliefs. Interrogators attempt to undermine the suspects' confidence in their own recollection of events, which would create sufficient self-doubt and confusion to cause them to adjust their perceptions of reality.

In contrast to the makers of coerced-compliant false confessions, those who make coerced-internalized false confessions only retract their confessions when they realize, or suspect, that they are in fact innocent. These retractions can take considerable time and, occasionally, may never occur if the original memory of events becomes permanently distorted.

9.4. Suggestibility and Compliance

Vitally important to an understanding of why false confessions can often prove so incriminating is an awareness of the theory of interrogative suggestibility *(54,55)*. At the heart of the theory is the way leading questions can produce distorted responses from suspects because they are phrased to suggest the expected response. Through this process people can come to accept a piece of postevent information and incorporate it into their memory, thus appearing to have "special knowledge" about the alleged offense. This special knowledge may seriously mislead the police and the courts to assume the suspect's guilt erroneously. Suggestibility correlates with anxiety, lack of assertiveness, poor self-esteem, and low intelligence *(56)*.

Compliance refers to the tendency of people to obey the instructions of others when they don't really want to, because they are either overeager to please or simply unable to resist the pressure *(57)*. The traits of both suggestibility and compliance are relevant to the issue of false confessions *(58)*.

9.5. Preventing False Confessions

It is a fundamental tenet of both American and English law that reliance should only be placed on confession evidence that is given freely and voluntarily. In considering the voluntary nature of a confession, several factors need to be considered. These include the vulnerability of the accused (through factors such as age, mental illness and handicap, physical illness or injury, and intoxication), the conditions of detention (lack of access to legal advice, failure to be given legal rights, and adequate rest periods during detention), and the characteristics of the interrogation (threats, physical abuse, and inducements).

In America, the most important legal development designed to protect the rights of suspects and deter police misconduct relates to the case of *Miranda v. Arizona*, which was decided in 1966 *(59)*. The effect of this judgment was to ensure that all criminal suspects in police custody must be warned against self-incrimination and made aware of their right to remain silent and to receive legal advice. These rights have to be actively waived by the accused before interrogation can commence, and any violations of the requirements render any subsequent confession inadmissible.

In the United Kingdom, statutory safeguards are provided by the Police and Criminal Evidence Act 1984 and the Codes of Practice set up under section 66 of this Act *(1)*, which regulate practice in respect to several matters, including the detention, treatment, and questioning of persons by police officers. Confessions will generally be inadmissible if the provisions of the Codes of Practice are breached by the police *(60,61)*.

The role of the forensic physician when assessing a suspect's fitness for interview is seen as fitting into this overall legal framework, the doctor's primary concern being to recognize any characteristics that might render the individual vulnerable to providing a false confession so that adequate safeguards can be put in place.

10. A Definition of "Fit for Interview"

Until recently, there has been no clear definition of what precisely is meant by the term *fit to be interviewed,* and this has led to confusion among those doctors called on to perform these assessments *(62).* To address this deficiency, Norfolk *(63)* proposed a definition that was used as the starting point for discussion by a subgroup set up by the Home Office Working Party on Police Surgeons in the United Kingdom. That working party made an interim recommendation *(64)* that has now been modified and included in the 2003 revision of the Police and Criminal Evidence Act Codes of Practice *(1),* thus providing the first Parliamentary approved definition of the term fitness for interview. The Codes of Practice state that:

A detainee may be at risk in an interview if it is considered that:

(a)   Conducting the interview could significantly harm the detainee's physical or mental state

(b)   Anything the detainee says in the interview about their involvement or suspected involvement in the offense about which they are being interviewed might be considered unreliable in subsequent court proceedings because of their physical or mental state.

Thus, a suspect with known ischemic heart disease who is experiencing chest pain satisfies the criteria of (a) above and clearly needs assessment and appropriate treatment before it is safe to conduct an interrogation.

The concept of unreliability may be harder to evaluate and will require consideration of the various vulnerability factors associated with false confessions. In making an assessment, the Codes of Practice require the doctor to consider the following:

1. How the detainee's physical or mental state might affect their ability to understand the nature and purpose of the interview, to comprehend what is being asked, and to appreciate the significance of any answers given and make rational decisions about whether they want to say anything.
2. The extent to which the detainee's replies may be affected by their physical or mental condition rather than representing a rational and accurate explanation of their involvement in the offense.
3. How the nature of the interview, which could include particularly probing questions, might affect the detainee.

10.1. Scheme of Examination

When assessing a detainee's fitness for interview, the traditional medical model of taking a history and then conducting an examination should be employed. As always, informed consent should be obtained and detailed and contemporaneous notes should be taken.

10.1.1. The History

As much background information as is practicable should be obtained and, when possible, an indication of how long any interview is likely to take. The demand characteristics of a long interview about a suspected murder will be much greater than a short interview about a shoplifting offense.

A general medical history should be taken, with inquiry made about significant illness and any prescribed medication. The detainee should be asked whether he or she has suffered from psychiatric illness, past or present, and specific inquiry should be made about alcohol and drug misuse. There should be questions about the person's educational background, because individuals with learning difficulties can be tough to recognize and inquiring about schooling may aid identification.

Ensure that the detainee has not been deprived of food or sleep, and inquire about significant social distractions (e.g., a single parent may make a false confession to obtain early release from custody and a speedy reunion with his or her child). Detainees should be asked whether they have been detained before and, if so, whether they have had unpleasant experiences while in custody in the past.

10.1.2. The Examination

The examination should include observations on the general appearance, physical examination as appropriate, and mental state examination. A functional assessment should be performed regarding whether the detainee is aware of the reason for arrest, his or her legal rights, and is capable of making a rational decision (able to choose between relevant courses of action) and of carrying out the chosen course of action.

Each examination needs to be tailored to the individual, but doctors should be able to assess the vulnerabilities of the detainees they have been asked to examine and thus ensure that any necessary safeguards are established before interrogation begins.

10.2. Alcohol and Fitness for Interview

It is generally accepted that severe alcohol intoxication renders a suspect unfit to be interviewed. However, there is much less agreement when it comes to deciding when somebody with mild or moderate intoxication should be considered fit to interview *(62,65)*. The customary view that intellectual processes are impaired at lower blood alcohol levels than sensory or motor processes has been challenged. Indeed, the opposite has been shown, with intellectual processes being more resistant to alcohol than sensory and motor skills *(66)*. Nonetheless, the effect alcohol can have on short-term memory should be remembered when advising the police on fitness. Research suggests that moderate quantities of alcohol impair the process of forming new memories *(67)*. Deterioration in performance of a task assessing short-term memory occurred at blood alcohol levels of 70 mg/100 mL in one study *(68)*, and a significant impairment of eyewitness memory has been demonstrated at average blood alcohol levels of 100 mg/100 mL *(69)*. When suspects mistrust their own memory of events, they are at increased risk of providing coerced–internalized false confessions *(52)*.

The ultimate decision regarding whether a suspect who has been drinking is fit for interview is best decided on the medical and functional assessment performed by the doctor rather than on arbitrarily defined "safe" blood alcohol levels *(70)*.

Alcohol withdrawal states and the complications of alcohol withdrawal can impair cognitive functioning and affect a suspect's ability to both cope with interrogative pressure and provide reliable testimony. Even the after effects of alcohol, or "hangover," impair critical task performance, such as aircraft operation, and can impair judgment *(71)*. Research evidence has also suggested that alcohol withdrawal can increase a suspect's suggestibility, although it is not totally clear whether this is a direct result of the alcohol withdrawal or is secondary effect of its treatment *(72)*.

10.3. Substance Misuse and Fitness for Interview

A substance misuser may be rendered unfit for interview by virtue of either intoxication or withdrawal. Generally speaking, intoxication is easy to recognize, and the police will usually wait until the intoxication has cleared before starting their questioning. However, problems may be encountered with hallucinogenic substances. For example, the mental state may fluctuate in the recovery stages of an LSD experience, which may not be immediately obvious to the interrogator *(73)*.

Withdrawal states can pose a bigger problem for the doctor assessing fitness for interview. Although most confessions made in these circumstances are reliable *(74)*, it should be recognized that the person suffering from drug withdrawal may be particularly vulnerable to providing a false confession. Such persons may believe that compliance will result in early release and that the risks entailed in providing a false confession may seem worthwhile in the presence of an overwhelming desire to re-establish access to their supply of drugs *(75)*.

Although symptoms of mild withdrawal from opiates, for example, is considered unlikely to be a barrier to interview *(62,73)*, the physical and mental distress occasioned by established withdrawal may seriously impair a suspect's fitness to undergo the somewhat threatening and difficult experience of police interrogation.

When faced with a suspect suffering from severe withdrawal, the doctor should consider advising that the interview be deferred until such time as the withdrawal has subsided or been adequately treated. If the doctor decides to treat the withdrawal state, consideration should be given to the risk that the therapeutic intervention, which may in itself have a bearing on fitness to interview. Arranging for therapy that the suspect has been receiving in the community to be continued in police custody is unlikely to influence fitness for interview *(76,77)*. However, when substitution therapy is initiated in custody or when symptomatic treatment alone is provided, the doctor may well need to assess the effect of the treatment before an interview occurs.

10.4. The Impact of Psychiatric Illnesses

There has been a considerable amount of research on the manner in which certain functional psychiatric illnesses can affect the reliability of testimony *(78,79)*. Thus, anxiety increases a suspect's suggestibility and depression can lead to feelings of guilt and poor self-esteem that render a suspect vulnerable to providing a false confession *(52)*. Psychiatric illness may also render a person unfit for interview by virtue of its effect on cognitive processes or because of associated thought disorder *(80,81)*. However, careful questioning that avoids the use of leading questions and coercive pressures can often elicit reliable testimony. That a suspect suffers from an illness, such as schizophrenia, does not necessarily mean that he or she is unfit for interview *(82)*; such an opinion would depend on the likely demand characteristics of the interview and the functional assessment by the doctor.

10.5. Learning Difficulties

The police rarely have difficulty recognizing moderate or severe learning difficulties, but borderline or low-to-normal intelligence may not be obvious even to trained observers *(83–85)*. It is important to identify people with learning difficulties—questions regarding reading and writing ability and the need for special help with education can be useful—because they will be particularly vulnerable in police custody. Such individuals may have difficulties in understanding their legal rights and in communicating with police officers. They are also more likely to be impressionable and acquiescent *(86)*.

10.6. The Effect of Physical Illnesses on Fitness for Interview

The presence of any physical illness renders an individual more vulnerable when faced with a stressful situation, such as a custodial interrogation. Features, such as anxiety or depression, affect a person's ability to function during the police interview, and physical illness—especially if severe—is as likely to cause anxiety and depression as any other form of stress *(87)*. The severity of the emotional response will depend on the nature of the illness itself, the personality of the individual, and social circumstances. Suspects who are already coping with physical illness are more likely to focus on the short-term consequences of their behavior than the long-term outcomes, thus increasing the risk that they might provide a false confession *(52)*.

Because the effect of physical illness on a person's coping strategy is not disease-specific, depending more on the actual or perceived severity of the illness rather than the nature of the illness itself, the actual diagnosis is unimportant. By contrast, there are many physical illnesses in which characteristic disturbances in cognitive functioning have been recognized *(88)*. With these illnesses, the nature and degree of the mental disturbance produced depends entirely on the diagnosis of the underlying condition. The more common of the conditions encountered in custody are discussed in the following subheadings.

10.6.1. Epilepsy

It is now clear, after long historical dispute, that a predisposition to epileptic fits does not mean *per se* that there will be associated intellectual impairment, personality disorder, or mental illness. Most patients with epilepsy remain mentally normal, although this does depend on the presence, site, and extent of any brain damage underlying the epilepsy *(89)*.

However, those patients with epilepsy without significant brain damage do, nonetheless, remain prone to cognitive impairment, particularly memory impairment, as a result of their epilepsy and its treatment. The potential impact of this cognitive impairment must be considered when assessing a patient with epilepsy's fitness for interview.

For example, problems with concentration, memory, and intellectual functioning can be seen when anticonvulsant drugs are administered in toxic doses or unsuitable combinations *(90)*. Suspicion should be raised when a suspect complains of mental lethargy or appears to be performing below expected levels, symptoms particularly associated with toxicity.

Further problems with the reliability of testimony from epileptics may be related to their personality. Patients with epilepsy are often overprotected in childhood by concerned parents and, later in life, can be exposed to profound social and occupational discrimination *(91)*. All these factors can lead to personality problems, which include feelings of insecurity, low self-esteem, and dependency. Individuals with these personality traits are likely to be highly suggestible and may strive to please interviewing officers by giving answers that seem plausible and consistent with the external cues provided, even though the responses are known to be untrue.

The neurophysiological consequences of an epileptic seizure can seriously distort an individual's perception of events occurring around the time of the seizure, thus rendering any subsequent account of that event potentially unreliable. Complex disturbances of thinking, memory, or awareness may feature as part of an aura preceding the actual seizure. These may include distortion sense of time, mental confusion, or feelings of depersonalization or déjà vu. The seizure may also be ushered in by distorted perceptions or actual hallucinations of sight, hearing, taste, or smell. When the ensuing fit is mild or abortive, the connection between these reported experiences and their epileptic causation may be missed *(91)*.

Typical absences, or petit mal epilepsy, is a disorder that usually starts in childhood, but the attacks can continue into adult life. Absence attacks are brief, with an abrupt onset and termination; several such absences may occur in quick succession, producing significant gaps in memory.

Further cognitive disturbances can follow in the wake of seizures, with clouding of consciousness and disorientation lasting for a few minutes or up to an hour or more, so that recollection for events occurring during the postictal period may also be unreliable *(89)*.

10.6.2. Head Injury

Head injuries may occur in several circumstances involving possible criminal offenses, such as road traffic accidents and assaults; therefore, it is not uncommon to encounter detainees with head injuries in police custody. The potential for the head injury to affect the person's ability to recall the details of the accident or assault can assume considerable importance.

Memory loss for events occurring around the time of the injury is likely to occur whenever there has been diffuse brain damage of a degree sufficient to cause concussion. In most cases, loss of consciousness will accompany the head injury, but this is not invariable, and it is possible for patients to display both retrograde and posttraumatic amnesia without losing consciousness *(88)*.

Retrograde amnesia refers to the loss of memory for events that immediately precede the head injury. Individuals can often indicate with fair precision the last event that they can clearly recollect. In road traffic accidents, the journey may be recalled up to a specific point, which allows an estimate of the extent of the pretraumatic gap to be made. Such amnesia is usually short in duration and can usually be counted in minutes or hours rather than days or weeks. Indeed, when the retrograde amnesia lasts for a long time the explanation often results from hysteria.

Retrograde amnesia may render a suspect unfit for interview immediately after the head injury, but the doctor should be aware that the extent of the amnesia can change with time. At first, it may be long, but it can then shrink over the next days and weeks, eventually ending up as a matter of minutes only. Recovery from retrograde amnesia tends to occur in chronological order, with items in the distant past recovering first.

By contrast, posttraumatic amnesia refers to the period from the moment of the injury until normal continuous memory returns, the length of the amnesia providing a good index, albeit in retrospect, of the severity of the brain damage *(92)*. It should be emphasized that the amnesia only ends when the person becomes able to give a clear and consecutive account of what is happening around him or her. Sometimes "islands of memory" will be exhibited, but these should not be taken as indicating the end of the amnesia. There is a similar danger in underestimating the duration of posttraumatic amnesia in those suspects who, although aware of things going on around them, are unable to recall these events at a later date *(88)*.

Several behaviors may be exhibited during the period of posttraumatic amnesia, ranging from apparent normality to obvious confusion. However, in general, behavior is unremarkable, and the doctor may be easily misled into believing that there is nothing amiss. The individuals themselves are usually unaware of the abnormal memory at the time and can give superficial or made-up explanations for any defects that are discovered. Occasionally, these false memories can appear most convincing *(93)*.

10.6.3. Migraine

Migraine is a common and sometimes incapacitating disorder, affecting approx 20% of women and 15% of men at some time in their lives *(94)*. Some degree of mental change is almost universal during attacks. Anxiety and irritability are common early in the attack and are often followed by drowsiness and lethargy. Cognitive impairment may occur. Cerebration is often slowed with poor concentration, and there may be marked impairment of memory *(88)*.

Detainees who claim that they suffered a migraine attack at or around the time of the alleged offense should be questioned closely about any cognitive impairment during previous attacks. However, it should be recognized that the pattern of any such impairment can change from attack to attack in the same person.

10.6.4. Hypothyroidism

A detainee who is being adequately treated for myxedema poses no particular problem for the physician assessing fitness for interview. However, an individual with undiagnosed or undertreated hypothyroidism may exhibit mental manifestations that are as important as the physical. The typical picture is of mental lethargy, general dulling of the personality, and slowing of all cognitive functions. In particular, the patient with hypothyroidism shows deficits in memory, abstraction, conceptual organization, and mathematical ability *(95)*.

10.6.5. Diabetes Mellitus

Although confusion is a prominent feature in patients who are slipping into hyperglycemic coma, this condition is rarely seen in police custody. Questions relating to fitness for interview and the potential reliability of a detainee's confession are more likely to involve those with hypoglycemia.

Episodes of hypoglycemia are associated with irritability, anxiety, and panic in the early stages. As the episode develops, the individual becomes disinhibited and may exhibit childish or aggressive behavior that often mimics drunkenness. Disorientation and mental confusion are common and, in severe cases, the person may pass into a coma. Anybody suffering from hypoglycemia will prove to be a poor witness to events that occur during the episode. Most will have complete amnesia for the content of the attack and occasionally for an additional period before the attack occurred when their behavior will have appeared to be normal *(96)*. The doctor should take a clear history of any hypoglycemic episodes that may have occurred before arrest and should consider checking the blood sugar of any diabetic about to be interviewed by the police. The manifestations of hypoglycemia with subsequent impaired intellectual function are extremely variable, and it has been recommended that the blood sugar should be kept at 6 mmol/L or more if a person with diabetes person is to give a statement or be interviewed *(97)*.

10.6.6. Dementia

Dementia is a large-scale problem in the elderly. It has been estimated that 5–8% of patients aged 65 yr and older suffer from dementia to an appreciable degree, with the proportion probably exceeding 20% in 80-yr-olds *(98)*. However, in many of these patients, dementia is not recognized until there is some form of crisis in their lives. Such a crisis may be precipitated by sudden illness, bereavement, or police arrest. Individuals seem able to develop strategies to cope with their daily tasks and thus appear to function normally until the crisis disrupts the status quo and exposes the degree of their dementia *(99)*.

Although there are many different causes of dementia, the clinical picture remains broadly similar, with any variation depending mainly on the age of onset of the illness, premorbid personality, and intelligence. In the custodial situation, the doctor is likely to encounter only those at an early stage of the disease. This is characterized by impaired memory, loss of the sense of time, and spatial disorientation, all of which can distort a suspect's recollection of events. This distortion may be compounded by the lack of judgment that is frequently displayed by those with dementia and that can cause the suspect to misjudge the importance of providing reliable testimony *(88)*. Therefore, it is important that the doctor be aware of the possibility that an elderly suspect may be suffering from dementia, even when there are reports of apparently normal social functioning before arrest. In such circumstances, recognition of the dementia can be facilitated by using a standard test of cognitive function, such as the Mini-Mental State Examination Score (*see* Appendix 4).

This test of cognitive function has been thoroughly validated *(100)*. It is called "mini" because it concentrates only on the cognitive aspects of mental functioning and excludes questions concerning mood, abnormal mental experiences, and the form of thinking. A score of 24 out of 30 was originally suggested as the lower limit of normal, but it has been repeatedly shown that performance on even this simple test is influenced considerably by age and by educational attainment. Hence, a well-educated young adult should perform flawlessly, whereas a normal elderly subject who left school at age 14 may score as low as 22 or 23. Given this proviso, the Mini-Mental State Examination is useful in quantifying cognitive impairment and is particularly useful for grading and monitoring the severity of dementia.

REFERENCES

1. Police and Criminal Evidence Act 1984 (s.60 (1)(a) and s.66) Codes of Practice A-F for England and Wales. Her Majesty's Stationery Office, Norwich, London, 2004.
2. British Medical Association's Medical Ethics Committee and Association of Forensic Physicians. Health Care of Detainees in Police Stations. British Medical Association, London, 2004.
3. Stark, M. M., Rogers, D. J., Norfolk, G. A. Good Practice Guidelines for Forensic Medical Examiners. Metropolitan Police. GPG Editors, Oxford, 2004.
4. Metropolitan Police, Medical Care of Prisoners-Person Ill or Injured. Special Notice 37/97. Metropolitan Police, London, 1997.
5. Payne-James, J. J. Work patterns of a forensic medical examiner for the Metropolitan Police. Police Surg. 42:21–24, 1992.
6. Young, S., Wells, D., Jackson, G. A tiered health care system for persons in police custody-the use of a forensic nursing service. J. Clin. Forensic Med. 1:21–25, 1994.

7. Smock, W. S. Development of a clinical forensic medicine curriculum for emergency physicians in the USA. J. Clin. Forensic Med. 1:27–30, 1994.

8. Hocking, G., Kalyanaraman, R., deMello, W. F. Better drug history taking: an assessment of the DRUGS mnemonic. J. R. Soc. Med. 91:305–306, 1998.

9. Howitt, J., Evans, V. The Safety and Security of the Administration of Medication in Police Custody. East Kilbride, Education and Research Committee of the Association of Forensic Physicians, 2004.

10. Howitt, J. Poor conditions of detention compromise ethical standards. J. R. Soc. Med. 88:40P–41P, 1995.

11. Brodie, M. J. Status epilepticus in adults. Lancet. 336:551–552, 1990.

12. Mathur, R., Bell, D. Asthma management in police study. J. Clin. Forensic Med. 3:133–140, 1996.

13. Heller, M. B., Vukmir, R. B. Glucagon for metabolic/endocrinologic emergencies: hypoglycaemia. In Picazo, J., ed., Glucagon in Acute Medicine. Pharmacological, Clinical and Therapeutic Implications. Kluwer Academic Publishers, London, 1992.

14. Payne-James, J. J. The role of cyanoacrylate tissue adhesive (Histoacryl blue) in forensic medical practice. Police Surg. 43:30-31, 1993.

15. Marks, P. V. Acute head injury: assessment and practical management. J. Clin. Forensic Med. 1:43–46, 1994.

16. Jennett, B., Teasdale, G. Aspects of coma after severe head injury. Lancet. 1:878–881, 1977.

17. National Institute for Clinical Excellence. Head injury. Triage, assessment, investigation and early management of head injury in infants, children and adults. Clinical Guideline 4. NICE, London, 2003.

18. Leigh, A., Johnson, G., Ingram, A. Deaths in Police Custody: Learning the Lessons. Police Research Series Paper 26. Police Research Group Publications, Home Office, London, 1998.

19. Norfolk, G. A., Rogers, D. J. Head Injury Warning. Education and Research Committee of the Association of Forensic Physicians, East Kilbride, 2004.

20. Payne-James, J. J., Keys, D. W., Wall, I., Dean, P. J. Prevalence of HIV factors for individuals examined in clinical forensic medicine. J. Clin. Forensic Med. 1:93–96, 1994.

21. UK Health Departments. Guidance for Clinical Health Care Workers: Protection Against Infection with Blood-borne Viruses. Department of Health, London, 1998.

22. Regier, D. A., Farmer, M. E., Rae, D. S., Comorbidity of mental disorders with alcohol and other drug abuse: results from the Epidemiologic Catchment Area (ECA) Study. JAMA. 264:2511–2518, 1990.

23. Krausz, M. Old problems-new perspectives. Eur. Addic. Res. 2:1–2, 1996.

24. Lehmann, A. F., Meyers, C. P., Corty, E. Classification of patients with psychiatric and substance abuse syndromes. Hosp. Commun. Psychiatry. 40:1019–1025, 1989.

25. Ingram, A., Johnson, G., Heyes, I. Self Harm and Suicide by Detained Persons: A Study. Police Research Group Publications, Home Office, London, 1997.

26. Norfolk, G. A. Deaths in police custody during 1994: a retrospective analysis. J. Clin. Forensic Med. 5:49–54, 1998.

27. Schnieden, V., Stark, M. M., Payne-James, J. J. Violence in clinical forensic medicine. Med. Sci. Law. 35:333–335, 1995.
28. Schnieden, V., Maguire, J. A Report on Violence at Work and its Impact on the Medical Profession within Hospitals and the Community. British Medical Association, London, 1993.
29. Royal College of Psychiatrists. Using the Mental Health Act-A Training Resource for Doctors. Gaskell, Royal College of Psychiatrists, p. 72, 1997.
30. Johns, A., Clarke, S., Stark, M. M. Management of potentially violent detainees. J. Clin. Forensic Med. 1:139–144, 1997.
31. Traub, S. J., Kohn, G. L., Hoffman, R. S., Nelson, L. S. Pediatric 'body packing'. Achives of Pediatric & Adolescent Medicine.157:1:174–177, 2003.
32. Association of Forensic Physicians and British Medical Association. Guidelines for Doctors Asked to Perform Intimate Body Searches. British Medical Association, London, 2004.
32a. Stark, M. M. Guidelines for Police Surgeons Asked to Perform Intimate Searches for Drugs. Education and Research Sub-Committee of the Association of Police Surgeons, Harrogate, North Yorkshire, 1997.
33. Heinemann, A., Miyaishi, S., Iwersen, S., Schmoldt, A., Puschel, K. Body-packing as cause of unexpected sudden death. Forensic Sci. Int. 92:1–10, 1998.
34. Glass, J. M., Scott, H. J. "Surgical mules": the smuggling of drugs in the gastrointestinal tract. J. R. Soc. Med. 88:450–453, 1995.
35. Das, D., Ali. B. Conservative management of asymptomatic cocaine body packers. Emer. Med. J. 20:172–174, 2003.
36. *F. v West Berkshire Health Authority.* 2 All ER 545, 1989.
37. Baldwin, J., McConville, M. Confessions in Crown Court Trials. Royal Commission on Criminal Procedure Research Study No. 5. Her Majesty's Stationery Office, London, 1980.
38. Wald, M., Ayres, R., Hess, D. W., Schantz, M., Whitebread, C. H. Interrogations in New Haven: the impact of Miranda. Yale Law J. 76:1519–1614, 1967.
39. *R. v Warickshall.* 1 Leach 263, 1783.
40. Inbau, F. E., Reid, J. E. Criminal Interrogations and Confessions, 2nd ed. Williams & Wilkins, Baltimore, MD, 1967.
41. Royal, R. F., Schutt, S. R. Gentle Art of Interviewing and Interrogation: A Professional Manual and Guide. Prentice Hall, Englewood Cliffs, NJ, 1976.
42. Walkley, J. Police Interrogation. A Handbook for Investigators. Police Review Publication, London, 1987.
43. Irving, B. Police Interrogation. A Case Study of Current Practice. Royal Commission on Criminal Procedure, Research Study No 2. Her Majesty's Stationery Office, London, 1980.
44. Irving, B. I., McKenzie, I. K. Police Interrogation: The Effects of the Police and Criminal Evidence Act. The Police Foundation, London, 1989.
45. Leiken, L. S. Police interrogation in Colorado: the implementation of Miranda. Denver Law J. 47:1–53, 1970.
46. Kennedy, L. 10 Rillington Place. Grafton, London, 1988.
47. Thomas, T. The Confait confessions. Policing. 3:214–225, 1987.

48. Kee, R. Trial and Error. The True Events Surrounding the Convictions and Trials of the Guildford Four and the Maguire Seven. Penguin, London, 1989.
49. Brandon, R., Davies, C. Wrongful Imprisonment. George Allen & Unwin,London, 1973.
50. Unreliable Evidence? Confessions and the Safety of Convictions. Justice, London, 1994.
51. Kassin, S. M., Wrightsman, L. S. The Psychology of Evidence and Trial Procedure. Sage Publications, London, 1985.
52. Gudjonsson, G. The Psychology of Interrogations, Confessions and Testimony. John Wiley & Sons, Chichester, 1992.
53. Wolchover, D., Heaton-Armstrong, A. On Confession Evidence. Sweet & Maxwell, London, p. 99, 1996.
54. Gudjonsson, G. H., Clark, N. K. Suggestibility in police interrogation: a social psychological model. Soc. Behav. 1:83–104, 1986.
55. Schooler, J. W., Loftus, E. F. Individual differences and experimentation: complementary approaches to interrogative suggestibility. Soc. Behav. 1:105–112, 1986.
56. Gudjonsson, G. Interrogative suggestibility-can it be recognised in custody? In Norfolk, G. A., ed., Fit to be Interviewed by the Police. Association of Police Surgeons, Harrogate, 1997, pp 12–14.
57. Gudjonsson, G. H. Compliance in an interrogation situation: a new scale. Pers. Ind. Diff. 10:535–540, 1989.
58. Groves, T. Explaining false confessions. Br. Med. J. 303:1087–1088, 1991.
59. Miranda v Arizona 384 US 436, 1966.
60. R v Kenny Crim. L. R. 284, 1994.
61. R v Cox Crim. L. R. 687, 1991.
62. Norfolk, G. A. Fitness to be interviewed and the appropriate adult scheme: a survey of police surgeons' attitudes. J. Clin. Forensic Med. 3:9–13, 1996.
63. Norfolk, G. A. "Fitness to be interviewed"-a proposed definition and scheme of examination. Med. Sci. Law. 37:228–234, 1997.
64. Norfolk, G. A. Fit to be interviewed-a police surgeon's perspective. In Norfolk, G.A., ed., Fit to be Interviewed by the Police, Association of Police Surgeons, Harrogate, 1997, pp 43–48.
65. Clarke, M. D. B. "Fit for Interview?" Police Surg. 40:15–18, 1991.
66. Carpenter, J. A. Effects of alcohol on some psychological processes. A critical review with special reference to automobile driving skill. Q. J. Stud. Alcohol. 23:274–314, 1980.
67. Loftus, E. F. "Did I really say that last night?" Alcohol, marijuana and memory. Psychol. Today. 92:42–56, 1980.
68. Carpenter, J. A., Ross, B. M. Effect of alcohol on short-term memory. Q. J. Stud. Alcohol. 26:561–579, 1965.
69. Yuille, J. C., Tollestrup, P. A. Some effects of alcohol on eyewitness memory. J. Appl. Psychol. 75:268–273, 1990.
70. Rogers, D. J., Stark, M. M., Howitt, J. B. The use of an alcometer in clinical forensic practice. J. Clin. Forensic Med. 2:177–183, 1995.

71. Yesavage, J. A., Leirer, V. O. Hangover effects on aircraft pilots 14 hours after alcohol ingestion: a preliminary report. Am. J. Psychiatry. 143:1546–1550, 1986.
72. Gudjonsson, G., Hannesdottir, K., Petursson, H., Bjornsson, G. The effects of alcohol withdrawal on mental state, interrogative suggestibility and compliance: an experimental study. J. Forensic Psych. 13:53–67, 2002.
73. Association of Police Surgeons and Royal College of Psychiatrists. Substance Misuse Detainees in Police Custody. Guidelines for Clinical Management (2nd ed.). Report of a Medical Working Group. Council Report CR81. Royal College of Psychiatrists, London, 2000.
74. Sigurdsson, J. F., Gudjonsson, G. H. Alcohol and drug intoxication during police interrogation and the reasons why suspects confess to the police. Addiction. 89:985–997, 1994.
75. Davison, S. E., Forshaw, D. M. Retracted confessions: through opiate withdrawal to a new conceptual framework. Med. Sci. Law. 33:285–290, 1993.
76. Stark, M. M. Management of drug misusers in police custody. J. R. Soc. Med. 87:584–587, 1994.
77. Zacny, J. P. Should people taking opioids for medical reasons be allowed to work and drive? Addiction. 91: 1581–1584, 1996.
78. Ross, D. F., Read, J. D., Toglia, M. P. (eds.) Adult Eyewitness Testimony. Cambridge University Press, Cambridge, 1994.
79. Gudjonsson, G. H. The vulnerabilities of mentally disordered witnesses. Med. Sci. Law. 35:101–106, 1995.
80. Bluglass, R., Bowden, P. Principles and Practice of Forensic Psychiatry. Churchill Livingstone, Edinburgh, 1990.
81. Rix, K. J. B. Fit to be interviewed by the police? Adv. Psychiatr Treat. 3:33–40, 1997.
82. Gudjonsson, G. "Fitness for interview" during police detention: a conceptual framework for forensic assessment. J. Forensic Psychiatry. 6:185–197, 1995.
83. Halstead, S. Forensic psychiatry for people with learning disability. Adv. Psychiatric Treat. 2:76–85, 1996.
84. Gudjonsson, G., Clare, I., Rutter, S., Pearse, J. The Royal Commission on Criminal Justice. Persons at Risk During Interviews in Police Custody: The Identification of Vulnerabilities. Research Study No. 12. Her Majesty's Stationery Office, London, 1993.
85. Lyall, I., Holland, A. J., Styles, P. Incidence of persons with a learning disability detained in police custody. A needs assessment for service development. Med. Sci. Law. 35:61–71, 1995.
86. Murphy, G., Clare, I. C. H. People with learning disabilities as offenders or alleged offenders in the UK criminal justice system. J. R. Soc. Med. 91:178–182, 1998.
87. Mayou, R. A. Emotional reactions to disorders. In Weatherall, D, J., Ledingham, J. G. G., Warrell, D. A., eds., Oxford Textbook of Medicine, 2nd ed. Oxford University Press, Oxford, 1987.
88. Lishman, W. A. Organic Psychiatry. The Psychological Consequences of Cerebral Disorder. 2nd ed. Blackwell Scientific Publications, Oxford, 1987.

89. Lishman, W. A. Specific conditions giving rise to mental disorder. In Weatherall, D. J., Ledingham, J. G. G., and Warrell, D. A., eds., Oxford Textbook of Medicine. 3rd ed. Oxford University Press, Oxford, 1996.

90. Williams, D. The psychiatry of the epileptic. Proc. R. Soc. Med. 56:707–710, 1963.

91. Laidlaw, J., Richens, A., Chadwick, D. (eds.) A Textbook of Epilepsy. 4th ed. Churchill Livingstone, Edinburgh, 1993.

92. Teasdale, G. M. Head injuries. In Weatherall, D. J., Ledingham, J. G. G., and Warrell, D. A., eds., Oxford Textbook of Medicine, 3rd ed. Oxford University Press, Oxford, 1996.

93. Whitty, C. W. M., Zangwill, O. L., eds. Amnesia. Butterworths, London, 1977.

94. Pearce, J. M. S. Headache. In Weatherall, D. J., Ledingham, J. G. G., and Warrell, D. A., eds., Oxford Textbook of Medicine. 3rd ed. Oxford University Press, Oxford, 1996.

95. Droba, M., Whybrow, P. C. Endocrine and metabolic disorders. In Kaplan, H. I., Sadock, B. J., eds., Comprehensive Textbook of Psychiatry, vol. 2, 5th ed. Williams and Wilkins, Baltimore, 1989.

96. Deary, I. J. Effects of hypoglycaemia on cognitive function. In Frier, B. M., Fisher, B. M., eds., Hypoglycaemia and Diabetes: Clinical and Physiological Aspects. Edward Arnold, London, 1993.

97. Levy, D. Management of diabetes in clinical forensic practice. J. Clin. Forensic Med. 3:31–36, 1996.

98. Hodges, J. R. Dementia, introduction. In Weatherall, D. J., Ledingham, J. G. G., Warrell, D. A., eds., Oxford Textbook of Medicine, 3rd ed. Oxford University Press, Oxford, 1996.

99. Pearce, J. Dementia. A Clinical Approach. Blackwell Scientific Publications, Oxford, 1984.

100. Folstein, M. F., Folstein, S. E., McHugh, P. R. "Mini-Mental State": a practical method for grading the cognitive state of patients for the clinician. J. Psychiatr. Res. 12:189–198, 1975

Chapter 9

Infectious Diseases

The Role of the Forensic Physician

Felicity Nicholson

1. INTRODUCTION

Infections have plagued doctors for centuries, in both the diagnosis of the specific diseases and the identification and subsequent management of the causative agents. There is a constant need for information as new organisms emerge, existing ones develop resistance to current drugs or vaccines, and changes in epidemiology and prevalence occur. In the 21st century, obtaining this information has never been more important. Population migration and the relatively low cost of flying means that unfamiliar infectious diseases may be brought into industrialized countries. An example of this was an outbreak of severe acute respiratory syndrome (SARS), which was first recognized in 2003. Despite modern technology and a huge input of money, it took months for the agent to be identified, a diagnostic test to be produced, and a strategy for disease reporting and isolation to be established. There is no doubt that other new and fascinating diseases will continue to emerge.

For the forensic physician, dealing with infections presents two main problems. The first problem is managing detainees or police personnel who have contracted a disease and may be infectious or unwell. The second problem is handling assault victims, including police officers, who have potentially been exposed to an infectious disease. The latter can be distressing for those involved, compounded, in part, from an inconsistency of management guidelines, if indeed they exist.

From: *Clinical Forensic Medicine: A Physician's Guide, 2nd Edition*
Edited by: M. M. Stark © Humana Press Inc., Totowa, NJ

With the advent of human rights legislation, increasing pressure is being placed on doctors regarding consent and confidentiality of the detainee. Therefore, it is prudent to preempt such situations before the consultation begins by obtaining either written or verbal consent from the detainee to allow certain pieces of information to be disclosed. If the detainee does not agree, then the doctor must decide whether withholding relevant details will endanger the lives or health of those working within custody or others with whom they may have had close contact (whether or not deliberate). Consent and confidentiality issues are discussed in detail in Chapter 2.

Adopting a universal approach with all detainees will decrease the risk to staff of acquiring such diseases and will help to stop unnecessary overreaction and unjustified disclosure of sensitive information. For violent or sexual assault victims, a more open-minded approach is needed (*see* also Chapter 3). If the assailant is known, then it may be possible to make an informed assessment of the risk of certain diseases by ascertaining his or her lifestyle. However, if the assailant is unknown, then it is wise to assume the worst. This chapter highlights the most common infections encountered by the forensic physician. It dispels "urban myths" and provides a sensible approach for achieving effective management.

2. UNIVERSAL PRECAUTIONS

The risk of exposure to infections, particularly blood-borne viruses (BBVs), can be minimized by adopting measures that are considered good practice in the United Kingdom, the United States, and Australia *(1–3)*.

Forensic physicians or other health care professionals should wash their hands before and after contact with each detainee or victim. Police officers should be encouraged to wash their hands after exposure to body fluids or excreta. All staff should wear gloves when exposure to body fluids, mucous membranes, or nonintact skin is likely. Gloves should also be worn when cleaning up body fluids or handling clinical waste, including contaminated laundry. Single-use gloves should only be used and must conform to the requirements of European Standard 455 or equivalent *(1–3)*. A synthetic alternative conforming to the same standards should also be available for those who are allergic to latex.

All staff should cover any fresh wounds (<24 hours old), open skin lesions, or breaks in exposed skin with a waterproof dressing. Gloves cannot prevent percutaneous injury but may reduce the chance of acquiring a blood-borne viral infection by limiting the volume of blood inoculated. Gloves should only be worn when taking blood, providing this does not reduce manual dexterity and therefore increase the risk of accidental percutaneous injury.

Ideally, a designated person should be allocated to ensure that the clinical room is kept clean and that Sharps containers and clinical waste bags are removed regularly. Clinical waste must be disposed of in hazard bags and should never be overfilled. After use, the clinical waste should be double-bagged and sealed with hazard tape. The bags should be placed in a designated waste disposal (preferably outside the building) and removed by a professional company.

When cells are contaminated with body fluids, a professional cleaning company should be called to attend as soon as possible. Until such time, the cell should be deemed "out of action."

2.1. Sharps Awareness

There is a legal requirement in the United Kingdom under the Environmental Protection Act (1990) and the Control of Substances Hazardous to Health Regulations 1994 to dispose of sharps in an approved container. In the United States, the Division of Health Care Quality Promotion on the Centers for Disease Control and Prevention (CDC) Web site provides similar guidance. In custody, where Sharps containers are transported off site, they must be of an approved type. In the United Kingdom, such a requirement is contained within the Carriage of Dangerous Goods (Classification, Packaging and Labelling) and Use of Transportable Pressure Receptacles Regulations 1996. These measures help to minimize the risk of accidental injury. Further precautions include wearing gloves when handling Sharps and never bending, breaking, or resheathing needles before disposal. Sharps bins should never be overfilled, left on the floor, or placed above the eye level of the smallest member of staff.

2.2. Contaminated Bedding

Any bedding that is visibly stained with body fluids should be handled with gloves. There are only three acceptable ways of dealing with contaminated bedding:

1. Laundering with a detergent at a minimum temperature of 71°C (160° F) or at a lower temperature (22–50°C) with water containing detergent and 50–150 ppm of chlorine bleach.
2. Dry cleaning at elevated temperatures/dry cleaning at cold temperatures followed by steam pressing.
3. Incineration.

It is not considered acceptable practice for detainees to share bedding.

2.3. Other Measures

It is not necessary for staff to wear masks or protective eyewear in the custodial setting because the risk of infection is low. However, single-use eyewash should be available in the clinical room or contained in other first aid kits located within the police station in case of accidental exposure. Contact lenses should be removed before eye washing.

3. FORMULATION OF GUIDELINES

An example of good practice is contained within the UK Health Department's 1998 document *(1)* which states: "that it is the responsibility of Health Authorities, Health Boards and NHS Trusts to create their own local guidelines to prevent the spread of BBVs in the health care setting." Such guidelines may not exist in other work places. If this is the case, then they should be formulated as soon as possible. Forensic physicians working for the Metropolitan Police in London can refer to the "Good Practice Guidelines" *(4)*. It is also prudent to prearrange a system of referral with the nearest hospital that has an accident and emergency department, a genitourinary department, and access to a specialist. The latter may be a consultant in virology, microbiology, infectious diseases, or genitourinary medicine. Similar guidance in the United States can be found in the *Guideline for Infection Control in Health Care Personnel (5).*

Most exposures to staff usually result from a failure to follow accepted practice; however, accidents can happen no matter how much care is taken. All forensic physicians and other health care professionals working in custody should understand what constitutes a risk. This involves taking a detailed history of the incident, including the type of exposure, the body fluids involved, and when the incident occurred.

This information can help to allay unnecessary anxiety from the outset and ensures that the victim is referred, if appropriate, to the designated hospital at the earliest opportunity. Knowledge of precise treatment protocols is not required, but it is helpful to be able to explain to the victim what to expect. For example, he or she will be asked to provide a voluntary baseline blood sample for storage and numerous follow-up samples for testing depending on the nature of the exposure. This is especially relevant for hepatitis B virus (HBV), hepatitis C virus (HCV), and human immunodeficiency virus (HIV). Occasionally, it may be necessary for samples to be obtained as long as 6 mo after the incident.

Sexual assault victims should ideally be referred to specialist centers, if available. A police station should be used only as a last resort because the environment is often hostile and there is no ready access to the necessary treatment and ongoing management (*see* Chapter 3).

4. ROUTES OF TRANSMISSION

Organisms may use more than one route of transmission. For ease of understanding, the infections discussed in this chapter are classified according to their primary route (i.e., transmission through blood and body fluids, through contact with lesions or organisms, through the respiratory route, or through the fecal–oral route).

5. TRANSMISSION THROUGH BLOOD AND BODY FLUIDS

The BBVs that present the most cross-infection hazard to staff or victims are those associated with persistent viral replication and viremia. These include HBV, HCV, hepatitis D virus (HDV), and HIV.

In general, risks of transmission of BBVs arise from the possible exposure to blood or other body fluids. The degree of risk varies with the virus concerned and is discussed under the relevant sections. Figure 1 illustrates the immediate management after a percutaneous injury, mucocutaneous exposure, or exposure through contamination of fresh cuts or breaks in the skin.

5.1. Hepatitis B

5.1.1. Epidemiology and Prevalence

HBV is endemic throughout the world, with populations showing a varying degree of prevalence. Approximately two thousand million people have been infected with HBV, with more than 350 million having chronic infection. Worldwide, HBV kills about 1 million people each year. With the development of a safe and effective vaccine in 1982, the World Health Organization (WHO) recommended that HBV vaccine should be incorporated into national immunization programs by 1995 in those countries with a chronic infection rate of 8% or higher, and into all countries by 1997. Although 135 countries had achieved this goal by the end of 2001, the poorest countries—often the ones with the highest prevalence—have been unable to afford it. In particular these include China, the Indian subcontinent, and Sub-Saharan Africa.

People in the early stages of infection or with chronic carrier status (defined by persistence of hepatitis B surface antigen [HBsAg] beyond 6 mo) can transmit infection. In the United Kindgom, the overall prevalence of chronic HBV is approx 0.2–0.3% *(6,7)*. A detailed breakdown is shown in Table 1.

5.1.2. Symptoms and Complications

The incubation period is approx 6 weeks to 6 months. As the name suggests, the virus primarily affects the liver. Typical symptoms include malaise, anorexia, nausea, mild fever, and abdominal discomfort and may last from 2 days to 3 weeks before the insidious onset of jaundice. Joint pain and skin rashes may also occur as a result of immune complex formation. Infections in the newborn are usually asymptomatic.

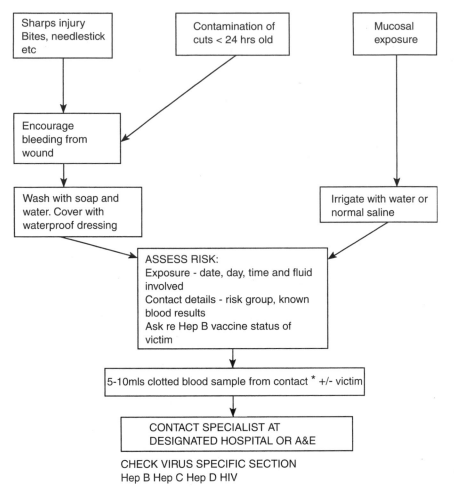

Fig. 1. Immediate management following occupational exposure to blood-borne viruses.

The majority of patients with acute HBV make a full recovery and develop immunity. After acute infection, approx 1 in 300 patients develop liver failure, which may result in death.

Chronic infection develops in approx 90% of neonates, approx 50% of children, and between 5 and 10% of adults. Neonates and children are usually

Table 1
Prevalence of Chronic Hepatitis B

• Blood-doning population	<1%
• Intravenous drug users	10–15%
• Homosexual/bisexuals	10–15%
• Institutionalized patients	no data available
• People from high-risk endemic areas (e.g., China and the Far East)	up to 30% of the population are carriers, and 75% have evidence of past infection; 5–10% are carriers (in Africa)

Table 2
Significance of Markers

Name	Infectivity	Immunity	Risk after needlestick
HBsAg	Yes	No	Only marker = 10–20%
HBeAg	Yes	No	With HBsAg = 30–40%
HBeA	Yes	Yes	With HBsAg = <10%
HBCA	No	Yes	0%
HBSA	No	Yes	0%

HBsAg, hepatitis B surface antigen; HbeAg, hepatitis B e antigen; HbeA, hepatitis B e antibody; HBCA, hepatitis B core antibody; HBSA, hepatitis B surface antibody.

asymptomatic. Adults may have only mild symptoms or may also be asymptomatic. Approximately 15–25% of chronically infected individuals (depending on age of acquisition) will develop cirrhosis over a number of years. This may also result in liver failure or other serious complications, including hepatocellular carcinoma, though the latter is rare. The overall mortality rate of HBV is estimated at less than 5%.

5.1.3. Period of Infectivity

A person is deemed infectious if HBsAg is detected in the blood. In the acute phase of the illness, this can be as long as 6 months. By definition, if HBsAg persists after this time, then the person is deemed a carrier. Carriers are usually infectious for life. The degree of infectivity depends on the stage of disease and the markers present Table 2.

5.1.4. Routes of Transmission

The major routes include parenteral (e.g., needlestick injuries, bites, unscreened blood transfusions, tattooing, acupuncture, and dental procedures where equipment is inadequately sterilized), mucous membrane exposure (including mouth, eyes, and genital mucous membranes), and contamination of broken skin (especially when <24 hours old).

5.1.5. At-Risk Groups

HBV is an occupational hazard for anyone who may come into contact with blood or bloodstained body fluids through the routes described. Saliva alone may transmit HBV. The saliva of some people infected with HBV contains HBV–DNA concentrations 1/1000–1/10,000 of that found in their serum (8). This is especially relevant for penetrating bite wounds. Infection after exposure to other body fluids (e.g., bile, urine, feces, and cerebrospinal fluid) has never been demonstrated unless the fluids are contaminated with blood.

Intravenous drug users who share needles or other equipment are also at risk. HBV can also be transmitted through unprotected sexual contact, whether homosexual or heterosexual. The risk is increased if blood is involved. Sexual assault victims should be included in this category.

Evidence has shown that the virus may also be spread among members of a family through close household contact, such as through kissing and sharing toothbrushes, razors, bath towels, etc. (9–11). This route of transmission probably applies to institutionalized patients, but there are no available data.

Studies of prisoners in western countries have shown a higher prevalence of antibodies to HBV and other BBVs than the general population (12–14); the most commonly reported risk factor is intravenous drug use. However, the real frequency of transmission of BBVs in British prisons is unknown owing to the difficulty in compiling reliable data.

HBV can be transmitted vertically from mother to baby during the perinatal period. Approximately 80% of babies born to mothers who have either acute or chronic HBV become infected, and most will develop chronic HBV. This has been limited by the administration of HBV vaccine to the neonate. In industrialized countries, all prenatal mothers are screened for HBV. Vaccine is given to the neonate ideally within the first 12 hours of birth and at least two more doses are given at designated intervals. The WHO recommends this as a matter of course for all women in countries where prevalence is high. However, the practicalities of administering a vaccine that has to be stored at the correct temperature in places with limited access to medical care means that there is a significant failure of vaccine uptake and response.

5.1.6. Disease Prevention

In industrialized countries, HBV vaccination is recommended for those who are deemed at risk of acquiring the disease. They include the following:

1. Through occupational exposure.
2. Homosexual/bisexual men.
3. Intravenous drug users.
4. Sexual partners of people with acute or chronic HBV.
5. Family members of people with acute or chronic HBV.
6. Newborn babies whose mothers are infected with HBV. If the mother is HBsAg positive, then hepatitis B-specific immunoglobulin (HBIG) should be given at the same time as the first dose of vaccine.
7. Institutionalized patients and prisoners.

Ideally, HBV vaccine should be administered before exposure to the virus. The routine schedule consists of three doses of the vaccine given at 0, 1, and 6 months. Antibody levels should be checked 8–12 weeks after the last dose. If titers are greater than 10 miU/mL, then an adequate response has been achieved. In the United Kingdom, this is considered to provide protection for 5–10 years. In the United States, if an initial adequate response has been achieved, then no further doses of vaccine are considered necessary.

Vaccine administration after exposure varies according to the timing of the incident, the degree of risk involved, and whether the individual has already been partly or fully vaccinated. An accelerated schedule when the third dose is given 2 months after the first dose with a booster 1 year later is used to prevent postnatal transmission. Where risks are greatest, it may be necessary to use a rapid schedule. The doses are given at 0, 7, and 21–28 days after presentation, again with a booster dose at 6–12 months. This schedule is currently only licensed with Engerix B.

HBIG may also be used either alone or in conjunction with vaccine. The exact dose given is age dependent but must be administered by deep intramuscular injection in a different site from the vaccine. In an adult, this is usually into the gluteus muscle.

HBIG is given in conjunction with the first dose of vaccine to individuals who are deemed at high risk of acquiring disease and the incident occurred within 72 hours of presentation. It is also used for neonates born to mothers who are HBeAg-positive.

Between 5 and 10% of adults fail to respond to the routine schedule of vaccine. A further full course of vaccine should be tried before deeming the patients as "nonresponders." Such individuals involved in a high-risk exposure should be given two doses of HBIG administered 1 mo apart. Ideally, the first dose should be given within 48 hours after exposure and no later than 2 weeks after exposure.

Other measures include minimizing the risk of exposure by adopting the safe working practices outlined in Subheading 2. Any potential exposures should be dealt with as soon as possible. In industrialized countries blood, blood products, and organs are routinely screened for HBV.

Intravenous drug users should be encouraged to be vaccinated and to avoid sharing needles or any other drug paraphernalia (*see* Subheading 6.9.2.).

5.1.7. Management in Custody

For staff or victims in contact with disease, it is wise to have a procedure in place for immediate management and risk evaluation. An example is shown in Fig. 1. Although forensic physicians are not expected to administer treatment, it is often helpful to inform persons concerned what to expect. Tables 3 and 4 outline treatment protocols as used in the United Kingdom.

Detainees with disease can usually be managed in custody. If the detainee is bleeding, then the cell should be deemed out of action after the detainee has left until it can be professionally cleaned. Contaminated bedding should be dealt with as described in Subheading 2.2. If the detainee has chronic HBV and is on an antiviral agent (e.g., Lamivudine), then the treatment course should be continued, if possible.

5.2. Hepatitis C

5.2.1. Epidemiology and Prevalence

HCV is endemic in most parts of the world. Approximately 3% (200 million) of the world's population is infected with HCV *(15)*. For many countries, no reliable prevalence data exist.

Seroprevalence studies conducted among blood donors have shown that the highest prevalence exists in Egypt (17–26%). This has been ascribed to contaminated needles used in the treatment of schistosomiasis conducted between the 1950s and the 1980s *(16)*.

Intermediate prevalence (1–5%) exists in Eastern Europe, the Mediterranean, the Middle East, the Indian subcontinent, and parts of Africa and Asia. In Western Europe, most of Central America, Australia, and limited regions in Africa, including South Africa, the prevalence is low (0.2–0.5%). Previously, America was included in the low prevalence group, but a report published in 2003 *(17)* indicated that almost 4 million Americans (i.e., 1.8% of the population) have antibody to HCV, representing either ongoing or previous infection. It also states that HCV accounts for approx 15% of acute viral hepatitis in America.

The lowest prevalence (0.01–0.1%) has been found in the United Kingdom and Scandinavia. However, within any country, there are certain groups

Table 3
Management After High-Risk Exposure
Contact in High-Risk Group or HBsAg-Positive Person With High-Risk Exposure

Vaccination status	HBSIG	Hepatitis B vaccine	Follow-up	Notes
Not vaccinated	• Yes if >3 d after exposure • No if <3 d	Yes Yes	AS via GP RDS via GP	Advise GP of timing
Vaccinated nonresponder	• Yes if within 3 d	No	Repeat HBSIG	Consider trying newer at 1 mo vaccines at later stage
Course completed. Levels <10 miU/mL	• No	Yes if primary course <3 yr ago	No	
Course completed within 3 yr Levels not checked[a] or course completed >73 yr, *see* Incomplete Course	• No	Yes	GP to check results of baseline blood test	If baseline antibodies >10 miU/mL advise RDS
Incomplete course (1 or 2 doses)	• Yes if within 3 d • No if <3 d.	Yes Yes	GP to check results of baseline blood test	>10 miU/mL advise RS <10 miU/mL advise RDS

[a]If <3 yr, *see*

GP, Family doctor; HBsAg, hepatitis B surface antigen; AS, accelerated schedule; RDS, rapid schedule; HBSIG, hepatitis B-specific immunoglobulin.

Table 4
Management After Low-Risk Exposure
Contact Is in Low-Risk Group or Known To Be HBsAg Negative and Has Had a Low-Risk Exposure

Vaccination status	HBSIG	Vaccine	Follow-up	Notes
Not vaccinated	No	Yes	RS via GP	
Vaccinated nonresponder	No	No		Consider using newer vaccines
Course completed	No	Yes if not checked or <3 yr since first course		
Incomplete course	No	Yes	GP to check results of baseline test	>10 IU complete RS

GP, Family doctor; HBsAg, hepatitis B surface antigen; HBSIG, hepatitis B-specific immunoglobulin; RS, routine schedule; IU, international unit.

246

Table 5
Prevalence of Hepatitis C

• General blood-doning population	0.06%
• Organ donors	0.72%
• Hemophiliacs	100%[a]
• Intravenous drug users	46–90%
• Homosexual/bisexuals	<5%

[a]Statistics applies to all who received blood products before the mid-1980s.

that have a higher chance of carrying HCV. These United Kingdom figures are given in Table 5.

5.2.2. Symptoms and Complications

After an incubation period of 6–8 weeks, the acute phase of the disease lasts approx 2–3 years. Unlike hepatitis A (HAV) or HBV, the patient is usually asymptomatic; therefore, the disease is often missed unless the individual has reported a specific exposure and is being monitored. Other cases are found by chance, when raised liver enzymes are found on a routine blood test.

A "silent phase" follows the acute phase when the virus lies dormant and the liver enzymes are usually normal. This period lasts approx 10–15 years. Reactivation may then occur. Subsequent viral replication damages the hepatocytes, and liver enzymes rise to moderate or high levels.

Eighty percent of individuals who are HCV antibody-positive are infectious, regardless of the levels of their liver enzymes. Approximately 80% of people develop chronic infection, one-fifth of whom progress to cirrhosis. There is a much stronger association with hepatocellular carcinoma than with HBV. An estimated 1.25–2.5% of patients with HCV-related cirrhosis develop liver cancer *(18)*. Less than 2% of chronic cases resolve spontaneously.

5.2.3. Routes of Transmission

Approximately 75% of cases are parenteral (e.g., needle-stick, etc.) *(19)*. Transmission through the sexual route is not common and only appears to be significant if there is repeated exposure with one or more people infected with HCV. Mother-to-baby transmission is considered to be uncommon but has been reported *(20)*. Theoretically, household spread is also possible through sharing contaminated toothbrushes or razors.

Because the disease is often silent, there is a need to raise awareness among the general population on how to avoid infection and to encourage high-risk groups to be tested. Health care professionals should also be educated to avoid occupationally acquired infection. An example of good practice is contained within the document *Hepatitis C Strategy for England*, issued by the UK Department of Health in 2002 *(18)*.

5.2.4. Risks From Exposure to an HCV RNA-Positive Person

Blood or blood-stained body fluids need to be involved for a risk to occur. Saliva alone is not deemed to be a risk. The risk from a single needlestick incident is 1.8% (range 0–7%). Contact through a contaminated cut is estimated at 1%. For penetrating bite injuries, there are no data, but it is only considered a risk if blood is involved. Blood or blood-stained body fluids have to be involved in transmission through mucous membrane exposure. This may account for the lower-than-expected prevalence among the gay population.

5.2.5. Management in Custody

5.2.5.1. Staff/Victims in Contact With Disease

Follow the immediate management flow chart, making sure all available information is obtained. Inform the designated hospital and/or specialist as soon as possible. If the contact is known and is believed to be immunocompromised and he or she has consented to provide a blood sample, it is important to tell the specialist, because the antibody tests may be spuriously negative. In this instance, a different test should be used (polymerase chain reaction [PCR], which detects viral RNA).

The staff member/victim will be asked to provide a baseline sample of blood with further samples at 4–6 weeks and again at 12 weeks. If tests are negative at 12 weeks but the risk was deemed high, then follow-up may continue for up to 24 weeks. If any of the follow-up samples is positive, then the original baseline sample will be tested to ascertain whether the infection was acquired through the particular exposure.

It is important to emphasize the need for prompt initial attendance and continued monitoring, because treatment is now available. A combination of Ribavirin (antiviral agent and interferon a-2b) *(18)* or the newer pegylated interferons *(15)* may be used. This treatment is most effective when it is started early in the course of infection.

5.2.5.2. Detainees With Disease

Unless they are severely ill, detainees can be managed in custody. Special precautions are only required if they are bleeding. Custody staff should wear gloves if contact with blood is likely. Contaminated bedding should be handled appropriately, and the cell cleaned professionally after use.

5.3. Hepatitis D (Δ Agent)

This defective transmissible virus was discovered in 1977 and requires HBV for its own replication. It has a worldwide distribution in association with HBV, with approx 15 million people infected. The prevalence of HDV is higher in southern Italy, the Middle East, and parts of Africa and South America, occurring in more than 20% of HBV carriers who are asymptomatic and more than 60% of those with chronic HBV-related liver disease. Despite the high prevalence of HBV in China and South East Asia, HDV in these countries is rare.

HDV is associated with acute (coinfection) and chronic hepatitis (super-infection) and can exacerbate pre-existing liver damage caused by HBV. The routes of transmission and at-risk groups are the same as for HBV. Staff/victims in contact with a putative exposure and detainees with disease should be managed as for HBV. Interferon-α (e.g., Roferon) can be used to treat patients with chronic HBV and HDV *(21)*, although it would not be practical to continue this treatment in the custodial setting.

5.4. Human Immunodeficiency Virus

5.4.1. Epidemiology and Prevalence

HIV was first identified in 1983, 2 years after the first reports were made to the CDC in Atlanta, GA, of an increased incidence of two unusual diseases (Kaposi's sarcoma and *pneumocystis carinii* pneumonia) occurring among the gay population in San Francisco. The scale of the virus gradually emerged over the years and by the end of 2002, there were an estimated 42 million people throughout the world living with HIV or acquired immunodeficiency syndrome (AIDS). More than 80% of the world's population lives in Africa and India. A report by The Joint United Nations Programme on HIV/AIDS and the WHO in 2002 stated that one in five adults in Lesotho, Malawi, Mozambique, Swaziland, Zambia, and Zimbabwe has HIV or AIDS. There is also expected to be a sharp rise in cases of HIV in China, Papua New Guinea, and other countries in Asia and the Pacific during the next few years.

In the United Kingdom, by the end of 2002, the cumulative data reported that there were 54,261 individuals with HIV, AIDS (including deaths from AIDS) reported, though this is likely to be an underestimate *(22)*.

From these data, the group still considered at greatest risk of acquiring HIV in the United Kingdom is homosexual/bisexual men, with 28,835 of the cumulative total falling into this category. Among intravenous drug users, the overall estimated prevalence is 1%, but in London the figure is higher at 3.7% *(6,23)*. In the 1980s, up to 90% of users in Edinburgh and Dundee were reported to be HIV positive, but the majority have now died. Individuals arriving from Africa or the Indian subcontinent must also be deemed a risk group because 80% of the world's total cases occur in these areas. The predominant mode of transmission is through unprotected heterosexual intercourse.

The incidence of mother-to-baby transmission has been estimated at 15% in Europe and approx 45% in Africa. The transmission rates among African women are believed to be much higher owing to a combination of more women with end-stage disease with a higher viral load and concomitant placental infection, which renders it more permeable to the virus *(24,25)*. The use of antiretroviral therapy during pregnancy, together with the advice to avoid breastfeeding, has proven efficacious in reducing both vertical and horizontal transmission among HIV-positive women in the western world. For those in third-world countries, the reality is stark. Access to treatment is limited, and there is no realistic substitute for breast milk, which provides a valuable source of antibodies to other life-threatening infections. Patients receiving blood transfusions, organs, or blood products where screening is not routinely carried out must also be included.

5.4.2. Incubation Period and Phases of Infection

The incubation is estimated at 2 weeks to 6 months after exposure. This depends, to some extent, on the ability of current laboratory tests to detect HIV antibodies or viral antigen. The development of PCR for viral RNA has improved sensitivity.

During the acute phase of the infection, approx 50% experience a seroconversion "flu-like" illness. The individual is infectious at this time, because viral antigen (p24) is present in the blood. As antibodies start to form, the viral antigen disappears and the individual enters the latent phase. He or she is noninfectious and remains well for a variable period of time (7–15 years). Development of AIDS marks the terminal phase of disease. Viral antigen reemerges, and the individual is once again infectious. The onset of AIDS has been considerably delayed with the use of antiretroviral treatment.

5.4.3. Routes of Transmission

Parenteral transmission included needlestick injuries, bites, unscreened blood transfusions, tattooing, acupuncture, and dental procedures where equipment is inadequately sterilized. Risk of transmission is increased with deep penetrating injuries with hollow bore needles that are visibly bloodstained, especially when the device has previously been in the source patient's (contact) artery or vein.

Other routes include mucous membrane exposure (eyes, mouth, and genital mucous membranes) and contamination of broken skin.

The higher the viral load in the contact, the greater the risk of transmission. This is more likely at the terminal stage of infection. HIV is transmitted mainly through blood or other body fluids that are visibly blood stained, with the exception of semen, vaginal fluid, and breast milk. Saliva alone is most unlikely to transmit infection. Therefore, people who have sustained penetrating bite injuries can be reassured that they are not at risk, providing the contact was not bleeding from the mouth at the time.

5.4.4. Risk of Seroconversion

The risk from a single percutaneous exposure from a hollow bore needle is low, and a single mucocutaneous exposure is even less likely to result in infection.

The risk from sexual exposure varies, although it appears that there is a greater risk with receptive anal intercourse compared with receptive vaginal intercourse *(26)*.

5.4.5. Body Fluids Containing HIV

High-risk fluids include blood, semen, vaginal fluid, and breast milk. There is little or no risk from saliva, urine, vomit, or feces unless they are visibly bloodstained. Other fluids that constitute a theoretical risk include cerebrospinal, peritoneal, pleural, synovial, or pericardial fluid.

5.4.6. Management in Custody of Staff/Victims in Contact With Disease

Management in custody of staff/victims in contact with disease includes following the immediate management flow chart (Fig. 1) and contacting the designated hospital/specialist with details of the exposure. Where possible, obtain a blood sample from the contact. Regarding HBV and HCV blood samples in the United Kingdom, they can only be taken with informed consent. There is no need for the forensic physician to go into details about the meaning of the test, but the contact should be encouraged to attend the genitourinary department (or similar) of the designated hospital to discuss the test results. Should the contact refuse to provide a blood sample, then any information about his or her lifestyle, ethnic origin, state of health, etc., may be useful for the specialist to decide whether postexposure prophylaxis (PEP) should be given to the victim. Where only saliva is involved in a penetrating bite injury, there is every justification to reassure the victim that he or she is not at risk. If in doubt, then always refer.

In the United Kingdom, the current recommended regime for PEP is Combivir (300 mg of Zidovudine twice daily plus 150 mg of Lamivudine twice daily) and a protease inhibitor (1250 mg of Nelfanivir twice daily) given for 4 weeks *(27)*. It is only given after a significant exposure to a high-risk fluid or any that is visibly bloodstained and the contact is known or is highly likely to be HIV positive. Ideally, treatment should be started within an hour after exposure, although it will be considered for up to 2 weeks. It is usually given for 4 weeks, unless the contact is subsequently identified as HIV negative or the "victim" develops tolerance or toxicity occurs. Weekly examinations of the "victim" should occur during treatment to improve adherence, monitor drug toxicity, and deal with other concerns.

Other useful information that may influence the decision whether to treat with the standard regimen or use alternative drugs includes interaction with other medications that the "victim" may be taking (e.g., phenytoin or antibiotics) or if the contact has been on antiretroviral therapy or if the "victim" is pregnant. During the second or third trimester, only Combivir would be used, because there is limited experience with protease inhibitors. No data exist regarding the efficacy of PEP beyond occupational exposure *(27)*.

PEP is not considered for exposure to low- or no-risk fluids through any route or where the source is unknown (e.g., a discarded needle). Despite the appropriate use and timing of PEP, there have been reports of failure *(28,29)*.

5.4.7. Management in Custody of Detainees With HIV

Unless they are severely ill, detainees can be kept in custody. Every effort should be made to continue any treatment they may be receiving. Apply universal precautions when dealing with the detainee, and ensure that contaminated cells and/or bedding are managed appropriately.

6. Transmission Through Contact With Lesions or Organisms

6.1. Varicella *(Chicken Pox)*

6.1.1. Epidemiology and Prevalence

Cases of this highly infectious disease occur throughout the year but are more frequent in winter and early spring. This seasonal endemicity is blurring with global warming. In the United Kingdom, the highest prevalence occurs in the 4- to 10-years age group. Ninety percent of the population over the age of 40 is immune *(30)*. A similar prevalence has been reported in other parts of Western Europe and the United States. In South East Asia, *Varicella* is mainly a disease of adulthood *(31)*. Therefore, people born in these countries who have moved to the United Kingdom are more likely to be susceptible to chicken pox.

There is a strong correlation between a history of chicken pox and serological immunity (97–99%). Most adults born and living in industrialized countries with an uncertain or negative history of chicken pox are also seropositive (70–90%). In March 1995, a live-attenuated vaccine was licensed for use in the United States and a policy for vaccinating children and susceptible health care personnel was introduced. In summer 2002, in the United Kingdom, GlaxoSmithKline launched a live-attenuated vaccine called Varilrix. In December 2003, the UK Department of Health, following advice from the Joint Committee on Vaccination and Immunisation recommended that the vaccine be given for nonimmune health care workers who are likely to have direct contact with individuals with chicken pox. Any health care worker with no previous history of chicken pox should be screened for immunity, and if no antibodies are found, then they should receive two doses of vaccine 4–8 weeks apart. The vaccine is not currently recommended for children and should not be given during pregnancy.

6.1.2. Incubation Period and Symptoms

Following an incubation period of 10–21 days (this may be shorter in the immunocompromised), there is usually a prodromal "flu-like" illness before the onset of the rash. This coryzal phase is more likely in adults. The lesions typically appear in crops, rapidly progressing from red papules through vesicles to open sores that crust over and separate by 10 days. The distribution of the rash is centripetal (i.e., more over the trunk and face than on the limbs). This is the converse of small pox. In adults, the disease is often more severe, with lesions involving the scalp and mucous membranes of the oropharynx.

6.1.3. Complications

In children, the disease is often mild, unless they are immunocompromised, so they are unlikely to experience complications. In adults (defined as 15 yr or older), the picture is rather different *(32)*. Secondary bacterial infection is common but rarely serious. There is an increased likelihood of permanent scarring. Hemorrhagic chicken pox typically occurs on the second or third day of the rash. Usually, this is limited to bleeding into the skin, but life-threatening melena, epistaxis, or hematuria can occur.

Varicella pneumonia ranges from patchy lung consolidation to overt pneumonitis and occurs in 1 in 400 cases *(33)*. It can occur in previously healthy individuals (particularly adults), but the risk is increased in those who smoke.

Immunocompromised people are at the greatest risk of developing this complication. It runs a fulminating course and is the most common cause of *Varicella*-associated death. Fibrosis and permanent respiratory impairment may occur in those who survive. Any suspicion of lung involvement is an indication for immediate treatment, and any detainee or staff member should be sent to hospital. Involvement of the central nervous system includes several conditions, including meningitis, Guillain-Barre, and encephalitis. The latter is more common in the immunocompromised and can be fatal.

6.1.4. Period of Infectivity

This is taken as 3 days before the first lesions appear to the end of new vesicle formation and the last vesicle has crusted over. This typically is 5–7 days after onset but may last up to 14 days.

6.1.5. Routes of Transmission

The primary route is through direct contact with open lesions of chicken pox. However, it is also spread through aerosol or droplets from the respiratory tract. Chicken pox may also be acquired through contact with open lesions of shingles (*Varicella zoster*), but this is less likely because shingles is less infectious than chicken pox.

6.1.6. At-Risk Groups

Nonimmune individuals are at risk of acquiring disease. Approximately 10% of the adult population born in the United Kingdom and less than 5% of adults in the United States fall into this category. Therefore, it is more likely that if chicken pox is encountered in the custodial setting, it will involve people born outside the United Kingdom (particularly South East Asia) or individuals who are immunocompromised and have lost immunity. Nonimmune pregnant women are at risk of developing complications.

Pneumonia can occur in up to 10% of pregnant women with chicken pox, and the severity is increased in later gestation *(34)*. They can also transmit infection to the unborn baby *(35)*. If infection is acquired in the first 20 weeks, there is a less than 3% chance of it leading to congenital *Varicella* syndrome. Infection in the last trimester can lead to neonatal *Varicella*, unless more than 7 days elapse between onset of maternal rash and delivery when antibodies have time to cross the placenta leading to either mild or inapparent infection in the newborn. In this situation, *Varicella* immunoglobulin (VZIG) should be administered to the baby as soon as possible after birth *(36)*.

6.1.7. Management in Custody

Staff with chicken pox should stay off work until the end of the infective period (approx 7–14 days). Those in contact with disease who are known to be nonimmune or who have no history of disease should contact the designated occupational health physician.

Detainees with the disease should not be kept in custody if at all possible (especially pregnant women). If this is unavoidable, then nonimmune or immunocompromised staff should avoid entering the cell or having close contact with the detainee.

Nonimmune, immunocompromised, or pregnant individuals exposed to chickenpox should seek expert medical advice regarding the administration of VZIG. Aciclovir (or similar antiviral agent) should be given as soon as possible to people who are immunocompromised with chicken pox. It should also be considered for anyone over 15 years old because they are more likely to develop complications.

Anyone suspected of severe complications should be sent straight to the hospital.

6.2. Herpes Zoster *(Shingles)*

6.2.1. Epidemiology

After chicken pox, the virus lies dormant in the dorsal root or cranial nerve ganglia but may re-emerge and typically involves one dermatome *(37)*. The site of involvement depends on the sensory ganglion initially involved. Shingles is more common in individuals over the age of 50 years, except in the immunocompromised, when attacks can occur at an earlier age. The latter are also more susceptible to secondary attacks and involvement of more than one dermatome. Bilateral *zoster* is even rarer but is not associated with a higher mortality.

In the United Kingdom, there is an estimated incidence of 1.2–3.4 per 1000-person years *(38)*.

6.2.2. Symptoms

There may be a prodromal period of paraesthesia and burning or shooting pains in the involved segment. This is usually followed by the appearance of a band of vesicles. Rarely, the vesicles fail to appear and only pain is experienced. This is known as *zoster sine herpete*. In individuals who are immunocompromised, disease may be prolonged and dissemination may occur but is rarely fatal.

Shingles in pregnancy is usually mild. The fetus is only affected if viremia occurs before maternal antibody has had time to cross the placenta.

6.2.3. Complications

The most common complication of shingles is postherpetic neuralgia, occurring in approx 10% of cases. It is defined as pain lasting more than 120 days from rash onset *(39)*. It is more frequent in people over 50 years and can lead to depression. It is rare in children, including those who are immunocompromised. Infection of the brain includes encephalitis, involvement of motor neurones leading to ptosis, paralysis of the hand, facial palsy, or contralateral hemiparesis. Involvement of the oculomotor division of the trigeminal ganglion can cause serious eye problems, including corneal scarring.

6.2.4. Period of Infectivity

Shingles is far less infectious than chicken pox and is only considered to be infectious up to 3 days after lesions appear.

6.2.5. Routes of Transmission

Shingles is only infectious after prolonged contact with lesions. Unlike chickenpox, airborne transmission is not a risk.

6.2.6. At-Risk Groups

Individuals who are immunocompromised may reactivate the dormant virus and develop shingles. People who have not had primary *Varicella* are at risk of developing chickenpox after prolonged direct contact with shingles. Despite popular belief, it is untrue that people who are immunocompetent who have had chicken pox develop shingles when in contact with either chicken pox or shingles. Such occurrences are merely coincidental, unless immunity is lowered.

6.2.7. Management in Custody

Staff with shingles should stay off work until the lesions are healed, unless they can be covered. Staff who have had chickenpox are immune (including pregnant women) and are therefore not at risk. If they are nonimmune (usually accepted as those without a history of chicken pox), they should avoid prolonged contact with detainees with shingles. Pregnant nonimmune women should avoid contact altogether.

Detainees with the disease may be kept in custody, and any exposed lesions should be covered. It is well documented that prompt treatment attenuates the severity of the disease, reduces the duration of viral shedding, hastens lesion healing, and reduces the severity and duration of pain. It also reduces the likelihood of developing postherpetic neuralgia *(40)*. Prompt treatment with Famciclovir (e.g., 500 mg three times a day for 7 days) should be initiated if the onset is 3 d ays or less. It should also be considered after this time if the detainee is over age 50 years. Pregnant detainees with shingles can be reassured that there is minimal risk for both the mother and the unborn child. Expert advice should be given before initiating treatment for the mother.

6.3. Scabies

6.3.1. Epidemiology

This tiny parasitic mite (*Sarcoptes scabiei*) has infested humans for more than 2500 years. Experts estimate that in excess of 300 million cases occur worldwide each year. The female mite burrows into the skin, especially around the hands, feet, and male genitalia, in approx 2.5 min. Eggs are laid and hatch into larvae that travel to the skin surface as newly developed mites.

6.3.2. Symptoms

The mite causes intense itching, which is often worse at night and is aggravated by heat and moisture. The irritation spreads outside the original point of infection resulting from an allergic reaction to mite feces. This irritation may persist for approx 2 weeks after treatment but can be alleviated by antihistamines.

Crusted scabies is a far more severe form of the disease. Large areas of the body may be involved. The crusts hide thousands of live mites and eggs, making them difficult to treat. This so-called Norwegian scabies is more common in the elderly or the immunocompromised, especially those with HIV.

6.3.4. Incubation Period

After a primary exposure, it takes approx 2–6 weeks before the onset of itching. However, further exposures reduce the incubation time to approx 1–4 days.

6.3.5. Period of Infectivity

Without treatment, the period of infectivity is assumed to be indefinite. With treatment, the person should be considered infectious until the mites and eggs are destroyed, usually 7–10 days. Crusted scabies is highly infectious.

6.3.6. Management in Custody

Because transmission is through direct skin-to-skin contact with an infected individual, gloves should be worn when dealing with individuals suspected of infestation. Usually prolonged contact is needed, unless the person has crusted scabies, where transmission occurs more easily. The risk of transmission is much greater in households were repeated or prolonged contact is likely.

Because mites can survive in bedding or clothing for up to 24 hour, gloves should also be worn when handling these items. Bedding should be treated using one of the methods in Subheading 2.2. Professional cleaning of the cell is only warranted in cases of crusted scabies.

6.3.7. Treatment

The preferred treatment for scabies is either permethrin cream (5%) or aqueous Malathion (0.5%) *(41)*. Either treatment has to be applied to the whole body and should be left on for at least 8 hours in the case of permethrin and 24 hours for Malathion before washing off. Lindane is no longer considered the treatment of choice, because there may be complications in pregnancy *(42)*.

Treatment in custody may not be practical but should be considered when the detainee is believed to have Norwegian scabies.

6.4. Head Lice

6.4.1. General Information

Like scabies, head lice occur worldwide and are found in the hair close to the scalp. The eggs, or nits, cling to the hair and are difficult to remove, but they are not harmful. If you see nits, then you can be sure that lice are also present. The latter are best seen when the hair is wet. The lice bite the scalp and suck blood, causing intense irritation and itching.

6.4.2. Route of Transmission

Head lice can only be passed from direct hair-to-hair contact.

6.4.3. Management in Custody

It is only necessary to wear gloves when examining the head for whatever reason. The cell does not need to be cleaned after use, because the lice live on or near skin. Bedding may be contaminated with shed skin, so should be handled with gloves and laundered or incinerated.

The presence of live lice is an indication for treatment by either physical removal with a comb or the application of an insecticide. The latter may be more practical in custody. Treatment using 0.5% aqueous Malathion should be applied to dry hair and washed off after 12 hours. The hair should then be shampooed as normal.

6.5. Crabs or Body Lice

6.5.1. General Information

Crabs or body lice are more commonly found in the pubic, axillary, chest, and leg hair. However, eyelashes and eyebrows may also be involved. They are associated with people who do not bath or change clothes regularly. The person usually complains of intense itching or irritation.

6.5.2. Routes of Transmission

The main route is from person to person by direct contact, but eggs can stick to fibers, so clothing and bedding should be handled with care (*see* Subheading 6.5.3.).

6.5.3 Management in Custody

Staff should always wear gloves if they are likely to come into contact with any hirsute body part. Clothing or bedding should be handled with gloves and either laundered or incinerated.

Treatment of a detainee in custody is good in theory but probably impractical because the whole body has to be treated.

6.6. Fleas

6.6.1. General Information

Fleas lay eggs on floors, carpets, and bedding. In the United Kingdom, most flea bites come from cats or dogs. The eggs and larvae fleas can survive for months and are reactivated in response to animal or human activity. Because animal fleas jump off humans after biting, most detainees with flea bites will not have fleas, unless they are human fleas.

6.6.2. Management in Custody

Treatment is only necessary if fleas are seen. After use, the cell should be vacuumed and cleaned with a proprietary insecticide. Any bedding should be removed wearing gloves, bagged, and either laundered or incinerated.

6.7. Bedbugs

6.7.1. General Information

Bedbugs live and lay eggs on walls, floors, furniture, and bedding. If you look carefully, fecal tracks may be seen on hard surfaces. If they are present for long enough, they emit a distinct odor. Bedbugs are rarely found on the person but may be brought in on clothing or other personal effects.

6.7.2. Symptoms

Bedbugs bite at night and can cause sleep disturbance.

6.7.3. Management in Custody

The detainee does not need to be treated, but the cell should deemed out of use until it can be vacuumed and professionally cleaned with an insecticide solution. Any bedding or clothing should be handled with gloves and disposed of as appropriate.

6.8. Methicillin-Resistant Staphylococcus aureus

6.8.1. Epidemiology

Staphylococcus aureus is commonly carried on the skin or in the nose of healthy people. Approximately 25–30% of the population is colonized with the bacteria but remain well *(43)*. From time to time, the bacteria cause minor skin infections that usually do not require antibiotic treatment. However, more serious problems can occur (e.g., infection of surgical wounds, drug injection sites, osteomyelitis, pneumonia, or septicemia). During the last 50 years, the bacteria have become increasingly resistant to penicillin-based antibiotics *(44)*, and in the last 20 years, they have become resistant to an increasing number of alternative antibiotics. These multiresistant bacteria are known as methicillin-resistant *S. aureus* (MRSA).

MRSA is prevalent worldwide. Like nonresistant staphylococci, it may remain undetected as a reservoir in colonized individuals but can also produce clinical disease. It is more common in individuals who are elderly, debilitated, or immunocompromised or those with open wounds. Clusters of skin infections with MRSA have been reported among injecting drug users (IDUs) since 1981 in America *(45,46)*, and more recently, similar strains have been found in the United Kingdom in IDUs in the community *(47)*. This may have particular relevance for the forensic physician when dealing with IDUs sores. People who are immunocompetent rarely get MRSA and should not be considered at risk.

6.8.2. Route of Transmission

The bacteria are usually spread via the hands of staff after contact with colonized or infected detainees or devices, items (e.g., bedding, towels, and soiled dressings), or environmental surfaces that have been contaminated with MRSA-containing body fluids.

6.8.3. Management in Custody

With either known or suspected cases (consider all abscesses/ulcers of IDUs as infectious), standard precautions should be applied. Staff should wear gloves when touching mucous membranes, nonintact skin, blood or other body fluids, or any items that could be contaminated. They should also be encouraged to their wash hands with an antimicrobial agent regardless of whether gloves have been worn. After use, gloves should be disposed of in a yellow hazard bag and not allowed to touch surfaces. Masks and gowns should only be worn when conducting procedures that generate aerosols of blood or other body fluids. Because this is an unlikely scenario in the custodial setting, masks and gowns should not be necessary. Gloves should be worn when handling bedding or clothing, and all items should be disposed of appropriately. Any open wounds should be covered as soon as possible. The cell should be cleaned professionally after use if there is any risk that it has been contaminated.

6.9. Other Bacteria Associated With Abscess Formation in IDUs

6.9.1. Epidemiology

During the last decade, there has been an increasing awareness of the bacterial flora colonizing injection sites that may potentially lead to life-threatening infection *(48)*. In 1997, a sudden increase in needle abscesses caused by a clonal strain of Group A *Streptococcus* was reported among hospitalized IDUs in Berne, Switzerland *(49)*. A recent UK study showed that the predominant isolate is *S. aureus*, with *Streptococcus* species forming just under one-fifth (50% β-hemolytic streptococci) *(50)*. There have also been reports of both nonsporing and sporing anerobes (e.g., *Bacteroides* and *Clostridia* species, including *Clostridia botulinum*) *(51,52)*.

In particular, in 2000, laboratories in Glasgow were reporting isolates of *Clostridium novyi* among IDUs with serious unexplained illness. By June 12, 2000, a total of 42 cases (18 definite and 24 probable) had been reported. A definite case was defined as an IDU with both severe local and systemic inflammatory reactions. A probable case was defined as an IDU who presented to the hospital with an abscess or other significant inflammation at an injecting site and had either a severe inflammatory process at or around an injection site or a severe systemic reaction with multiorgan failure and a high white cell count *(53)*.

In the United Kingdom, the presence of *C. botulinum* in infected injection sites is a relatively new phenomenon. Until the end of 1999, there were no cases reported to the Public Health Leadership Society. Since then, the number has increased, with a total of 13 cases in the United Kingdom and Ireland being reported since the beginning of 2002. It is believed that these cases are associated with contaminated batches of heroin. Simultaneous injection of cocaine increases the risk by encouraging anerobic conditions. Anerobic flora in wounds may have serious consequences for the detainee, but the risk of transmission to staff is virtually nonexistent.

6.9.2. Management in Custody

Staff should be reminded to wear gloves when coming into contact with detainees with infected skin sites exuding pus or serum and that any old dressings found in the cell should be disposed of into the yellow bag marked "clinical waste" in the medical room. Likewise, any bedding should be bagged and laundered or incinerated after use. The cell should be deemed out of use and professionally cleaned after the detainee has gone.

The health care professional managing the detainee should clean and dress open wounds as soon as possible to prevent the spread of infection. It may also be appropriate to start a course of antibiotics if there is abscess formation or signs of cellulites and/or the detainee is systemically unwell. However, infections can often be low grade because the skin, venous, and lymphatic systems have been damaged by repeated penetration of the skin. In these cases, signs include lymphedema, swollen lymph glands, and darkly pigmented skin over the area. Fever may or may not be present, but septicemia is uncommon unless the individual is immunocompromised (e.g., HIV positive). Co-Amoxiclav is the preferred treatment of choice because it covers the majority of staphylococci, streptococci, and anerobes (the dose depends on the degree of infection).

Necrotizing fasciitis and septic thrombophlebitis are rare but life-threatening complications of intravenous drug use. Any detainee suspected of either of these needs hospital treatment. Advice about harm reduction should also be given. This includes encouraging drug users to smoke rather than inject or at least to advise them to avoid injecting into muscle or skin. Although most IDUs are aware of the risk of sharing needles, they may not realize that sharing any drug paraphernalia could be hazardous. Advice should be given to use the minimum amount of citric acid to dissolve the heroin because the acid can damage the tissue under the skin, allowing bacteria to flourish. Drugs should be injected at different sites using fresh works for each injection. This is particularly important when "speedballing" because crack cocaine creates an anerobic environment. Medical help should be requested if any injection site become painful and swollen or shows signs of pus collecting under the skin. Because intravenous drug users are at increased risk of acquiring HBV and HAV, they should be informed that vaccination against both diseases is advisable.

Another serious but relatively rare problem is the risk from broken needles in veins. Embolization can take anywhere from hours to days or even longer if it is not removed. Complications may include endocarditis, pericarditis, or pulmonary abscesses *(54,55)*. IDUs should be advised to seek medical help as soon as possible, and should such a case present in custody, then send the detainee straight to the hospital.

6.10. Management of Human and Dog Bites

6.10.1. Introduction

The forensic physician may encounter bites in the following four circumstances:

1. During the examination of assault victims (both children and adults) where presentation is more likely to be late.
2. Among police officers bitten during the arrest of a detainee.
3. In detainees during the arrest if dogs have been used.
4. Where detainees have been involved in a fight either around the time of arrest or earlier.

A detailed forensic examination of bites is given in Chapter 4. With any bite that has penetrated the skin, the goals of therapy are to minimize soft tissue deformity and to prevent or treat infection.

6.10.2. Epidemiology

In the United Kingdom and the United States, dog bites represent approximately three-quarters of all bites presenting to accident and emergency departments *(56)*. A single dog bite can produce up to 220 psi of crush force in addition to the torsional forces as the dog shakes its head. This can result in massive tissue damage. Human bites may cause classical bites or puncture wounds (e.g., impact of fists on teeth) resulting in crush injuries.

6.10.3. Rates and Risks of Infection

An estimated 10–30% of dog bites and 9–50% of human bites lead to infection. Compare this with an estimated 1–12% of nonbite wounds managed in accident and emergency departments.

The risk of infection is increased with puncture wounds, hand injuries, full-thickness wounds, wounds requiring debridement, and those involving joints, tendons, ligaments or fractures.

Comorbid medical conditions, such as diabetes, asplenia, chronic edema of the area, liver dysfunction, the presence of a prosthetic valve or joint, and an immunocompromised state may also increase the risk of infection.

6.10.4. Other Complications of Bites

Infection may spread beyond the initial site, leading to septic arthritis, osteomyelitis, endocarditis, peritonitis, septicemia, and meningitis. Inflammation of the tendons or synovial lining of joints may also occur. If enough force is used, bones may be fractured or the wounds may be permanently disfiguring.

6.10.5. Initial Management

Assessment regarding whether hospital treatment is necessary should be made as soon as possible. Always refer if the wound is bleeding heavily or fails to stop when pressure is applied. Penetrating bites involving arteries, nerves, muscles, tendons, the hands, or feet, resulting in a moderate to serious facial wound, or crush injuries, also require immediate referral.

If management within custody is appropriate, ask about current tetanus vaccine status, HBV vaccination status, and known allergies to antibiotics.

Wounds that have breached the skin should be irrigated with 0.9% (isotonic) sodium chloride or Ringer's lactate solution instead of antiseptics, because the latter may delay wound healing.

A full forensic documentation of the bite should be made as detailed in Chapter 4.

Note if there are clinical signs of infection, such as erythema, edema, cellulitis, purulent discharge, or regional lymphadenopathy. Cover the wound with a sterile, nonadhesive dressing. Wound closure is not generally recommended because data suggest that it may increase the risk of infection. This is particularly relevant for nonfacial wounds, deep puncture wounds, bites to the hand, clinically infected wounds, and wounds occurring more than 6–12 hours before presentation. Head and neck wounds in cosmetically important areas may be closed if less than 12 hours old and not obviously infected.

6.10.6. Pathogens Involved

1. Bacteria
   - Dog bites—*Pasteurella canis, Pasteurella multocida, S. aureus*, other staphylococci, Streptococcus species, *Eikenella corrodens*, Corynebacterium species, and anerobes, including *Bacteroides fragilis* and *Clostridium tetani*
   - Human bites—Streptococcus species, *S. aureus, E. corrodens*, and anerobes, including bacteroides (often penicillin resistant), Peptostreptococci species, and *C. tetani*. Tuberculosis (TB) and syphilis may also be transmitted.
2. Viruses
   - Dog bites—outside of the United Kingdom, Australia, and New Zealand, rabies should be considered. In the United States, domestic dogs are mostly

vaccinated against rabies *(57)*, and police dogs have to be vaccinated, so the most common source is from racoons, skunks, and bats.
• Human bites—HBV, HBC, HIV, and herpes simplex.

6.10.7. Antibiotic Prophylaxis

Antibiotics are not generally needed if the wound is more than 2 days old and there is no sign of infection or in superficial noninfected wounds evaluated early that can be left open to heal by secondary intention in compliant people with no significant comorbidity *(58)*. Antibiotics should be considered with high-risk wounds that involve the hands, feet, face, tendons, ligaments, joints, or suspected fractures or for any penetrating bite injury in a person with diabetes, asplenia, or cirrhosis or who is immunosuppressed.

Coamoxiclav (amoxycillin and clavulanic acid) is the first-line treatment for mild–moderate dog or human bites resulting in infections managed in primary care. For adults, the recommended dose is 500/125 mg three times daily and for children the recommended does is 40 mg/kg three times daily (based on amoxycillin component). Treatment should be continued for 10–14 days. It is also the first-line drug for prophylaxis when the same dose regimen should be prescribed for 5–7 days. If the individual is known or suspected to be allergic to penicillin, a tetracycline (e.g., doxycycline 100 mg twice daily) and metronidazole (500 mg three times daily) or an aminoglycoside (e.g., erythromycin) and metronidazole can be used. In the United Kingdom, doxycycline use is restricted to those older than 12 years and in the United States to those older than 8 years old. Specialist advice should be sought for pregnant women.

Anyone with severe infection or who is clinically unwell should be referred to the hospital. Tetanus vaccine should be given if the primary course or last booster was more than 10 years ago. Human tetanus immunoglobulin should be considered for tetanus-prone wounds (e.g., soil contamination, puncture wounds, or signs of devitalized tissue) or for wounds sustained more than 6 hours old. If the person has never been immunized or is unsure of his or her tetanus status, a full three-dose course, spaced at least 1 month apart, should be given.

6.10.8. Management of Suspected
Viral Infections From Human Bites

Penetrating bite wounds that involve only saliva may present a risk of HBV if the perpetrator belongs to a high-risk group. For management, *see* Subheadings 5.1.6. and 5.1.7. HCV and HIV are only a risk if blood is involved. The relevant management is dealt with in Subheadings 5.2.5. and 5.4.6.

7. Infections Transmitted Through the Respiratory Route
7.1. General Information

Respiratory tract infections are common, usually mild, and self-limiting, although they may require symptomatic treatment with paracetamol or a nonsteroidal antiinflammatory. These include the common cold (80% rhinoviruses and 20% coronaviruses), adenoviruses, influenza, parainfluenza, and, during the summer and early autumn, enteroviruses. Special attention should be given to detainees with asthma or the who are immunocompromised, because infection in these people may be more serious particularly if the lower respiratory tract is involved.

The following section includes respiratory pathogens of special note because they may pose a risk to both the detainee and/or staff who come into close contact.

7.2. Meningococcal Meningitis (Neisseria meningitidis)
7.2.1. General Information and Epidemiology

There are five serogroups of *Neisseria meningitidis*: A, B, C, W135, and Y. The prevalence of the different types varies from country to country. There is currently no available vaccine against type B, but three other vaccines (A+C, C, and ACWY) are available. Overall, 10% of the UK population carry *N. meningitidis* (25% in the 15–19 age group) *(59)*.

In the United Kingdom, most cases of meningitis are sporadic, with less than 5% occurring as clusters (outbreaks) amongst school children. Between 1996 and 2000, 59% of cases were group B, 36% were group C, and W135 and A accounted for 5%. There is a seasonal variation, with a high level of cases in winter and a low level in the summer. The greatest risk group are the under 5 year olds, with a peak incidence under 1 year old. A secondary peak occurs in the 15- to 19-year-old age group. In Sub-Saharan Africa, the disease is more prevalent in the dry season, but in many countries, there is background endemicity year-round. The most prevalent serogroup is A.

Routine vaccination against group C was introduced in the United Kingdom November 1999 for everybody up to the age of 18 years old and to all first-year university students. This has since been extended to include everyone under the age of 25 years old. As a result of the introduction of the vaccination program, there has been a 90% reduction of group C cases in those younger than under 18 years and an 82% reduction in those under 1 year old *(60,61)*.

An outbreak of serogroup W135 meningitis occurred among pilgrims on the Hajj in 2000. Cases were reported from many countries, including the United Kingdom. In the United Kingdom, there is now an official requirement to be vaccinated with the quadrivalent vaccine (ACWY Vax) before going on a pilgrimage (Hajj or Umra), but illegal immigrants who have not been vaccinated may enter the country *(62)*.

7.2.2. Symptoms

After an incubation period of 3–5 days *(63,64)*, disease onset may be either insidious with mild prodromal symptoms or florid. Early symptoms and signs include malaise, fever, and vomiting. Sever headache, neck stiffness, photophobia, drowsiness, and a rash may develop. The rash may be petechial or purpuric and characteristically does not blanche under pressure. Meningitis in infants is more likely to be insidious in onset and lack the classical signs. In approx 15–20% of cases, septicemia is the predominant feature. Even with prompt antibiotic treatment, the case fatality rate is 3–5% in meningitis and 15–20% in those with septicemia. *(65)*.

7.2.3. Period of Infectivity

A person should be considered infectious until the bacteria are no longer present in nasal discharge. With treatment, this is usually approx 24 hour.

7.2.4. Routes of Transmission

The disease is spread through infected droplets or direct contact from carriers or those who are clinically ill. It requires prolonged and close contact, so it is a greater risk for people who share accommodation and utensils and kiss. It must also be remembered that unprotected mouth-to-mouth resuscitation can also transmit disease.

7.2.5. Management in Custody

It is not possible to tell if a detainee is a carrier. Nevertheless, the risk of acquiring infection even from an infected and sick individual is low, unless the individual has carried out mouth-to-mouth resuscitation. Any staff member who believes he or she has been placed at risk should report to the occupational health department (or equivalent) or the nearest emergency department at the earliest opportunity for vaccination.

If the detainee has performed mouth-to-mouth resuscitation, prophylactic antibiotics should be given before receiving vaccination. Rifampicin, ciprofloxacin, and ceftriaxone can be used, however, ciprofloxacin has numerous advantages *(66)*. Only a single dose of 500 mg (adults and children older than 12 years) is needed and has fewer side effects and contraindications than rifampicin. Ceftriaxone has to be given by injection and is therefore best avoided in the custodial setting. If the staff member is pregnant, advice should be sought from a consultant obstetrician, because ciprofloxacin is not recommended *(67)*.

For anyone dealing regularly with illegal immigrants (especially from the Middle East or Sub-Saharan Africa) (e.g., immigration services, custody staff at designated stations, medical personnel, and interpreters), should consider being vaccinated with ACWY Vax. A single injection provides protection for 3 years. Detainees suspected of disease should be sent directly to the hospital.

7.3. Tuberculosis

7.3.1. Prevalence and Epidemiology

Human TB is caused by infection with *Mycobacterium tuberculosis, Mycobacterium bovis, or Mycobacterium africanum*. It is a notifiable disease under legislation specific to individual countries; for example, in the United Kingdom, this comes under the Public Health (Control of Disease) Act of 1984. In 1993, the WHO declared TB to be a global emergency, with an estimated 7–8 million new cases and 3 million deaths occurring each year, the majority of which were in Asia and Africa. However, these statistics are likely to be an underestimate because they depend on the accuracy of reporting, and in poorer countries, the surveillance systems are often inadequate because of lack of funds.

Even in the United Kingdom, there has been an inconsistency of reporting particularly where an individual has concomitant infection with HIV. Some physicians found themselves caught in a dilemma of confidentiality until 1997, when the codes of practice were updated to encourage reporting with patient consent *(68)*.

With the advent of rapid identification tests and treatment and the use of Bacillus Calmette-Guérin (BCG) vaccination for prevention, TB declined during the first half of the 20th century in the United Kingdom. However, since the early 1990s, numbers have slowly increased, with some 6800 cases reported in 2002 *(69)*. In 1998, 56% of reported cases were from people born outside the United Kingdom and 3% were associated with HIV infection *(70,71)*.

London has been identified as an area with a significant problem. This has been attributed to its highly mobile population, the variety of ethnic groups, a high prevalence of HIV, and the emergence of drug-resistant strains (1.3% in 1998) (PHLS, unpublished data—Mycobnet).

A similar picture was initially found in the United States, when there was a reversal of a long-standing downward trend in 1985. However, between 1986 and 1992, the number of cases increased from 22,201 to 26,673 *(72)*. There were also serious outbreaks of multidrug-resistant TB (MDR-TB) in hospitals

Table 6
Symptoms of Tuberculosis

• Cough lasting >3 wk	• Fatigue
• Anorexia and weight loss	• Fever and night sweats
• Mild hemoptysis (rusty colored)	• Cough with phlegm
• Swollen lymph glands	

in New York City and Miami *(73)*. Factors pertinent to the overall upswing included the emergence of HIV, the increasing numbers of immigrants from countries with a high prevalence of TB, and perhaps more significantly, stopping categorical federal funding for control activities in 1972. The latter led to a failure of the public health infrastructure for TB control. Since 1992, the trend has reversed as the CDC transferred most of its funds to TB surveillance and treatment program in states and large cities. From 1992 to 2001, the annual decline averaged by 7.3% *(74)*, but the following year this was reduced to 2%, indicating that there was no room for complacency. The WHO has been proactive and is redirecting funding to those countries most in need. In October 1998, a global partnership called Stop TB was launched to coordinate every aspect of TB control, and by 2002, the partnership had more than 150 member states. A target was set to detect at least 70% of infectious cases by 2005.

The acquisition of TB infection is not necessarily followed by disease because the infection may heal spontaneously. It may take weeks or months before disease becomes apparent, or infection may remain dormant for years before reactivation in later life especially if the person becomes debilitated or immunocompromised. Contrary to popular belief, the majority of cases of TB in people who are immunocompetent pass unnoticed. Of the reported cases, 75% involve the lung, whereas nonrespiratory (e.g., bone, heart, kidney, and brain) or dissemination (miliary TB) are more common in immigrant ethnic groups and individuals who are immunocompromised *(75)*. They are also more likely to develop resistant strains. In the general population, there is an esti-mated 10% lifetime risk of TB infection progressing to disease *(76)*.

There has been an increase in the number of cases of TB associated with HIV owing to either new infection or reactivation. TB infection is more likely to progress to active TB in HIV-positive individuals, with a greater than 50% lifetime risk *(77)*. TB can also lead to a worsening of HIV with an increase in viral load *(78)*. Therefore, the need for early diagnosis is paramount, but it can be more difficult because pulmonary TB may present with nonspecific features (e.g., bilateral, unilateral, or lower lobe shadowing) *(79)*.

7.3.2. Symptoms of Pulmonary TB

After an incubation period of 4–12 weeks, symptoms may develop (*see* Table 6).

7.3.3. Routes of Transmission

The main route is airborne through infected droplets, but prolonged or close contact is needed. Nonrespiratory disease is not considered a risk unless the mycobacterium is aerosolized under exceptional circumstances (e.g., during surgery) or there are open abscesses.

7.3.4. Period of Infectivity

A person is considered infectious as long as viable bacilli are found in induced sputum. Untreated or incompletely treated people may be intermittently sputum positive for years.

After 2 weeks of appropriate treatment, the individual is usually considered as noninfectious. This period is often extended for treatment of MDR-TB or for those with concomitant HIV. Patient compliance also plays an important factor.

7.3.5. At-Risk Groups

The risk of infection is directly proportional to the degree of exposure. More severe disease occurs in individuals who are malnourished, immunocompromised (e.g., HIV), and substance misusers.

People who are immunocompromised are at special risk of MDR-TB or Mycobacterium avium intracellulare (MAI).

7.3.6. Management in Custody

Staff with disease should stay off work until the treatment course is complete and serial sputum samples no longer contain bacilli. Staff in contact with disease who have been vaccinated with BCG are at low risk of acquiring disease but should minimize their time spent in the cell. Those who have not received BCG or who are immunocompromised should avoid contact with the detainee wherever possible. Detainees with MAI do not pose a risk to a staff member, unless the latter is immunocompromised. Any staff member who is pregnant, regardless of BCG status or type of TB, should avoid contact.

Anyone performing mouth-to-mouth resuscitation with a person with untreated or suspected pulmonary TB should be regarded as a household contact and should report to occupational health or their physician if no other route exists. They should also be educated regarding the symptoms of TB. Anyone who is likely to come into repeated contact with individuals at risk of

TB should receive BCG (if he or she has not already done so), regardless of age, even though there is evidence to suggest that BCG administered in adult life is less effective. This does not apply to individuals who are immunocompromised or pregnant women. In the latter case, vaccination should preferably be deferred until after delivery.

Detainees with disease (whether suspected or diagnosed) who have not been treated or treatment is incomplete should be kept in custody for the minimum time possible. Individuals with TB who are immunocompromised are usually too ill to be detained; if they are, they should be considered at greater risk of transmitting disease to staff. Any detainee with disease should be encouraged to cover his or her mouth and nose when coughing and sneezing.

Staff should wear gloves when in contact with the detainee and when handling clothing and bedding. Any bedding should be bagged after use and laundered or incinerated. The cell should be deemed out of action until it has been ventilated and professionally decontaminated, although there is no hard evidence to support that there is a risk of transmission from this route *(70)*.

7.4. Severe Acute Respiratory Syndrome

7.4.1. General Information

On March 14, 2003, the WHO issued a global warning to health authorities about a new atypical pneumonia called SARS. The earliest case was believed to have originated in the Guandong province of China on November 16, 2002. The causative agent was identified as a new Corona virus—SARS–CoV *(80,81)*. By the end of June 2003, 8422 cases had been reported from 31 different countries, with a total of 916 deaths. Approximately 92% of cases occurred in China (including Hong Kong, Taiwan, and Macao). The case fatality rate varied from less than 1% in people younger than 24 years, 6% in persons aged 25–44 years, 15% in those aged 44–64 years, and more than 50% in persons 65 years or older. On July 5, 2003, the WHO reported that the last human chain of transmission of SARS had been broken and lifted the ban from all countries. However, it warned that everyone should remain vigilant, because a resurgence of SARS is possible. Their warning was well given because in December 2003, a new case of SARS was detected in China. At the time of this writing, three more cases have been identified. Knowledge about the epidemiology and ecology of SARS–CoV and the disease remains limited; however, the experience gained from the previous outbreak enabled the disease to be contained rapidly, which is reflected in the few cases reported since December 2003. There is still no specific treatment or preventative vaccine that has been developed.

7.4.2. Incubation Period and Symptoms

The incubation period is short, approx 3–6 days (maximum 10 days), and, despite the media frenzy surrounding the initial outbreak, SARS is less infectious than influenza. The following clinical case definition of SARS has been developed for public health purposes *(82)*.

A person with a history of any combination of the following should be examined for SARS:

- Fever (at least 38°C); and
- One of more symptoms of lower respiratory tract illness (cough, difficulty in breathing, or dyspnea); and
- Radiographic evidence of lung infiltrates consistent with pneumonia or respiratory distress syndrome or postmortem findings of these with no identifiable cause; and
- No alternative diagnosis can fully explain the illness.

Laboratory tests have been developed that include detection of viral RNA by PCR from nasopharyngeal secretions or stool samples, detection of antibodies by enzyme-linked immunosorbent assay or immunofluorescent antibody in the blood, and viral culture from clinical specimens.

7.4.3. Route of Transmission

Available information suggests that close contact via aerosol or infected droplets from an infected individual provide the highest risk of acquiring the disease. Most cases occurred in hospital workers caring for an index case or his or her close family members.

7.4.4. Management in Custody

Despite the re-emergence of SARS, it is highly unlikely that a case will be encountered in the custodial setting in the near future. However, forensic physicians must remain alert for the SARS symptoms and keep up-to-date with recent outbreaks. Information can be obtained from the WHO on a daily basis from its Web site. If SARS is suspected, medical staff should wear gloves and a surgical mask when examining a suspected case; however, masks are not usually available in custody. Anyone suspected of SARS must be sent immediately to the hospital, and staff who have had prolonged close contact should be alerted as to the potential symptoms.

8. INFECTIONS TRANSMITTED THROUGH THE FECAL–ORAL ROUTE

8.1. General Considerations

The most consistent feature of diseases transmitted through the fecal–oral route is diarrhea (*see* Table 7). Infective agents include bacteria, viruses,

Table 7

Common Causes of Infective Diarrhea

Cause	Symptoms	Incubation	Infectivity	Notes
Campylobacter	C, F, N, V, BD	1–10 days	Untreated, 7 weeks	Requires antibiotics. Seek advice. Acute phase exclude from custody.
Escherichia coli O157:H7	BD (or WD) F unusual	3–8 days	Up to 7 days	Person to person spread. Can be serious with TTP, HUS, dehydration. Seek advice.
Norwalk virus	N, V, D, A P, mild F	24–48 hours	Up to 48 hours after diarrhea stops	Mild to moderate. Self-limiting.
Rotavirus	F, V, WD	24–72 hours	Up to 8 days. Up to 30 d in immuno-compromised	Symptomatic treatment. Persists in environment.
Salmonella	H, AP, D, N, F ± V	6–72 hours	1 day to 1 week	Persistent carriage can occur. Requires antibiotics. Seek advice.
Shigella	DY/WD, F, N (C,V)	12–96 hours	Up to 4 weeks	Usually mild in United Kingdom. Can be severe in IC. Requires antibiotics in custody. Take advice. Person to person spread.

AP, abdominal pain; BD, bloody diarrhea; C, cramps; D, diarrhea; DY, dysentery (blood and mucus); F, fever; H, headache; HUS, hemolytic–uremic syndrome; IC, immunocompromised; N, nausea; TTP, thrombotic thrombocytopenic purpura; V, vomiting; WD, watery diarrhea.

and protozoa. Because the causes are numerous, it is beyond the remit of this chapter to cover them all. It is safest to treat all diarrhea as infectious, unless the detainee has a proven noninfectious cause (e.g., Crohn's disease or ulcerative colitis).

All staff should wear gloves when in contact with the detainee or when handling clothing and bedding, and contaminated articles should be laundered or incinerated. The cell should be professionally cleaned after use, paying particular attention to the toilet area.

8.3. Hepatitis A

8.3.1. Epidemiology and Prevalence

This viral hepatitis occurs worldwide, with variable prevalence. It is highest in countries where hygiene is poor and infection occurs year-round. In temperate climates, the peak incidence is in autumn and winter, but the trend is becoming less marked.

All age groups are susceptible if they are nonimmune or have not been vaccinated. In developing countries, the disease occurs in early childhood, whereas the reverse is true in countries where the standard of living is higher.

In the United Kingdom, there has been a gradual decrease in the number of reported cases from 1990 to 2000 (83,84). This results from, in part, improved standards of living and the introduction of an effective vaccine. The highest incidence occurs in the 15- to 34-year-old age group. Approximately 25% of people older than 40 years have natural immunity, leaving the remainder susceptible to infection (85).

Small clusters occur from time to time, associated with a breakdown in hygiene. There is also an increasing incidence of HAV in gay or bisexual men and their partners (86). An unpublished study in London in 1996 showed a seroprevalence of 23% among gay men (Young Y et al., unpublished).

8.3.2. Symptoms

The clinical picture ranges from asymptomatic infection through a spectrum to fulminant hepatitis. Unlike HBV and HCV, HAV does not persist or progress to chronic liver damage. Infection in childhood is often mild or asymptomatic but in adults tends to be more severe.

After an incubation period of 15–50 days (mean 28 days) symptomatic infection starts with the abrupt onset of jaundice anything from 2 days to 3 weeks after the anicteric phase. It lasts for approximately the same length of time and is often accompanied by a sudden onset of fever.

HAV infection can lead to hospital admission in all age groups but is more likely with increasing age as is the duration of stay.

The overall mortality is less than 1%, but 15% of people will have a prolonged or relapsing illness within 6–9 months (CDC fact sheet). Fulminant hepatitis occurs in less than 1% of people but is more likely to occur in individuals older than 65 years or in those with pre-existing liver disease. In patients who are hospitalized, case fatality ranges from 2% in 50–59 years olds to nearly 13% in those older than 70 years *(84)*.

8.3.3. Period of Infectivity

The individual is most infectious in the 2 weeks before the onset of jaundice, when he or she is asymptomatic. This can make control of infection difficult because the disease is not recognized.

8.3.4. Routes of Transmission

The main route is fecal–oral through the ingestion of contaminated water and food. It can also be transmitted by personal contact, including homosexuals practicing anal intercourse and fellatio. There is a slight risk from blood transfusions if the donor is in the acute phase of infection. It should not be considered a risk from needlestick injuries unless clinical suspicion of HAV is high.

8.3.5. Risk Groups

Risk groups include homeless individuals, homosexuals, IDUs, travellers abroad who have not been vaccinated, patients with chronic liver disease and chronic infection with HBV and HCV, employees and residents in daycare centers and hostels, sewage workers, laboratory technicians, and those handling nonhuman primates.

Several large outbreaks have occurred among IDUs, some with an epidemiological link to prisons *(87,88)*. Transmission occurs during the viremic phase of the illness through sharing injecting equipment and via fecal–oral routes because of poor living conditions *(89)*. There have also been reports of HAV being transmitted through drugs that have been carried in the rectum. A study in Vancouver showed that 40% of IDUs had past infection of HAV, and they also showed an increased prevalence among homosexual/bisuexual men *(90)*.

8.3.6. Management in Custody

Staff with disease should report to occupational health and stay off work until the end of the infective period. Those in contact with disease (either through exposure at home or from an infected detainee) should receive prophylactic treatment as soon as possible (*see* Subheading 8.3.7.).

Table 8
Suspicion of Exotica?
History and Examination Aide Memoir

- Has the detainee traveled to Africa, South East Asia, the Indian subcontinent, Central/South America, or the Far East in the last 6–12 months?
- Ascertain whether he or she received any vaccinations before travel and, if so, which ones.
- Ask if he or she took malaria prophylaxis, what type, and whether he or she completed the course.
- Ask if he or she swam in any stagnant lakes during the trip.
- If the answer to any of the above is yes, ask if he or she has experienced any of the following symptoms:
  - A fever/hot or cold flushes/shivering.
  - Diarrhea ± abdominal cramps ± blood or slime in the stool.
  - A rash.
  - Persistent headaches ± light sensitivity.
  - Nausea or vomiting.
  - Aching muscles/joints.
  - A persistent cough (dry or productive) lasting at least 3 weeks.
- Take temperature.
- Check skin for signs of a rash and note nature and distribution.
- Check throat.
- Listen carefully to the lungs for signs of infection/consolidation.

To minimize the risk of acquiring disease in custody, staff should wear gloves when dealing with the detainee and then wash their hands thoroughly. Gloves should be disposed of only in the clinical waste bags.

Detainees with disease should be kept in custody for the minimum time possible. They should only be sent to the hospital if fulminant hepatitis is suspected. The cell should be quarantined after use and professionally cleaned. Any bedding or clothing should be handled with gloves and laundered or incinerated according to local policy. Detainees reporting contact with disease should be given prophylactic treatment as soon as possible (*see* Subheading 8.3.7.).

8.3.7. Prophylaxis and Treatment

Contacts of HAV should receive HAV vaccine (e.g., Havrix Monodose or Avaxim) if they have not been previously immunized or had disease. Human normal immunoglobulin (HNIG), 500 mg, deep intramuscular in gluteal muscle should be used in the following circumstances:

Table 9
Tropical Diseases That Present With Fever

Disease	Countries	Incubation	Transmission	Management
Dengue	Most hot climates	3–14 days	Mosquito No person-to-person in UK	Symptomatic
Hantavirus	Eastern Europe	2 days–8 weeks	No person-to-person in UK	Symptomatic
Lassa Fever	West Africa			Hospital
Malaria	Sub-Saharan Africa, Southeast Asia, South America	7 days–1 years	Mosquito	No person-to-person in UK. Requires urgent treatment. Hospital.
Typhoid	Hot climates	Up to 72 hours	Oral–fecal	Requires antibiotics.
Yellow Fever	Sub-Saharan Africa, parts of South America	3–6 days No person-to-person in UK	Mosquito	Hospital

UK, United Kingdom.

Table 10
Tropical Diseases That Present With Diarrhea

Disease	Incubation	Infectivity	Transmission	Management
Amoebic dysentery	Days to months	1 Year	Oral–fecal	Requires antibiotics
Cholera	Hours–5 days	3–5 days after recovery	Oral–fecal; vomit.	Requires antibiotics
Giardia	3–25 days	Months	Oral–fecal	Treat with tinidazole
Malaria	7 days –1 years	None	No person-to-person	Urgent treatment. Hospital.
Typhoid	Up to 72 hours	Days to weeks	Oral–fecal	Requires antibiotics

- The contact is older than 50 years.
- Has cirrhosis or pre-existing HBV, HBC, or HDV.
- Contact has occurred more than 8 d but less than 28 days from exposure.

Staff at higher risk of coming in to contact with HAV should consider being vaccinated before exposure. Two doses of vaccine given 6–12 months apart give at least 10 years of protection.

There is no specific treatment for HAV, except supportive measures and symptomatic treatment.

9. EXOTICA

Although the chance of encountering a tropical disease in custo1dy is small, it is worth bearing in mind. It is not necessary for a forensic physician to be able to diagnose the specific disease but simply to recognize that the detainee/staff member is ill and whether he or she needs to be sent to the hospital (*see* Tables 8–10).

This is best achieved by knowing the right questions to ask and carrying out the appropriate examination. Tables 8–10 should be used as an aide to not missing some more unusual diseases.

REFERENCES

1. UK Health Guidelines. Guidance for Clinical Health Care Workers: Protection Against Infection with Blood-borne Viruses; Recommendations of the Expert Advisory Group on AIDS and the Advisory Group on Hepatitis. [HSC 1998/063], NHS Executive, London, UK, 1998.
2. Guidelines for Hand Hygiene in Health Care Settings. Recommendations of the Healthcare Infection Control Practices Advisory Committee and the HICPAC/ SHEA/APIC/IDSA Hand Hygiene Task Force. MMWR Mob. Mortal. Wkly. Rep. 51:1–44, 2002.
3. National Model Regulations for the Control of Workplace Hazardous Substances. Commonwealth of Australia, National Occupational Health and Safety Committee. [NOHSC:1005], 1994.
4. Nicholson F. Chapter 4: Infectious diseases and an at risk exposure. In: Stark M. M., Rogers, D.J., Norfolk, G. A. eds., Good Practice Guidelines for Forensic Medical Examiners, 2nd Ed. Metropolitan Police. GPG Editors, Oxford, UK, 2004.
5. Bolyard, E, A., Tablan, O. C., Williams, W. W., Pearson, M. L., Shapiro, C. N., Deitchman, S. D., and the Hospital Infection Control Practices Advisory Committee. Guideline for infection control in health care personnel. Am. J. Infect. Control. 26:289–354, 1998.
6. Prevalence of HIV and hepatitis infections in the United Kingdom 2000. Annual report of the Unlinked Anonymous Prevalence Monitoring Programme. Report from the Unlinked Anonymous Surveys Steering Group. Department of Health, London, UK, 2001.

7. A Strategy for Infectious Diseases-Progress Report. Blood-borne and sexually transmitted viruses: hepatitis. Department of Health, London, UK, 2002.

8. Perspectives in disease prevention and health promotion update. Universal precautions for prevention of transmission of human immuno-deficiency virus, hepatitis B virus and other bloodborne pathogens in health-care settings. Morb. Mortal. Wkly. Rep. 37:377–388, 1988.

9. Martinson, F. E., Weigle, K.A., Royce, R. A., Weber, D. J., Suchindran, C. M., Lemon, S. M. Risk factors for horizontal transmission of hepatitis B in a rural district in Ghana. Am. J. Epidemiol. 147:478–487, 1998.

10. Verma, G., Dalai, P., Bapat, M., Rathi, P., Abraham, P. Familial clustering of hepatitis B infection: study of a family. Indian J. Gastroenterol. 22:22–23, 2003.

11. Erol, S., Ozkurt, Z., Ertek, M., Tasyaran, M. A. Intrafamilial transmission of hepatitis B in the Eastern Anatolian region of Turkey. Euro. J. Gastroenterol. Hepatol. 15: 345–349, 2003.

12. Hutchinson, S., Goldberg, D., Gore, S. et al. Hepatitis B outbreak at Glenochil prison during January to June 1993. Epidemiol. Infect. 121:185–191,1998.

13. European Network for HIV/AIDS and Hepatitis Prevention in Prisons. Second annual report. The Network, Bonn and Marseille, May 1998.

14. Weild, A. R., Gill, O. N., Bennett, D., Livingstone, S. J. M., Parry, J. V., Curran, L. Prevalence of HIV, hepatitis B and hepatitis C antibodies in prisoners in England and Wales; a national survey. Communicable Dis. Public Health. 3:121–126, 2000.

15. Alter, M. J. The epidemiology of acute and chronic hepatitis C. Clin. Liver Dis. 1: 559–562, 1997.

16. Frank, C., Mohamed, M. K., Strickland, G. T. The role of the parenteral antischistosomal therapy in the spread of hepatitis C virus in Egypt. Lancet. 355:887–891, 2000.

17. Chronic Hepatitis C: Disease Management. NIH publication No. 03-4230. February 2003.

18. Hepatitis C strategy for England. Department of Health, London, UK, August 14, 2002.

19. Gish, R. G., Lau, J. Y. N. Hepatitis C virus: eight years old. Viral Hepatitis Rev. 3:17–37, 1997.

20. Ramsay, M. E., Balogun, M. A., Collins, M., Balraj, V. Laboratory surveillance of hepatitis C virus in England and Wales: 1992–1996. Communicable Dis. Public Health. 1:89–94, 1998.

21. Hepatitis D. Sean Lacey, Assistant Professor, Dept. of Medicine, Case Western Reserve University. http://www.emedicine@topic994.htm. Accessed Feb. 2004. Last update September 6, 2001.

22. Cumulative UK Data to end of December 2002. AIDS/HIV quarterly surveillance tables provided by the PHLS AIDS centre (CDSC) and the Scottish centre for Infection and Environmental Health. No 57: 02/4. February 2003.

23. HIV and AIDS in the UK in 2001. Communicable Disease Surveillance Centre. An update. November 2002.

24. International Perinatal HIV Group. Mode of vertical transmission of HIV-1. A metanalysis of fifteen prospective cohort studies. N. Engl. J. Med. 340:977–987, 1999.

25. Duong, T., Ades, A., Gibbs, D. M., et al. Vertical transmission rate for HIV in the British Isles estimated on Surveillance data. Br. Med. J. 319:1227–1229, 1999.

26. Limb, S., Kawar, M., Forster, G. E. HIV post-exposure prophylaxis after sexual assault: the experience of a sexual assault service in London. Int. J. STDS AIDS. 13:602–605, 2002.

27. HIV Post-Exposure Prophylaxis: Guidance from the UK Chief Medical Officer's Expert Advisory Group on AIDS. UK Health Department, London, UK, 2000.

28. Jochimsen, E. M. Failures of zidovudine post exposure prophylaxis. Am. J. Med. 102:52–55, 1997.

29. Hawkins, D. A., Asboe, D., Barlow, K., Evans, B. Seroconversion to HIV-1 following a needlestick injury despite combination post-exposure prophylaxis. J. Infect. 43:12–15, 2001.

30. Salisbury, D. M., Begg, N. T. Department of Health, Immunisation Against Infectious Disease. United Kingdom: Her Majesty's Stationery Office, London, UK, 1996.

31. Sinha, D. P. Chickenpox—disease predominantly affecting adults in rural West Bengal, India. Int. J. Epidemiol. 5:367–374, 1996.

32. Centers for Disease Control and Prevention. Prevention of *varicella*: recommendations of the Advisory Committee on Immunization Practices. Morb. Mortal. Wkly. Rep. 45:1–36, 1996.

33. Fairley, C. K., Miller, E. *Varicella-zoster* virus epidemiology. A changing scene? J. Infect. Dis. 174 (Suppl 3):314–319, 1996.

34. Smego, R. A., Asperilla, M. O. Use of Acyclovir for *varicella* pneumonia during pregnancy. Obstet. Gynecol. 78:1112–1116, 1991.

35. Pastuszak, A. L., Levy, M., Schick, B., et al. Outcome after maternal varicella infection in the first 20 weeks of pregnancy. N. Engl. J. Med. 330:901–905, 1994.

36. Miller, E., Cradoc-Watson, J. E., Ridehalgh, M. K. Outcome in newborn babies given anti-*varicella zoster* immunoglobulin after perinatal maternal infection with *varicella zoster* virus. Lancet. 2:371–373, 1989.

37. Gilden, D. H., Vafai, A., Shtram, Y., et al. *Varicella-zoster* virus DNA in human sensory ganglia. Nature. 306:478–80, 1983.

38. Dworkin, R. H., Schmader, K. E. Epidemiology and natural history of herpes zoster and post herpetic neuralgia. In: Watson, C. P. N., Gershon, A. A., eds., Herpes Zoster and Postherpetic Neuralgia. 2nd Ed. Elsevier Press, New York, NY, 2001, pp. 39–64.

39. Desmond, R. A., Weiss, H. L., Arani, R. B., et al. Clinical applications for change-point analysis of herpes zoster pain. J. Pain Sys. Manage. 23:510–516, 2002.

40. Gnann, J. W. Jr., Whitley, R. J. Herpes Zoster. N. Engl. J. Med. 347:340–346, 2002.

41. Haustein, U. F., Hlawa, B. Treatment of scabies with permethrin versus lindane and benzoyl benzoate. Acta Derm. Venereol. (Stock). 69:348–351, 1989.

42. Brown, S., Becher, J., Brady, W. Treatment of ectoparasitic infections; review of the English-language literature. 1982–1992. Clin. Infect. Dis. 20 (Suppl 1):S104–S109, 1995.

43. Klutymans, J., Van Belkum, A., Verbrugh, H. Nasal carriage of Staphylococcus aureus: epidemiology and control measures. Infect. Dis. Clin. North Am. 3:901–913, 1989.

44. Lowry, F. D. Staphylococcus aureus infections. N. Engl. J. Med. 339:520–532, 1998.
45. Centers for Disease Control and Prevention. Community-acquired methicillin-resistant Staphylococcus aureus infections—Michigan. Morb. Mortal. Wkly. Rep. 30:185–187, 1981.
46. Saravolatz, L. D., Markowitz, N., Arking, L., Pohlod, D., Fisher, E. Methicillin-resistant Staphylococcus aureus, Epidmiologic observations during a community acquired outbreak. Ann. Intern. Med. 96:11–16, 1982.
47. Health Protection Agency. Emergence of PVL-producing strains of Staphylococcus aureus. Commun. Dis. Rep. CDR Wkly. [serial online]. 13: 2003. Available at Website: (http://www.phls.org.uk/publications). Accessed in Jan. 2004.
48. Summanen, P. H., Talan, D. A., Strong, C., et al. Bacteriology of skin and soft tissue infections: comparison of infections in intravenous drug users and individuals with no history of intravenous drug use. Clin. Infect. Dis. 20(Suppl 2):S279–S282, 1995.
49. Bohlen, L. M., Muhlemann, K., Dubuis, O., Aebi, C., Tauber, M. G. Outbreak among drug users caused by a clonal strain of group a streptococcus. Dispatches—emerging infectious diseases. Available at Website: (http://www.cdc.gov). Accessed March 2003.
50. Lettington, W. Bacteriological skin and subcutaneous infections in injecting drug users—relevance for custody. J. Clin. Forensic Med. 9:65–69, 2002.
51. Passaro, D. J., Werner, S. B., McGee, J., MacKenzie, W. R., Vugia, D. J. Wound botulism associated with black tar heroin among injecting drug users. JAMA. 279, 859–63, 1998.
52. Brazier, J.S., Duerden, B. I., Hall, V., et al. Isolation and identification of clostridium spp from infections associated with injection of drugs: experiences of a microbiological investigation team. J. Med. Microbiol. 51:985–989, 2002.
53. Greater Glasgow Health Board, SCIFH. Unexplained illness among drug injectors in Glasgow. Eurosurveillance 4: 500518, August 6, 2001.
54. Kuylaylat, M. N., Barakat, N., Stephan, R. N., Gutierrez, I. Embolization of illicit needle fragments. J. Emerg. Med. 11:403–408, 1993.
55. Ngaage, D. L., Cowen, M. E. Right ventricular needle embolus in an injecting drug user: the need for early removal. Emerg. Med. J. 18:500–501, 2001.
56. Spanierman, C. Departments of Emergency Medicine and Pediatrics, Lutheran General Hospital of Oak Brook, Advocate Health System. eMedicine-Human Bites, Available at Website: (http://www.emedicine.com/ped/topic246.htm). Accessed in Feb 2004.
57. Presutti, J. P. Prevention and treatment of dog bites. Am. Fam. Physician. 63:1567–1572, 2001.
58. Revis, D. R., Jr., Seagel, M. B. Human bites. Department of Plastic Surgery, University of Florida College of Medicine, eMedicine-Human Bites. Available at Website: (http://www.emedicine.com/ent/topic728.htm). Accessed in Feb 2004.
59. Guidelines for public health management of meningococcal diseases in the UK. Communicable Disease and Public Health. PHLS. 5:187–204, 2002.
60. Miller, E., Salisbury, D., Ramsay, M. Planning, registration and implementation of an immunisation campaign against meningococcal serogroup C disease in the UK: a success story. Vaccine. 20 (Suppl 1):S58–S67, 2001.

61. Ramsay, M., Andrews, N., Kaczmarski, E., Miller, E. Efficacy of meningococcal serogroup C conjugate vaccine in teenagers and toddlers in England. Lancet. 357:195–196, 2001.
62. PHLS. Quadrivalent meningoimmunisation required for pilgrims to Saudi Arabia. Commun. Dis. Rep. CDR Wkly. 11:8/11/2001. http://www.phls.org.uk/publications. Accessed on May 11, 2004.
63. Boutet, R., Stuart, J. M., Kaczmarski, E., Gray, S. J., Jones, M., Andrews, N. Risk of laboratory-acquired meningococcal disease. J. Hosp. Infect. 49:282–284, 2001.
64. Orr, H., Kaczmarski, E., Sarangi, J., Pankhania, B., Stuart, J. Cluster of meningococcal disease in rugby match spectators. Commun. Dis. Public Health. 4:316–317, 2001.
65. Salisbury, D. M., Begg, N. T. Immunisation against Infectious Disease. Her Majesty's Stationery Office, London, UK, 1996.
66. CDSC. Ciprofloxacin as a chemoprophylactic agent for meningococcal disease—low risk of anaphylactoid reactions. Commun. Dis. Rep. Wkly. 11:2001.
67. Joint Formulary Committee 2002–03. British National Formulary. British Medical Association and Royal Pharmaceutical Society of Great Britain, London, UK, 2003.
68. Omerod, L. P., Watson, J. M., Pozniak, A., et al. Notification of tuberculosis an updated code of practice for England and Wales. J. Royal Coll. Phys. Lond. 31:299–303, 1997.
69. Statutory notifications to the Communicable Disease Surveillance Centre. Preliminary annual report on tuberculosis cases reported in England, Wales, and N. Ireland. http://www.hpa.org.UK/infections. Accessed in Dec. 2003.
70. The Interdepartmental Working Group on Tuberculosis. The prevention and control of tuberculosis in the United Kingdom: UK guidance on the prevention and control of transmission of 1. HIV-related tuberculosis 2. Drug-resistant, including multiple drug-resistant, tuberculosis. Department of Health, Scottish Office, The Welsh Office, Scotland, 1998.
71. Joint Tuberculosis Committee of the British Thoracic Society. Control and prevention of tuberculosis in the United Kingdom: Code of Practice 2000. Thorax. 55:887–901, 2000.
72. Cantwell, M. F., Snider, D. E., Cauthen, G. M., Onorato, I. M. Epidemiology of tuberculosis in the United States, 1985 through 1992. JAMA. 272:535–539, 1994.
73. Centers for Disease Control. Nosocomial transmission of multi-drug resistant tuberculosis among HIV-infected persons—Florida, New York, 1988–1991. Morb. Mortal. Wkly. Rep. 40:585–591, 1991.
74. Navin, T. R., McNabb, S. J. N., Crawford, J. T. The Continued Threat of Tuberculosis. Emerg. Infect. Dis. [serial online]. Available at Website:(http://www.cdc.gov/ncidod/EID/vol8no11/02–0468). Accessed November 2002.
75. Sepkowitz, D. V. Chapter 5: Tuberculosis in HIV-Infected Individuals. In: Lutwick, Larry I., ed., Tuberculosis—A Clinical Handbook. Chapman & Hall Medical, London, UK, 1995.
76. Murray, J. F. The White Plague: down and out, or up and coming? Am. Rev. Resp. Dis. 140:1788–1795.
77. Selwyn, P. A., Hartel, D., Lewis, V. A., et al. A prospective study of the risk of tuberculosis among intravenous drug users with human immunodeficiency virus infection. N. Engl. J. Med. 320:545–550, 1989.

78. Wallis, R. S., Vjecha, M., Amir-Tahmasseb, M., et al. Influence of tuberculosis on human immunodeficiency virus (HIV-1): enhanced cytokine expression and elevated B_2-microglobulin in HIV-1 associated tuberculosis. J. Infect. Dis. 167:43–48, 1993.

79. Long, R., Maycher, B., Scalcini, M., Manfreda, J. The chest roenterogram in pulmonary tuberculosis patients seropositive for human immunodeficiency virus type 1. Chest. 99:123–127, 1991.

80. Peiris, J. S. M., Lais, T., Poon, L. L. M., et al. Coronavirus as a possible cause of severe acute respiratory syndrome. Lancet. 361:1319–1325, 2003.

81. Donnelly, C. A., Ghani, A. C., Leung, G. M., et al. Epidemiological determinants of spread of causal agents of severe acute respiratory syndrome in Hong Kong. Lancet. 361:761–766, 2003.

82. Alert, verification and public health management of SARS in post-outbreak period. World Health Organization. Available at Website: (http://www.who.int/csr/sars/postoutbreak/en/). Accessed 14, 2003.

83. Gay, N. J., Morgan-Capner, P., Wright, J., Farrington, C. P., Miller, E. Age-specific antibody prevalence to hepatitis A in England: implications for disease control. Epidemiol. Infect. 113:113–120, 1994.

84. Crowcroft, N. S., Walsh, B., Davison, K. L., Gungabissoon, U., PHLS Advisory Committee on Vaccination and Immunisation. Guidelines for the control of hepatitis A infection. Commun. Dis. Public Health. 4:213–227, 2001.

85. Irwin, D. J., Millership, S. Control of a community hepatitis A outbreak using hepatitis A vaccine. Commun. Dis. Public Health. 2:184–187, 1999.

86. Katz, M. H., Hsu, L., Wong, E., Liska, S., Anderson, L., Janssen, R. S. Seroprevalence of and risk factors for hepatitis A infection among young homosexual and bisexual men. J. Infect. Dis. 175:1225–1229, 1997.

87. Harkess, J., Gildon, B., Istre, G. R. Outbreaks of hepatitis A among illicit drug users, Oklahoma, 1984–1987. Am. J. Public Health. 79:463–466, 1989.

88. Hutin, Y. J., Bell, B. P., Marshall, K. L., et al. Identifying target groups for a potential vaccination program during a hepatitis A community outbreak. Am. J. Public Health. 89:918–19, 1999.

89. Hutin, Y. J., Sabin, K. M., Hutwagner, L. C., et al. Multiple modes of hepatitis A transmission among metamphetamine users. Am. J. Epidemiol. 152:186–192, 2000.

90. Ochnio, J. J., Patrick, D., Hom, T. G., et al. Past infection with hepatitis A among Vancouver Street youth, injection drug users and men who have sex with men; implications for vaccination programmes. Can. Med. Assoc. J. 165:293–297, 2001.

Chapter 10

Substance Misuse

Margaret M. Stark and Guy Norfolk

1. INTRODUCTION

The number of individuals passing through the criminal justice system with substance misuse problems is increasing, and doctors should be aware of current drug trends in their area.

In the United States, there is a well-established program of research drug-testing urine samples of people arrested by the police—known as the Arrestee Drug Abuse Monitoring Program (ADAM), which recently replaced the Drug Use Forecasting Program, which was originally established in 1988. Data from urinalyses performed in 2000 show that 64% or more of adult male arrestees had recently used at least one of the following drugs: cocaine, marijuana, opiates, methamphetamine or phencyclidine *(1)*. Marijuana was the drug most commonly used, followed by cocaine.

The New English and Welsh Arrestee Drug Abuse Monitoring (NEW-ADAM) program is a national research study of interviews and voluntary urine tests designed to establish the prevalence of drug use among arrestees. Summary results of the first two years of the NEW-ADAM program *(2)* show that 69% of urine samples from arrestees tested positive for one or more illegal drugs and 36% tested positive for two or more substances. In particular, 38% of arrestees tested positive for opiates and/or cocaine.

2. General Principles (3)

2.1. History and Examination

A detailed history of recent drug use, including alcohol, must be obtained to establish whether the individual is a currently dependent or recreational user

From: *Clinical Forensic Medicine: A Physician's Guide, 2nd Edition*
Edited by: M. M. Stark © Humana Press Inc., Totowa, NJ

Table 1
Substance Misuse—History

- Period of regular use
- The quantity used per day on a "typical" day
- The frequency of use
- Route of administration
- The amount used in the last 24 h
- Time of the last dose
- Prescribed drugs
- Experience of withdrawal

Table 2
Substance Misuse—Examination

• Blood pressure	• Yawning
• Pulse rate	• Lachyrmation
• Temperature	• Rhinorrhea
• Pupil size	• Gooseflesh
• Pupillary reaction to light	• Sweating
• Conscious level (lethargy/stupor/coma)	• Bowel sounds
• Glasgow Coma Scale	• Presence of needle tracks
• Orientated in time, place, and person	• Restlessness/agitation
• Speech	• Disordered perceptions
• Pallor	• Coordination
• Flushed	• Gait
• Tremor at rest	• Romberg's
	• Auscultation of the chest

(Table 1). Street names of substances will vary from country to country, within regions in the same country, with the cultural background of the user, and with time. The examination should look for signs of intoxication, withdrawal, or previous drug use (Table 2). Baseline parameters are useful for re-examination if the detainee is kept in custody. Purity of illicit substances will vary between countries and from year to year; this may be reflected in the drug history obtained, with increasing amounts ingested as drug purity diminishes. Averaged figures from recent seizures (police and customs) available from the United States in 2001 show purity for cocaine at 69%, heroin 50%, and methamphetamine 40% (4), compared with UK figures in 2000 of cocaine 52%, heroin 47%, and amphetamine 5% (5). There were significant differences between the purity of drugs seized by customs and the police, showing the extent to which certain drugs are cut prior to distribution by dealers.

2.2. *Harm Minimization*

Information and advice should be given to the detainee by the physician on reducing the harm from continued drug misuse. Advice can be provided on a range of issues *(3,6)*:

- Blood-borne viruses (BBVs), including hepatitis B and C and HIV awareness.
- The availability of hepatitis B vaccination.
- The hazards of injecting substances and the greater safety of smoking rather than injecting
- If the individual must inject the preference for hitting a vein rather than injecting into the muscle or skin.
- Avoidance of "shared works," such as needles, syringes, spoons, etc.
- To use different sites for injecting.
- To attend for medical assistance if any pain, redness, or pus collects under the skin at an injection site.
- Information regarding the local services involved in drug counseling and treatment can also be offered.
- Other general health problems may require treatment/referral.

Substance misusers who inject may have experienced a broken needle at some time in their injecting career *(7)*. Central embolization may occur within a few hours up to several days, and this can lead to potentially fatal consequences, including pericarditis, endocarditis, and pulmonary abscesses. Needle fragments must be removed as soon as possible to avoid future complications. This may be done by the users themselves or necessitate attendance at the accident and emergency department.

Brief interventions, whereby it is possible to provide advice about the risks inherent in a range of patterns of substance use and to advise reducing or stopping use as part of screening and assessment, are useful with alcohol consumption *(8)*. A person's motivation to change is important in determining the likelihood of success of any intervention *(9)*, and such motivation may alter depending on a variety of factors. For example, negative life events, such as being arrested for an acquisitive crime motivated by a need to finance a drug habit, can introduce conflict in the detainee's mind about substance misuse and may increase the likelihood of successful intervention.

Arrest referral schemes are partnership initiatives set up to encourage drug misusers brought into contact with the police service to voluntarily participate in confidential help designed to address their drug-related problems. Early evaluation of such projects in the United Kingdom provides good evidence that such schemes can be effective in reducing drug use and drug-related crime *(10)*. In the United States, it has also been recognized that point of arrest is an appropriate stage of intervention for addressing substance misuse (1).

2.3. Prescribing

Although prompt treatment to limit or prevent the withdrawal syndrome is desirable, no central nervous system (CNS) depressant medication should be given if there is evidence of intoxication with other drugs (e.g., alcohol), because many substances have an additive effect. Consideration of whether the detainee is fit for detention is the priority. Most individuals are not detained in police custody for long, and, therefore, medical treatment may not be required. This is particularly so if there is any question that the detainee may have recently ingested substances, the full effects of which may not as yet be obvious. Reassessment after a specific period should be recommended, depending on the history given by the detainee and the examination findings.

Details of medication should be verified whenever possible. It is good practice for all new substitute opiate prescriptions to be taken initially under daily supervision (11). In the custodial situation, if the detainee is on a supervised therapy program, one can be reasonably sure the detainee is dependent on that dose; the detainee may of course be using other illicit substances as well. Recent urine test results may be checked with the clinic to see whether methadone or other drugs are detected on screening.

Particularly with opiate substitution treatment, in the absence of withdrawal signs, confirmation of such treatment should be sought before authorizing continuation. The prescribed dose of opiate substitution therapy may not necessarily indicate accurately the actual amount taken each day if not supervised, because part or all of the dose may be given to other individuals. If there is doubt about the daily dose, it can be divided and given every 12 h. It should be remembered that giving even a small amount of opiates to a nondependent individual may be fatal. Cocaine abuse accelerates the elimination of methadone; therefore, higher doses of methadone must be prescribed to individuals on maintenance regimes who continue to abuse cocaine (12). Any decision to prescribe should be made on the assessment of objective signs as opposed to subjective symptoms, and a detailed record of the history and examination should be made contemporaneously.

Good practice dictates that where treatment can be verified, it should be continued as long as it is clinically safe to do so. Evidence from the National Treatment Outcome Research Study (NTORS), a prospective study of treatment outcome among substance misusers in the United Kingdom, has shown substantial reduction across a range of problem behaviors 4–5 years after patients were admitted to national treatment programs delivered and it is important not to disrupt such programs *(13)*.

2.4. Medical Complications of Substance Misuse

Medical complications of substance misuse may give an indication of a problem in the absence of acute symptoms or signs of intoxication. Intravenous injection may result in superficial thrombophlebitis, deep vein thrombosis, and pulmonary embolus and chronic complications of limb swelling and venous ulcers. If injection occurs accidentally into an artery, vascular spasm may occur and result in ischemia, which, if prolonged, can lead to gangrene and amputation.

Cellulitis and abscesses may be seen around injection sites, and deep abscesses may extend into joints, producing septic arthritis. Self-neglect, malnutrition, and dental decay may occur, as may infectious diseases, such as hepatitis B and C, human immunodeficiency virus (HIV), and the acquired immunodeficiency syndrome (AIDS).

Skin manifestations of drug addiction may be seen more commonly in opiate rather than stimulant users, even though stimulant users inject more frequently *(14)*. This is partly because stimulants do not cause histamine release and, therefore, are seldom associated with pruritus and excoriations and also because cutaneous complications are frequently caused by the adulterants injected along with the opiates, rather than the drugs themselves. Fresh puncture sites, tattoos used to cover needle tracks, keloid formation, track marks from chronic inflammation, ulcerated areas and skin popping resulting in atrophic scars, hyperpigmentation at sites of healed abscess, puffy hands (lymphedema with obliteration of anatomic landmarks and pitting edema absent), and histamine-related urticaria (opiates act on mast cells resulting in histamine release) may be seen.

3. SPECIFIC DRUGS

The classification of drugs into their physiological or psychological actions (e.g., stimulants and sedatives), is unsatisfactory because a single drug may have several actions; it is preferable to classify drugs according to their pharmacodynamic actions (Table 3) *(15)*

3.1. Opiate Intoxication and Withdrawal

The characteristics of the medical syndromes in opiate intoxication, overdose, and withdrawal are given in Table 4. Opiates, such as heroin, may be taken orally, more usually injected, or smoked—chasing the dragon. The start

Table 3
Drugs of Misuse: How They Work

Mechanism	Transmitter
Mimicking (substituting for) natural transmitters	
• Opioids	Endorphin/encephalon
• Alcohol	GABA-A/endorphins
• Benzodiazepines	GABA-A
• Cannabis	Anandamide (?)
• LSD	5-HT (1,2 receptors)
Increasing endogenous transmitter release	
• Cocaine	Dopamine
• Amphetamine	Dopamine
• Ecstasy	5-HT/dopamine
• Solvents	Noradrenaline (?)
Blocking natural transmitters	
• Alcohol	Glutamate
• Barbiturates	Glutamate

GABA-A, γ-aminobutyric acid A type receptor; 5-HT, serotonin.
Adapted from ref. *15*.

of withdrawal will vary in time with the different opioid drugs, and it should be remembered that the severity of withdrawal symptoms is influenced greatly by psychological factors *(16)*; the environment of a police cell is likely to exacerbate these symptoms.

Chronic administration of opiate drugs results in tolerance (Table 5) to effects such as euphoria mediated by the opiate receptors and to the effects on the autonomic nervous system mediated by the noradrenergic pathways. Tolerance to heroin can develop within 2 weeks of commencing daily heroin use, occurs more slowly with methadone, and may go as quickly as it develops. With abrupt withdrawal of opiates, there is a "noradrenergic storm," which is responsible for many of the opiate withdrawal symptoms (Table 6). Cyclizine may be taken intravenously in large doses with opiates, because it is reported to enhance or prolong opioid effects, also resulting in intense stimulation, hallucinations, and seizures; tolerance and dependence on cyclizine may also result *(17)*. Many opiate users are also dependent on benzodiazepines, and concurrent benzodiazepine withdrawal may increase the severity of opiate withdrawal *(18)*.

Table 4
Medical Syndromes in Heroin Users

Syndrome (onset and duration)	Characteristics
Opiate intoxication	Conscious, sedated "nodding"; mood normal to euphoric; pinpoint pupils
Acute overdose	Unconscious; pinpoint pupils; slow shallow respirations
Opiate withdrawal	
• Anticipatory 3–4 h after the last fix (as acute effects of heroin subside)	Fear of withdrawal, anxiety, drug-craving, drug-seeking behavior
• Early 8-10 h after last fix	Anxiety, restlessness, yawning, nausea, sweating, nasal stuffiness, rhinorrhea, lacrimation, dilated pupils, stomach cramps, increased bowel sounds, drug-seeking behavior
• Fully developed 1-3 d after last fix	Severe anxiety, tremor, restlessness, pilo-erection (cold-turkey), vomiting, diarrhea, muscle spasms (kicking the habit), muscle pain, increased blood pressure, tachycardia, fever, chills, impulse-driven drug-seeking behavior
• Protracted abstinence	Hypotension, bradycardia, insomnia, loss of energy and appetite, stimulus-driven opiate cravings

From ref. *15a.*

3.1.1. Treatment of Opiate Withdrawal

Symptomatic treatment of the opiate withdrawal syndrome can often be achieved using a combination of drugs, such as benzodiazepines for anxiety and insomnia; loperamide or diphenoxylate and atropine for diarrhea; promethazine, which has antiemetic and sedative properties; and paracetamol or nonsteroidal antiinflammatories for generalized aches.

Substitution treatment may be required in more severe cases of opiate dependence using a choice of methadone, buprenorphine, or dihydrocodeine. Because street heroin varies in purity, the starting dose cannot be accurately estimated on the basis of the amount of street drug used. Therefore, substitution therapy should be titrated against the symptoms and signs of withdrawal. For example, dihydrocodeine may be commenced in a dose of 120 mg three times a day, with the dose being increased if the patient has demonstrable clinical signs of opiate withdrawal *(19)*.

Clonidine and lofexidine act as presynaptic α_2-adrenergic agonists, which inhibit the noradrenergic storm associated with opiate withdrawal. Although

Table 5
Diagnostic Criteria for Opioid Dependence and Severity of Opioid Dependence

1. Opioids are taken in larger amounts or over a longer period that the person intended.
2. A desire for the drug persists, or the patient has made one or more unsuccessful effort to cut down or to control opioid use.
3. A great deal of time is spent in activities necessary to obtain opioids (such as theft), taking the drug, or recovering from its effects.
4. The patient is frequently intoxicated or has withdrawal symptoms when expected to fulfill major role obligations at work, school or home (e.g., does not go to work, goes to school or work "high," is intoxicated while taking care of children) or when opioid use is physically hazardous (such as driving under the influence).
5. Important social, occupational, or recreational activities are given up or reduced.
6. Marked tolerance; needs greatly increased amounts of the drug—at least 50% increase—to achieve the desired effect or a notably diminished effect occurs with continued use of the same amount.
7. Has characteristic withdrawal syndrome.
8. Opioids are often taken to relieve or avoid withdrawal symptoms.

In addition, some symptoms of the disturbance have persisted for at least a month or have occurred repeatedly over a longer period.

Severity

Mild	Few, if any symptoms are present in excess of those required to make the diagnosis, and the symptoms result in no more than mild impairment in occupational functioning or in usual social activities or relationships with others.
Moderate	Functional impairment of symptoms is between mild and severe.
Severe	Many symptoms are present in excess of those required to make the diagnosis, and the symptoms greatly interfere with occupational functioning or usual social activities or relationship with others.
Partial remission	During the past 6 mo, there has been some use of the substance and some symptoms of dependence.
Full remission	During the past 6 mo, either there has been no use of opioids, or opioids have been used and there were no symptoms of dependence.

From ref. *15a*.

Table 6
DSM-IV Diagnostic Criteria for Opioid Withdrawal

A. Either of the following:
- Cessation of (or reduction in) opioid use that has been heavy and prolonged (several weeks or longer)
- Administration of an opioid antagonists after a period of opioid use

B. Three (or more) of the following, developing within minutes to several days after Criterion A:

• Dysphoric mood	• Lacrimation or rhinorrhea
• Nausea or vomiting	• Diarrhea
• Muscle aches	• Fever
• Pupillary dilation, piloerection, or sweating	• Yawning
	• Insomnia

C. The symptoms in Criterion B cause clinically significant distress or impairment in social, occupational, or other important areas of functioning.

D. The symptoms are not due to a general medical condition and are not better accounted for by another mental disorder.

From ref. *165.*

clonidine is effective in reducing most withdrawal symptoms, the drug has side effects of hypotension, sedation, and psychiatric problems, which render it unsuitable for use in police custody. By contrast, lofexidine has been used in detoxification from opiates with fewer side effects *(20)*.

Maternal opiate withdrawal syndrome may be life threatening for the fetus, and special care should be taken to ensure that a pregnant, opiate-dependent woman's medication is continued while she is in custody. There should be a low threshold for referral for hospital assessment, especially in the third trimester.

3.1.2. Buprenorphine (Subutex®)

Buprenorphine is an opioid with mixed agonist-antagonist properties that may be abused or used as an alternative to methadone in detoxification from opiates *(21)*. It is taken sublingually, and self-administration of the drug in the custodial environment must be personally supervised by the doctor who should observe the patient for 5 min to ensure that the drug has fully dissolved *(22)*. An unusual property of buprenorphine is that after chronic administration the onset of the abstinence syndrome is delayed. Heroin addicts who are dependent on a small dose of opiate can be transferred onto buprenorphine, which can be withdrawn fairly easily because of the delayed onset of the abstinence

Table 7
Half-Lives and Observation Times Required After Acute Narcotic Overdose

Opioid	Duration of action via iv route	t 1/2	Observation time
Methadone (Dolophine, Amidone)	May be days	15–72	24–36
Morphine	Usually 2-4 h	3	6
Heroin	Usually 2-4 h	v. short	6
Codeine	2–4 h (oral)	3	6

Note: Generally, if a patient remains asymptomatic 6 hours after the administration of naloxone they may be discharged.
From ref. *23a*.

syndrome. However, if it is given to an individual dependent on large doses of opiates, the antagonist properties precipitate withdrawal symptoms *(23)*.

3.1.3. Naloxone

Naloxone is an opioid antagonist that reverses the effects of severe intoxication (Table 7). The use of naloxone may precipitate withdrawal in addicted patients, but in initial doses of 0.4–0.8 mg, it is relatively safe, with little risk of vomiting, seizures, hypotension, hypertension, or cardiac arrest *(24)*. The half-life of naloxone is shorter than that of most opiates; therefore, a period of observation in the hospital is required after administration. It is recommended to give half the dose intravenously and half intramuscularly (absorption is slower and the antidotal activity prolonged); this is useful, because individuals often discharge themselves once awakened. In the prehospital environment, naloxone should only be given where there is life-threatening opiate poisoning with a respiratory rate lower than 8/min, a Glasgow Coma Scale less than 8, or when the airway is at risk *(25)*. Heroin may be taken in combination with cocaine ("speedball"), and the use of naloxone in this situation may precipitate ventricular dysrhythmias *(26)*.

3.2. Benzodiazepines

Benzodiazepines produce physical and psychological dependence and are therefore only recommended for limited periods *(27)*. The drugs are commonly misused either illicitly, which usually involves high doses, or by persistent therapeutic use at a lower dose. The pharmacological properties of the benzodiazepines are hypnotic, anxiolytic, muscle relaxant, and anticonvulsant and are produced by enhancing γ-aminobutyric acid (GABA) transmission *(28)*.

Table 8
Manifestations of Sedative-Hypnotic Drug Intoxication and Withdrawal

Mild	Sedation, disorientation, slurred speech, ataxia, nystagmus
Severe	Coma, hypoventilation, hypotension, hypothermia, depressed or absent corneal, gag and deep tendon reflexes
Withdrawal	Anxiety, insomnia, irritability, agitation, anorexia, tremor, seizures

Manifestations of intoxication and withdrawal are given in Table 8. Tolerance usually develops after continuous use, slowly for those drugs that have a long half-life but more quickly for the short-acting drugs *(29)*. Benzodiazepines are well absorbed from the gastrointestinal tract after oral administration; food can delay the rate but not the extent of absorption.

Side effects of use include daytime drowsiness, aggravation of depression, and antcrograde amnesia *(30)* at therapeutic doses, the risk increasing at high dosages. Amnesic effects may be associated with inappropriate behaviors and other paradoxic behavioral responses, such as increased aggression, excitement, confusion, and restlessness *(31,32)*. Rage reactions with violent behavior are most likely in people with a history of aggressive behavior or unstable emotional behavior. Anxiolytics lower tolerance to alcohol and in high doses produce mental confusion similar to alcohol intoxication. The interaction between alcohol and benzodiazepines results in a potentiation of the CNS effects. However, in general, they have a high toxic–therapeutic ratio, and doses 15–20 times the therapeutic dose may not cause serious side effects *(33)*.

Sudden cessation of benzodiazepines can lead to a recognized withdrawal syndrome *(34)* with anxiety symptoms, disordered perceptions, and major complications, such as seizures and psychosis *(35)*. A long-acting benzodiazepine, such as diazepam or chlordiazepoxide, is preferable in treating symptoms of withdrawal and preventing the major complications.

Flumazenil is a specific benzodiazepine antagonist used for the reversal of benzodiazepine-induced sedation and coma. When overdosage is suspected, it can be used in patients who would otherwise need intubation and ventilation *(36)*, but care should be taken when mixed overdoses are suspected *(37)*. Complications, such as convulsions, dysrhythmias, heart block, and cardiac arrest, suggest that its use in the prehospital environment should not be encouraged *(38)*.

Table 9
Manifestations of Solvent Intoxication and Abuse

Mild	Euphoria; disinhibition; dizziness; slurred speech; lack of coordination; sneezing and coughing
Moderate	Lethargy, stupor; hallucinations; nausea, vomiting; diarrhea; nystagmus; ataxia; tremors; myalgias; paresthesia
Severe	Coma; seizures
Chronic	Cerebellar syndrome: ataxia, nystagmus, tremor (toluene); fatigue, difficulty in concentrating; Parkinsonism (toluene); peripheral neuropathy: symmetrical, motor, mainly involving hands and feet (*n*-hexane and naphtha)

Adapted from ref. *33.*

3.3. Barbiturates

Barbiturates are used in the treatment of epilepsy and for the induction of anesthesia. They became less commonly misused after the introduction of benzodiazepine drugs but may be used by polydrug users. Mild intoxication may result in slurred speech, oversedation, ataxia, and nystagmus, although severe intoxication may present with coma, absent reflexes, hypothermia, hypotension, and respiratory depression. There is a narrow margin between therapeutic dose and serious toxicity. Physical and psychological dependence occurs, and the withdrawal syndrome is similar to that of benzodiazepine withdrawal, with a greater risk of seizures. Benzodiazepines may be used to prevent the withdrawal syndrome associated with barbiturates *(35).*

3.4. Solvents

Volatile substance abuse (VSA) is the deliberate inhalation of fumes given off by volatile substances (solvents) to achieve intoxication and can occur at any age but is a particular problem among adolescents. Adhesives, aerosols, anesthetics, dry cleaning agents, fuel gases, nail varnish, and paint stripper are among the substances inhaled *(39),* either directly from their containers, from a plastic bag placed over the nose and mouth, from impregnated rags, or sprayed directly into the mouth.

Regular users may have nasal sores, known as "glue-sniffer's rash" (perioral dermatitis), and have the odor of solvents on their breath. Acute effects begin within minutes *(40)* and may last 15–45 minutes; persistent abnormalities may occur in severe chronic abusers (Table 9) *(41).*

Table 10
Deaths From Volatile Substance Misuse

Acute	Direct	• Immediate	• Postponed
	Indirect	• Trauma	• Aspiration
		• Asphyxia	• Drowning
Delayed	Direct	• Liver failure	• Renal failure
		• Liver tumors	• Bone marrow depression
		• CNS involvement	

From ref. *42*.

Most acute direct VSA-related deaths result from cardiac dysrhythmias owing to "sensitization" of the myocardium to adrenaline; deaths may also occur from indirect effects or may be delayed (Table 10) *(42)*. Animal experiments confirm that myocardial sensitivity may continue for hours after the initial inhalant exposure *(43)*. Tolerance may develop, and psychological dependence after long-term use and a withdrawal syndrome similar to delirium tremens has been described *(44)*.

3.5. Lysergic Acid Diethylamide

Lysergic acid diethylamide (LSD) is usually taken orally in a dose of 20–100 mg, with sympathomimetic effects occurring in 5–10 minutes and psychological effects in 30–0 minutes *(45)*. There is a recovery period of 10–12 hours, where there may be periods of normal perception and cognition alternating with degrees of intoxication, which may affect fitness for interview.

Acute effects include tachycardia, hypertension, pyrexia, dilated pupils with both anisocoria (unequal size) and hippus (spasmodic rhythmical dilation and constriction), dry mouth, sweating, flushing, tremor, and hyper-reflexia. Emotional lability, euphoria and anxiety, distortion of time, visual and auditory illusions (although true hallucinations can occur), and synesthesia, with a mixing of the sensory input—"seeing" sounds or "hearing" smells—may all occur *(46)*.

Both enjoyable and unpleasant effects, a "bad trip" may occur in a first-time user or with repeated use *(47)*. Five major categories of psychiatric adverse effects have been described, which include anxiety and panic attacks, self-destructive behavior, hallucinations, acute psychosis, and major depressive reactions *(48)*. Polydrug users may use benzodiazepines to alleviate anxiety and panic attacks.

Chronic toxic effects include a prolonged psychosis, major depressive illness, disruption of personality, and post-hallucinogen perceptual disorder *(48)* characterized by flashbacks even months or years after LSD use.

Table 11
Effects of MDMA (Ecstasy)

Psychological	Euphoria, heightened awareness, improved sense of communication
Neuropsychiatric	Anxiety, insomnia, depression, paranoia, confusion, panic attacks, psychosis
Chronic	Depression, drowsiness, anxiety, panic disorder, aggressive outbursts, psychosis, memory disturbance
Medical	Tachycardia, hypertension, dry throat, bruxism, trismus, sweating, pyrexia, nausea, vomiting, anorexia, loss of coordination with ataxia, dilated pupils, nystagmus, hot and cold flushes, hyperreflexia

Physical dependence does not occur, and psychological dependence is uncommon and short-lived. Tolerance does occur in the chronic abuser, but a few days' abstinence will restore full CNS sensitivity to the drug.

3.6. Phencyclidine

Phencyclidine, known as "angel dust," is usually smoked, although it can be taken orally, intravenously, or by nasal inhalation. It is commonly used as an additive to other drugs, such as cannabis or LSD, and the symptoms and signs may vary greatly (49). At low doses, euphoria, relaxation, and an altered body image may occur, but at higher doses, there may be agitation, bizarre behavior, and a paranoid psychosis (50). Analgesia occurs, which may lead to self-injury. Physical effects include nystagmus (lateral and vertical), and with severe intoxication there is adrenergic stimulation with hypertension, tachycardia, flushing, hyperthermia, and cholinomimetic stimulation with sweating, hypersalivation, miosis, dystonia, ataxia, and myoclonus eventually resulting in coma, respiratory arrest, and circulatory collapse (51). Death may also result from intoxication or from violent behavior. Chronic effects of phencyclidine abuse include memory impairment, personality changes, and depression; however, there is probably no physical dependence.

3.7. Ecstasy

3,4-Methylenedioxymethamphetamine (MDMA), or "ecstasy," is commonly taken in an oral dose of 75–120 mg as a recreational drug within the dance culture or "rave" scene for its central stimulant and psychedelic effects (Table 11) (52). The effects last for 4–6 hours, with tolerance developing to the acute effects. However, physical and psychological dependence do not occur.

Adverse effects such as a polydipsia, hyponatremia, and catatonic stupor have been reported (53,54). An acute rise in antidiuretic hormone (arginine vasopressin) accompanied by a small fall in plasma sodium has been shown after MDMA ingestion. Therefore, in view of the risk of hyponatremia, individuals who take such drugs should avoid drinking fluid in excess of the body's requirement. This may be difficult because MDMA reduces the perception of thirst and impairs judgment *(55)*, and people tend to overcompensate and consciously overdrink.

Regular users may habitually use chewing gum to overcome the effects on the jaw muscles. The clenching of teeth in the acidic environment caused by carbonated (fizzy) drinks will result in an increased likelihood of tooth wear on the back teeth *(56)*. Other adverse effects have been described, including jaundice and hepatotoxicity *(57)*; flashbacks and psychosis *(58)*; pneumomediastinum *(59)*; urinary retention *(60)*; hyperthermia; coagulopathy *(61)*; rhabdomyolysis; and cardiovascular complications resulting in death *(62–64)*. Development of chronic paranoid psychosis has been described after heavy misuse of the drug *(65)*, and the serotonin syndrome *(66)* (altered mental state, hyperthermia, and autonomic dysfunction) has also been reported following MDMA ingestion *(67)*. Evidence is emerging of possible long-term damage to the brain in the form of serotonin neural injury, which may result in depression, anxiety, and memory disorders *(68)*. However, there are other factors, such as other concomitant drug use, that complicate the issue.

3,4-Methylenedioxyamphetamine is an analog of MDMA with similar effects. 3,4-Methylenedioxyamphetamine and paramethoxyamphetamine may also be used as recreational drugs. Overdose may result in severe sympathetic stimulation and death *(69)*.

3.8. Cocaine and Crack

Cocaine occurs naturally in the leaves of the coca plant *Erythroxylum coca*, which grows predominantly in South America. Cocaine hydrochloride is a white powder that is usually snorted but can be taken orally. Crack is prepared by mixing cocaine hydrochloride with sodium bicarbonate and water and heating it. The cocaine base precipitates out and forms small "rocks" as it cools. Crack may be smoked in a pipe or heated on foil with the vapor inhaled. Both crack and cocaine may be injected.

The onset-of-action and plasma half-life varies depending on the route of use, rapidly if taken intravenously or smoked compared with when it is snorted. The duration of effects will also vary with administration route *(70)*. Ingestion of stimulant drugs, such as cocaine or amphetamine, result in activation of the sympathetic nervous system with resulting euphoria followed by irritability, depression, insomnia, and paranoia (Table 12).

Tolerance occurs to the psychological effects but not to the effects on the heart. Deaths may occur, most commonly from cardiac dysrhythmias, myocardial infarction, agitated delirium, and stroke. Chronic effects include per-

Table 12
Effects of Cocaine and Amphetamine Intoxication

Initial low dose	Euphoria, insomnia, dry mouth, hyperthermia, tachycardia, hypertension, increased respiration, sweating, dilated pupils
With increasing dose	Irritability, impulsivity, aggressiveness, agitated delirium, paranoia, delusions, seizures

foration of the nasal septum and rhinorrhea, and long-term use may result in a range of psychiatric problems and vascular diseases *(71)*.

Cocaine produces a physical and psychological dependence, the severity of which will vary depending on the method of administration, being more severe if the drug is smoked or injected than if snorted. Dependence may result in a particular strong craving for the drug, followed by a withdrawal syndrome, or "crash," with irritability, insomnia, depression, and anxiety on cessation. In conditions of police custody, the depression and inability to sleep may lead to acts of self-harm and suicide, and close supervision may be required, with consideration given to prescribing hypnotics and antidepressants.

3.9. Amphetamine

Amphetamine is usually found as a white powder, amphetamine sulphate, and can be taken nasally, orally, or intravenously. Clinical effects are similar to those of cocaine (Table 12), although amphetamine has a longer half-life of 10–15 h, so the duration of euphoria is longer. "Ice" is a pure form of methamphetamine hydrochloride (98–100% pure), which is usually smoked like crack cocaine.

Tolerance occurs with long-term use. "Speed runs" describe repeated use over a period of days, with several grams of amphetamine used daily. At the end of the "run," the user may sleep for several days. Alcohol, sedative-hypnotic drugs, and heroin may be used to reduce the anxiety caused by amphetamine or, alternatively, amphetamine may be used to reduce the sedative effects of such drugs. Psychological dependence occurs, and psychosis may occur, which resolves when the drug is stopped. However, it is possible that amphetamine use may trigger latent schizophrenia.

3.10. Khat

Khat consists of the young leaves of the *Catha edulis* plant; it is usually chewed for its stimulant effect when fresh but may be drunk as an infusion of leaves. In the United Kingdom, it is sold legally (it is illegal in the United States) and is used by Somali populations *(72,73)*. The main component is cathinone, with effects similar to those of amphetamine, resulting in euphoria, increased alertness, and anorexia *(74)*. There may also be mood lability, anxiety, and insomnia *(75)*.

Heavy khat consumption may result in mania-like symptoms, paranoia, and an acute schizophrenia-like psychosis, usually resolving within weeks of cessation of use *(76,77)*. Although there is no specific physical withdrawal syndrome, depression, hypersomnia, and loss of energy may occur when khat use is stopped *(75)*.

3.11. Marijuana

Marijuana is the most commonly used illicit drug in the United Kingdom (with 11% of 16–59 years olds having used it in the last year; *see* ref. *78*) and United States. It is obtained from the Cannabis sativa plant, and the principal active ingredient, accounting for the majority of effects, is Δ-9-tetrahydrocannabinol (THC). There are several forms, including hashish (a resin), herbal cannabis (a green-colored preparation made from the leaves of the plant), and cannabis oil. "Skunk" is a term used to describe a potent form of the cannabis plant with high levels of THC *(79)*, which is grown indoors using hydroponic techniques, in nutrient-rich liquids rather than soil, under grow lights, or in greenhouse conditions. The onset of effects is reported as being more rapid, and the hallucinogenic properties are heightened. Psychotic episodes may be precipitated by relatively small quantities *(80)*.

Cannabis is usually smoked but can be ingested as "cannabis cookies." One "joint" typically contains 10–30 mg of THC and has an onset of action of 10–20 minutes, with effects lasting 2–3 hours *(50)*. The acute effects of cannabis are given in Table 13 *(81)*.

Tolerance develops to many effects of cannabis, including the "high" with chronic use, and an abstinence syndrome has been described with disturbed sleep, decreased appetite, restlessness, irritability, and sweating. Withdrawal symptoms are usually mild and short-lived, although they may be more severe in heavy regular users *(82)*.

3.12. Anabolic Steroids

Anabolic steroids may be taken orally or intramuscularly by body builders or other individuals who want to enhance their physical appearance. Research has shown that injections of testosterone enanthate increase muscle size and strength, especially when combined with exercise *(83)*. To achieve the desired effect, different steroids are taken in cycles, with rest periods in between, a regime known as "stacking," or, alternatively, increasing doses of the same steroid are taken, a so-called drug pyramid *(84)*. Most of the steroids sold in the United Kingdom are counterfeit rather than produced by legitimate pharmaceutical companies. Consequently, they may contain a different steroid from the

Table 13

Pharmacological Actions of Cannabis in Man (in Therapeutic Dosage Range)

Central nervous system

Psychological effects	Euphoria, dysphoria, anxiety, depersonalization, precipitation/aggravation of psychotic states
Effects on perception	Heightened sensory perception, distortion of space and time sense, misperceptions, hallucinations
Effects on cognition and psychomotor performance	Fragmentation of thoughts, mental clouding, memory impairment, global impairment of performance especially in complex and demanding tasks
Effects on motor function	Increased motor activity followed by inertia and incoordination, ataxia, dysarthria, tremulousness, weakness and muscle twitching
Analgesic effects	Similar in potency to codeine (nonopioid mechanism)
Tolerance	To most behavioral and somatic effects, including the euphoria with chronic use
Dependence/abstinence syndrome	Rarely observed; symptoms include disturbed sleep, decreased appetite, restlessness, irritability, and sweating

Cardiovascular system

Heart rate	Tachycardia with acute dosage; bradycardia with chronic use
Peripheral circulation	Vasodilation, conjunctival redness, postural hypotension

Respiratory system

Ventilation	Small doses stimulate; large doses suppress
Bronchodilatation	Coughing but tolerance develops

Adapted from ref. *81.*

one indicated on the bottle, and scant reliance can be placed on the reported dose because they may have little or no steroid in them at all *(85)*.

General effects of anabolic steroids *(86)* include baldness, acne (typically affecting the shoulders and upper back), raised blood pressure and heart rate, fluid retention, and a reduction in high-density lipoprotein cholesterol. Long-term effects include an increased risk of thrombosis. Gynecomastia may occur, and the prostate gland may swell, resulting in impaired micturition. Most of these effects are dose dependent and more likely with prolonged administration.

While the drug is being taken, there is a significant reduction in testosterone production by the testes so that sperm output and quality are decreased, and a return to normal can take many months after drug use is stopped. The effect on sex drive is variable, but overall it seems that the sex drive increases at the beginning of a steroid-using cycle, and then decreases to below normal after several weeks of use. Drive may remain below normal levels even after the drug is stopped, until such time as the testes start producing testosterone again. There may also be a reduction in size of the testicles *(87)*.

In women, menstrual irregularities are reported, with permanent enlargement of the clitoris. There may also be growth of facial and body hair, male pattern baldness, and decreased breast size. Abuse of sex steroids by recreational body builders may be an unrecognized cause of subfertility *(88)*.

Liver function tests may show abnormalities that usually return to normal once the drug is stopped. Drug-induced jaundice can be caused by temporarily impaired excretory function, and peliosis hepatitis, in which the liver tissue is replaced by blood-filled cysts, may occur, as can liver tumors *(89)* and Wilms' tumor.

Initial use may result in stimulatory effects, such as increased confidence, decreased fatigue, heightened motivation, agitation, irritability, and insomnia, which may progress to argumentative and aggressive behavior and major mood disturbances including depression, mania, and hypomania *(90,91)*. "Roid rage," which may be associated with violent crimes *(92)*, requires a high dose of steroids over several weeks, as may occur when "stacking."

3.13. Other Body-Building Drugs

Other drugs may be used by body builders *(93)*, including tamoxifen to reduce or prevent gynecomastia; diuretics to counteract the fluid retention caused by anabolic steroids; thyroxine to increase the rate of metabolism, which might theoretically increase the ability of anabolic steroids to boost physical strength *(94)*; and β human chorionic gonadotrophin to alleviate testicular atrophy *(95)*. Nalbuphine (Nubain) is an opioid agonist/antagonist analgesic used for the treatment of moderate-to-severe pain, and dependence has been reported associated with anabolic steroid use *(96)*.

Furthermore, there has been a case report of a 21-year-old body builder who was admitted after taking excessive amounts of insulin intravenously; apparently, insulin is advertised in body-building magazines as having anabolic properties *(97)*. The recreational use of caffeine to toxic levels has been reported in a body builder who presented with a grand mal seizure *(98)*. Clenbuterol, which is a sympathomimetic agonist (used as a oral bronchodilator in some European countries but not licensed for human use in the United Kingdom or United States) is said to have an "anabolic-like" effect but at high dose may cause cardiac dysrhythmias, tremor, and serious hypokalemia *(99)*.

3.14. γ-Hydroxy Butyrate

γ-hydroxy butyrate (GHB) is a naturally occurring substance in the human brain structurally related to GABA that may be a neurotransmitter *(100)*. It has been used as an anesthetic (although it has little analgesic effect), to alleviate narcolepsy, and to treat alcohol and opiate dependence *(101)*. There have been reports of abuse in the United Kingdom and United States within the dance scene and gay clubs and with body builders because it is said to promote slow-wave sleep during which growth hormone is secreted *(102)*. It is available as a colorless, odorless liquid, powder, or a capsule to be taken orally; it is rarely injected. GHB is rapidly absorbed, with peak plasma concentrations occurring 20–45 minutes after oral administration. It has a half-life of 30 minutes *(103)*, and effects can last from 45 minutes to 8 h *(104)*.

Initial effects include euphoria followed by profound sedation, confusion, agitation, amnesia, nausea, vomiting, diarrhea, ataxia, seizures, hypotonia, tremor, vertigo and dizziness, bradycardia, hypotension, hypothermia, coma *(105)*, and respiratory collapse.

There is a narrow margin between intoxication and coma *(106)*, and the clinical effects are potentiated by use of other CNS depressant drugs, such as alcohol, opiates, benzodiazepines, and neuroleptics *(107)*. Tolerance and physical dependence after high-dose use can develop with a withdrawal syndrome, which may include insomnia, muscular cramping, tremor, and anxiety *(101)*. Symptoms of withdrawal from GHB are broadly similar to those for alcohol although of a more rapid onset. A rapid deterioration into delirium may occur in more frequent high-dose dependent users. Withdrawal is not associated with seizures, but if suspected, hospital admission should be considered *(108)*.

3.15. Ketamine

Ketamine is a commercially available anesthetic for intravenous and intramuscular use. It contains analgesic properties and is available on the street in powder, tablet, and liquid form; it can be smoked or taken intranasally ("snorted"), orally, intramuscularly, or intravenously *(109)*. The onset of effects depends on the route of administration; when taken orally, effects start within 20 minutes and can last up to 3 hours, whereas given intravenously, effects will be seen within 30 seconds and last about 30 minutes *(110)*. Tolerance develops after repeated use, with a decreased duration of effect *(111)*.

Physical effects may include a cocaine-like "rush," hypertension, dysrhythmias, nausea, and vomiting, slurred speech, nystagmus, lack of coordination, and seizures. On recovery, "emergence phenomena" may occur, with psychological dissociation or out of body (flying or floating) sensations, confusion, hallucinations, synesthesia, and depersonalization *(112)*. Such dissociative states may result in the individual becoming divorced from reality, and these effects, coupled with possible loss of coordination and pronounced analgesia, can result in serious accidents to users. A dose-dependent depression of respiration may occur *(113)*, and this can be a particular problem when taken with other respiratory depressant drugs, such as benzodiazepines and alcohol, occasionally resulting in death *(114)*.

3.16. Alkyl Nitrites

The alkyl nitrites are volatile yellowish clear liquids that have a distinctive sweet smell. All the nitrites have vasodilatory properties and are used as a euphoric relaxant within the dance culture and to relax the anal sphincter and enhance sexual performance. The effect of inhaling the vapor, usually from the bottle or poured onto a cloth, is instantaneous and short-lived, resulting in a "rush," but adverse effects, such as dizziness, flushing, tachycardia and palpitations, headache, cold sweats, and hypotension, may occur *(115,116)*. Swallowing of volatile nitrites as opposed to inhaling them may result in severe methemoglobinemia *(117)*.

4. ALCOHOL

Crime statistics show a clear association between heavy drinking and criminal behavior, the association being most marked in relation to violent crimes. One review found that the incidence of alcohol-related violent crime ranged from 24 to 85%, which contrasted dramatically with the 12–38% incidence of alcohol-related nonviolent crime *(118)*. Although some have confirmed the association between alcohol and crime *(119,120)*, a direct causal link between the two has been disputed *(121)*. Nonetheless, alcohol assumes an importance in clinical forensic medicine because of its link with criminal activity and by virtue of the significant role it plays in a large number of assessments regarding fitness for detention *(122–124)*. Accordingly, a thorough understanding of the metabolism, effects, and problems associated with alcohol is essential for any doctor practicing in this field, not least because those detainees with alcohol problems, particularly those with gross intoxication, are an extremely vulnerable group for whom police custody may be inappropriate (125).

4.1. The Metabolism of Alcohol

Ethanol, hereafter referred to as alcohol, is produced by the fermentation of sugar by yeast, a process that halts at a concentration of alcohol by volume of approx 15% because of the death of yeast above these levels. As a rough guide, one measure of spirits, one glass of wine, or one half-pint of beer contain 1 U, or 8 g, of alcohol. However, there is a variation in the alcohol content of different drinks (126), and any accurate assessment of intake must bear this in mind. In the European Union, there is now international agreement about the labeling of alcohol content, with the alcohol content of beverages being referred to by the percentage alcohol by volume (percent v/v) (127). This is equivalent to the number of milliliters of pure alcohol per 100 mL of the drink. In the United States, alcoholic strengths are measured in terms of percentage proof. US proof spirit contains 50% of alcohol by volume, so to convert US proof to percent v/v, one simply divides by two.

Most people who have alcohol in the body have drunk it, although it can be absorbed into the systemic circulation through the lungs (blood alcohol concentrations of up to 50 mg/100 mL have been achieved after breathing alcohol/air mixtures for several hours) (128). Little or no alcohol is absorbed through the intact skin of adults.

Once ingested, alcohol is subsequently absorbed into the body by a process of passive diffusion that occurs across the mucosal surfaces of the gastrointestinal tract (129). As liquids pass quickly through the mouth and esophagus, little absorption occurs until alcohol has reached the stomach. The rate of absorption is maximal in the duodenum, because its mucosa is thinner and blood supply more abundant than that of the stomach. Accordingly, any condition that delivers alcohol into the small intestine more quickly than normal, such as gastrectomy, will lead to more rapid absorption and an earlier, higher peak blood alcohol level (130).

As soon as alcohol enters the bloodstream, mechanisms for its removal come into action. Approximately 5–10% of the total amount absorbed is excreted unchanged in breath, urine, and sweat (129), an important factor that allows the estimation of blood alcohol concentrations from the levels in urine and breath. The remaining 90–95% of alcohol is oxidized in the liver by alcohol dehydrogenase to form acetaldehyde, and this is further metabolized to acetate (acetic acid). Because alcohol dehydrogenase becomes satu-

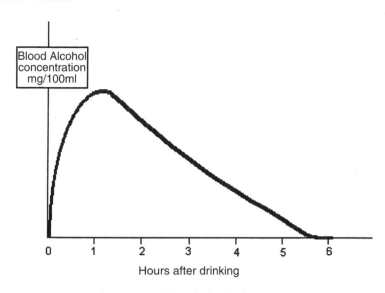

Fig. 1. The blood alcohol curve.

rated at relatively low alcohol concentrations, it soon reaches its maximum working rate, and alcohol elimination proceeds at this constant rate *(131)*.

The rate of absorption is much faster than the rate of elimination, giving rise to the characteristic blood alcohol curve, as described by several researchers (Fig. 1) *(132–134)*. Generally speaking, the peak blood alcohol concentration is reached 30–60 minutes after drinking, although the range may be anything from 20 minutes to 3 hours. However, the peak blood alcohol concentration, the time taken to reach the peak, the area under the blood alcohol curve, and the time taken to reach a zero blood alcohol level varies from person to person and within the same person over time *(135)*. Indeed, several factors can influence the kinetics of alcohol.

4.1.1. Sex and Weight

Alcohol is highly hydrophilic, so once it enters the systemic circulation, it is distributed evenly throughout total body water (V_d, or the volume of distribution). In general, the larger the person the larger the V_d, so that if two different sized males drink the same quantity of alcohol, a higher peak concentration will be reached in the lighter of the two because he will have a smaller V_d for the alcohol to distribute itself throughout. Similarly, because women have more body fat compared with men, and fat contains no water, higher peak alcohol levels are achieved in women than in men of the same weight. The V_d of alcohol for adult males has been shown to be approx 0.70, compared with 0.60 for adult females *(129)*.

4.1.2. Duration of Drinking

If a volume of alcohol is consumed over a prolonged period, it may be eliminated almost as quickly as it is absorbed, giving rise to a much lower peak alcohol concentration.

4.1.3. Nature of the Drink Consumed

The rate of alcohol absorption increases with the concentration of the ingested solution to levels between 10 and 20%, at which point absorption is maximal. Because alcohol is absorbed by passive diffusion, the rate of absorption is slower with drinks of lesser strength because of a lower concentration gradient. Furthermore, the larger volumes involved may also delay gastric emptying and further slow absorption. By contrast, when the alcohol concentration of drinks exceeds 20%, the alcohol irritates the gastric mucosa and pyloric sphincter, causing increased secretion of mucus and delayed gastric emptying, thus slowing absorption.

4.1.4. Food in the Stomach

Studies have shown that eating a full meal before drinking can reduce the peak alcohol level by an average of 9–23% *(129,136–138)*. The presence of food in the stomach reduces the rate of gastric emptying, dilutes the alcohol that enters the stomach, and limits the contact between the alcohol and the gastric mucosa. Alcohol absorption is slowed for all these reasons.

4.1.5. Physiological Factors and Genetic Variation

Factors, such as stomach wall permeability, blood supply to the alimentary tract, and the rate of gastric emptying, vary from person to person and from time to time in the same person. All of these affect the shape of the blood alcohol curve.

4.1.6. Drugs

The interaction between alcohol and drugs, either prescribed or illicit, is important because many detainees take other drugs in conjunction with alcohol *(2)*. Generally, the most important interactions involve drugs altering the way a subject responds to a given amount of alcohol in the blood, for example, because the drug has CNS depressant effects that add to those of alcohol.

Table 14
Drugs That Affect the Rate of Stomach Emptying
and So Influence the Rate of Alcohol Absorption

- Drugs that slow gastric emptying:
  - Drugs with anticholinergic actions, such as: atropine; chlorpromazine; tricyclic antidepressants
  - Drugs with an adrenergic action, such as: amphetamines
  - Drugs with an opioid action, such as: antidiarrheal medicines; codeine and dihydrocodeine; diamorphine (heroin); methadone; dextropropoxyphene (in co-proxamol)
- Drugs that hasten stomach emptying, such as: metoclopramide; cisapride; erythromycin

Adapted from ref. *128.*

However, several drugs may influence the rate of alcohol absorption by virtue of their affect on the rate of gastric emptying (Table 14).

4.1.7. Rate of Elimination

The rate of elimination of alcohol has been determined experimentally. Reported values range from approx 10 mg/100 mL of blood per hour (mg/dL/h) to 25 mg/dL/h, with an average of 15–18.6 mg/dL/h *(131,139)* (approximately equivalent to the elimination of 1 U of alcohol per hour in a 70-kg male). Habituation to alcohol is the single most important factor affecting the rate of elimination. One recent study reported the rate of ethanol disappearance in 22 alcoholics as ranging from 13 to 36 mg/dL/h, with an average of 22 mg/dL/h *(140)*. The increased rate of elimination is believed to be because chronic alcoholics have facilitated liver enzyme systems.

4.2. Effects of Alcohol

Alcohol acts as a CNS depressant, which, in small doses interferes with cortical function, but in larger doses may depress medullary processes. The apparent stimulatory effects of alcohol occur because it acts first on the so-called higher centers of the brain that govern inhibition *(141)*.

Although there is general agreement on the sequence of clinical effects caused by drinking alcohol, the blood alcohol concentrations at which these effects occur vary in different subjects. The difference in susceptibility is most marked between habituated and nonhabituated drinkers, but tolerance to the effects remains variable even within these broad categories *(142,143)*.

Table 15
Sequence of Central Nervous Depressant Effects of Alcohol

Stage of influence	Blood alcohol concentration mg/100 mL	Clinical effect
Sobriety	10–50	• Often no obvious effect; may feel "relaxed"
Euphoria	30–120	• Mild euphoria with increased talkativeness • Decreased inhibitions • Increased self-confidence • Impaired fine motor skills
Excitement	90–200	• Emotional instability • Poor sensory perception • Impaired memory and comprehension • Incoordination and loss of balance
Drunkenness	150–300	• Disorientation, mental confusion • Disturbances of vision (e.g., diplopia) • Decreased pain sense • Increased incoordination with staggering gait • Slurred speech
Stupor	250–400	• General inertia approaching paralysis • Marked lack of response to stimuli • Inability to stand or walk • Vomiting, incontinence of urine and feces
Coma	350–500	• Coma and anesthesia • Depressed or absent reflexes • Cardiovascular and respiratory depression • Possible death
Death	Over 450	• Death from respiratory depression

Table 15 provides a guide to the general effects. It should be noted that the effects are more pronounced when blood alcohol levels are rising than when falling. This is known as the Mellanby effect and is believed to result from an acute tolerance to alcohol that develops during intoxication *(144)*. Some specific effects are discussed.

4.2.1. Nystagmus

Because the eye is effectively part of the CNS, it is one of the easiest parts of the body to examine to detect the effects of alcohol; the most extensively studied ocular effect of alcohol intoxication is nystagmus. Alcohol can cause nystagmus through at least two mechanisms. By acting on the vestibular system, it can cause positional alcohol nystagmus (PAN) *(145)*, detected when the patient is lying supine with the head turned to either the left or right. Horizontal gaze nystagmus (HGN) results from the inhibition of the smooth pursuit system and the impaired ability to maintain eccentric gaze *(146)* brought about by alcohol's effect on ocular movements via neural mechanisms *(147)*.

Positional alcohol nystagmus occurs in two stages *(148)*. The first stage, PAN I, is associated with acute elevation of blood alcohol, tending to occur approx 30 minutes after alcohol ingestion. In PAN I, the fast phase of nystagmus is in the direction toward which the head is turned. PAN II normally occurs at approx 5–6 hours after drinking and is characterized by nystagmus in the opposite direction to that seen in PAN I.

HGN is a jerky eye movement noted when gaze is directed to one side. The fast phase of HGN is in the direction of gaze, and it becomes intensified at a more eccentric gaze position *(147)*. Although HGN can be seen in normal individuals at extreme lateral gaze *(149)*, when detected at lesser deviations, it is considered pathological. An angle of onset of 40° or less from the midline is a sensitive indicator of a blood alcohol level in excess of 100 mg/100 mL *(143)*. Although some authors have maintained that blood alcohol levels of more than 80 mg/100 mL are consistently associated with HGN *(150)*, others have found that it is absent in just less than 40% of drivers with an average blood alcohol of 120 mg/100 mL (range 9–218 mg/100 mL) *(151)*. Because HGN may be noted in several pathological conditions, including the ingestion of sedative and tranquilizing drugs *(152)*, its presence should not be taken as proof of alcohol intoxication. It is perhaps for these reasons that the Kansas Supreme Court, when assessing the admissibility of HGN evidence in drink driving prosecutions decided that "the reliability of HGN evidence is not currently a settled proposition in the scientific community" *(153)*.

4.2.2. Pupillary Changes

In the early stages of alcoholic intoxication the pupils are said to dilate, often becoming pinpoint as the level of intoxication advances, particularly when the state of coma is reached *(154)*. However, some commentators report the pupils as being normal-sized in alcohol intoxication *(155)*, with current advice favoring the view that pupil size may be normal or dilated *(156)*.

Alcohol may slow the pupillary response to light, such an effect being one of the more reliable eye signs of intoxication, albeit a difficult one to detect clinically *(151,157)*.

4.2.3. Slurred Speech

Speech production is a complex motor activity. Because it requires a high degree of coordination, it can be a sensitive index of alcohol intoxication

(158). Reliable changes in speech are produced at blood alcohol levels above 100 mg/100 mL, although the effects of lower blood alcohol levels have been variable *(159).*

4.2.4. Cardiovascular Effects

Moderate doses of alcohol cause a slight increase in blood pressure and pulse rate *(160,161).* However, the most prominent effect with higher doses is a depression of cardiovascular functions. This depression is probably a combination of central effects and direct depression of the myocardium *(144).*

4.2.5. Metabolic Effects

Forensic physicians must be aware that severe hypoglycemia may accompany alcohol intoxication because of inhibition of gluconeogenesis. Alcohol-induced hypoglycemia, which develops within 6–36 hours of heavy drinking, typically occurs in an undernourished individual or one who has not eaten for the previous 24 hours. The usual features of hypoglycemia, such as flushing, sweating, and tachycardia, are often absent, and the person may present in coma.

4.3. Death From Alcohol Poisoning

Alcohol intoxication may result in death owing to respiratory or circulatory failure or as a result of aspiration of stomach contents in the absence of a gag reflex. Levels of blood alcohol above 500 mg/100 mL are considered to be "probably fatal" *(162),* although survival at much higher concentrations is now well documented. In 1982, for example, the case of a 24-year-old woman with a blood alcohol level of 1510 mg/100 mL was reported. She had gone to the hospital complaining of abdominal pain and was noted to be conscious but slightly confused. Two days later, her pain had eased, her blood alcohol level fallen, and she was able to leave the hospital and return home *(163).*

Death associated with blood alcohol levels below 350 mg/100 mL suggests that other complicating factors are present. Most commonly, this will be an interaction between alcohol and some other drug that has also been ingested.

4.4. Diagnosis of Intoxication

The terms *alcohol intoxication* and *drunkenness* are often used interchangeably. However, a distinction between these terms is justified because people may exhibit behavioral changes associated with drunkenness when they believe they have consumed alcohol but actually have not *(164).* Thus, the diagnostic features of alcoholic intoxication developed by the American Psychiatric Association include a requirement that there must have been recent ingestion of alcohol (Table 16) *(165).*

Table 16
Diagnostic Criteria for Alcohol Intoxication—DSM-IV

- Recent ingestion of alcohol
- Clinically significant maladaptive behavioral or psychological changes (e.g. inappropriate sexual or aggressive behavior, mood lability, impaired judgment, impaired social or occupational functioning) that developed during, or shortly after, alcohol ingestion.
- One (or more) of the following signs, developing during, or shortly after, alcohol use:
  - slurred speech
  - unsteady gait
  - impairment in attention or memory
  - incoordination
  - nystagmus
  - stupor or coma
- The symptoms are not due to a general medical condition and are not better accounted for by another mental disorder.

DSM-IV, *Diagnostic and Statistical Manual of Mental Disorders*, 4th ed.

Table 17
Pathological States Simulating Alcohol Intoxication

- Severe head injuries
- Metabolic disorders (e.g., hypoglycemia, hyperglycemia, uremia, hyperthyroidism)
- Neurological conditions associated with dysarthria, ataxia, tremor, drowsiness (e.g., multiple sclerosis, intracranial tumors, Parkinson's disease, epilepsy, acute vertigo)
- The effects of drugs, either prescribed or illicit (e.g., insulin, barbiturates, benzodiazepines, cocaine)
- Psychiatric disorders (e.g., hypomania, general paresis)
- High fever
- Carbon monoxide

The fourth edition of the *Diagnostic and Statistical Manual of Mental Disorders* (DSM-IV) criteria requires that medical conditions likely to account for the observed condition must be excluded before the diagnosis of alcohol intoxication is made. This is particularly important when assessing an intoxicated detainee in police custody. Indeed, the doctor's first duty in examining such individuals should be to exclude pathological conditions that may simulate intoxication *(154)* (Table 17), because failure to do so may lead to deaths in police custody *(166)*.

4.5. Alcohol Dependence

Alcohol abuse and dependence is a major risk factor for serious health, social, and economic problems *(167)*. Early identification of those who are dependent on alcohol increases the possibility of successful treatment, and brief intervention by the forensic physician seems both feasible and acceptable *(124,168)*. Although not yet validated in police custody, brief interventions show a high acceptance among drinkers in licensed premises *(169)*.

However, obtaining accurate and reliable information about a person's drinking habits can be extremely difficult because heavy drinkers tend to underestimate or deliberately lie about their alcohol consumption *(170)*. Use of the Alcohol Use Disorders Identification Test identifies persons whose alcohol consumption has become harmful or hazardous to health *(171)*; self-report questionnaires, such as the Michigan Alcohol Screening Test *(172,173)* and CAGE *(174,175)* may help to identify those with alcohol dependency and should prevent the doctor falling into the trap of assuming that alcohol abuse is synonymous with alcohol dependence (Appendix 5). DSM-IV *(165)* distinguishes between these two diagnostic categories. The main features differentiating alcohol dependence from alcohol abuse are evidence of tolerance, the presence of withdrawal symptoms, and the use of alcohol to relieve or avoid withdrawal. Treatment may be required for detainees who show signs of alcohol dependence. However, there is no need to treat those who simply abuse alcohol and who do not have a history of alcohol withdrawal.

4.6. Alcohol Withdrawal

Many alcoholics develop symptoms of withdrawal when in custody. Their acquired tolerance to and physical dependence on alcohol is a manifestation of compensatory neuropsychological changes that offset the drug's CNS depressant effects. When alcohol intake is abruptly stopped on incarceration, the compensatory changes give rise to signs and symptoms of withdrawal *(176)*. The severity of the symptoms depends mainly on the amount and duration of alcohol intake, although other factors, such as concurrent withdrawal from other drugs, like benzodiazepines, may contribute to the clinical picture *(177)*.

Alcohol withdrawal may present as a mild picture of uncomplicated alcohol withdrawal or as the more severe syndrome of alcohol withdrawal delirium (DSM-IV criteria).

4.6.1. Uncomplicated Alcohol Withdrawal

This is the most frequent and benign type, usually occurring some 12–48 hours after alcohol intake is reduced, although it can develop as early as 6 hours after drinking has stopped. The essential features are a coarse tremor of the hands, tongue, and eyelids, together with at least one of the following:

- Nausea and vomiting.
- Malaise and weakness.
- Autonomic hyperactivity (raised blood pressure and tachycardia).
- Anxiety, depressed mood, and irritability.
- Transient hallucinations and illusions.
- Headache and insomnia.

If symptoms are mild, it is safe to recommend simple observation, but significant tremor and agitation will usually require sedation. The drugs of choice are long-acting benzodiazepines, which will not only treat alcohol withdrawal symptoms but will also prevent later complications *(178)*. The starting dosages depend on the severity of the withdrawal, but 20 mg of chlordiazepoxide, or 10 mg of diazepam, both given four times a day, will generally be appropriate *(179)*.

Usually the benzodiazepines should not be started until such time as the blood alcohol level has reached zero *(180)*. However, detained persons with marked alcohol dependence may develop withdrawal symptoms before this point is reached. In these circumstances, it is both safe and reasonable to initiate therapy when the blood alcohol level has reached 80 mg/100 mL or thereabouts.

4.6.2. Alcohol Withdrawal Delirium

The essential diagnostic feature of this disorder is a delirium that develops after recent cessation of or reduction in alcohol consumption. Traditionally referred to as delirium tremens, this withdrawal state typically begins 72–96 hours after the last drink, so it is uncommon within the normal span of detention in police custody. The delirium is characterized by impaired attention and memory, disorganized thinking, disorientation, reduced level of consciousness, perceptual disturbances, and agitation. Vivid, and often terrifying, hallucinations may occur. Usually these are visual, but other sensory modalities (e.g., auditory or tactile) may be involved. The disorder usually coexists with other features of alcohol withdrawal, for example, autonomic hyperactivity, which is usually severe.

Alcohol withdrawal delirium is a medical emergency with a mortality rate of approx 5%. Once diagnosed, the detained person with delirium requires urgent hospitalization.

4.6.3. Complications of Alcohol Withdrawal

Several complications of alcohol withdrawal have been recognized, any one of which may be encountered when alcoholics are detained in police custody *(176)*.

4.6.3.1. Withdrawal Seizures

Seizures are typically single and generalized. They usually occur between 6 and 48 hours after the last drink and although in themselves are not life threatening, their importance lies in the fact that about one-third of those with seizures will go on to develop alcohol withdrawal delirium.

4.6.3.2. Alcoholic Hallucinosis

This is an infrequent disorder that tends to occur at about the age of 40 years in those who have been drinking heavily for more than 10 years. The essential features are vivid and persistent hallucinations, which develop shortly (usually within 48 hours) after cessation of alcohol intake. The hallucinations may be auditory or visual, and their content is usually unpleasant and disturbing. The disorder may last several weeks or months and is quite different from the fleeting hallucinations observed in other forms of alcohol withdrawal.

4.6.3.3. Cardiac Arrhythmias

The frequency of tachyrhythmias in alcohol withdrawal is high, probably because of high adrenergic nervous system activity. Sudden deaths in alcohol withdrawal most likely result from such dysrhythmias. Adequate sedation will play a part in preventing such unwanted occurrences happening in police custody, although those with severe alcohol withdrawal are best admitted to the hospital, where they can be placed on a cardiac monitor.

4.6.3.4. Metabolic Disorders

Wernicke's encephalopathy is an acute, potentially reversible neurologic disorder that is believed to result from a deficiency of thiamine and is often secondary to chronic alcohol abuse. Features include disturbance of consciousness (ranging from mild confusion to coma), ophthalmoplegia, nystagmus, and ataxia. The disorder has a high mortality and can lead to death within 24 hours. If untreated, it can progress to Korsakoff's psychosis. This is a chronic condition that usually presents as impairment of short-term memory with inability to learn new information and compensatory confabulation. Korsakoff's psychosis probably represents irreversible brain damage secondary to the combined toxicity of alcohol and metabolic derangement resulting from thiamine deficiency.

REFERENCES

1. National Institute of Justice. 2000 Arrestee Drug Abuse Monitoring: Annual Report. U.S. Department of Justice, Office of Justice Programs, Washington D.C., 2000.

2. Bennett, T. and Holloway K. Drug use and offending: summary results of the first two years of the NEW-ADAM programme. Findings 179. Home Office Research, Development and Statistics Directorate. London: Home Office. Detailed report available online—Holloway, K. and Bennett, T. The results of the first two years of the NEW-ADAM programme. Home Office Online Report 19/04. Research, Development and Statistics Directorate. London: Home Office, 2004.
3. Association of Police Surgeons and Royal College of Psychiatrists. Substance Misuse Detainees in Police Custody. Guidelines for Clinical Management, 2nd Ed. Report of a Medical Working Group. Council Report CR81. London: Royal College of Psychiatrists, 2000.
4. Drug Enforcement Administration. Illegal Drug Price and Purity Report. Drug Intelligence Report. US Department of Justice. Drug Enforcement Administration, 2003
5. Corkery, J. M. Drug Seizure and Offender Statistics, United Kingdom 2002. Home Office, London, 2002.
6. Nicholson, F. Infectious diseases and an at risk exposure. In: Stark M.M., Rogers D.J., Norfolk G.A. eds., Good Practice Guidelines for Forensic Medical Examiners–Metropolitan Police. GPG Editors, Oxford, 2004.
7. Norfolk, G. A., and Gray S. F. Intravenous drug users and broken needles—a hidden risk? Addiction. 98:1163–1166, 2003.
8. Wallace, P., Cutler, S., Haines, A. Randomised controlled trial of general practitioner intervention in patients with excessive alcohol consumption. Br. Med. J. 297:663–668, 1988.
9. Porchaska, J. O., and Clemente. C. C. The Transtheoretical Approach: Crossing Traditional Boundaries of therapy, Dow-Jones-Irwin, Homewood, IL, 1984.
10. Edmunds, M., May, T., Hearnden, I., Hough, M. Arrest Referral: Emerging Lessons from Research. Home Office Drugs Prevention Initiative Paper 23. Home Office, London, 1998.
11. Department of Health. The Scottish Office Department of Health. Welsh Office. Department of Health and Social Services, Northern Ireland. Drug Misuse and Dependence—Guidelines on Clinical Management. Her Majesty's Stationery Office, London, 1999.
12. Tennant, F. and Shannon, J. Cocaine abuse in methadone maintenance patients is associated with low serum methadone concentrations. J. Addict. Dis. 14:67–74, 1995.
13. Gossop, M., Marsden, J., Stewart, D., Kidd, T. The National Treatment Outcome Research Study (NTORS): 4-5 year follow-up results. Addiction. 98:291–303, 2003.
14. Karch, S. B. Medical consequences of opiate abuse. In: Karch, S. B., ed., The Pathology of Drug Abuse. CRC Press, Boca Raton, 2002, pp. 392–400.
15. Nutt, D. J. Addiction: brain mechanisms and their treatment implications. Lancet. 347:31–36, 1996.

15a. Ling, W. and Wesson, D. R. Drugs of abuse: opiates, in addiction medicine (Special Edition). West. J. Med. 152: 565–572, 1990.

16. Phillips, G. T., Gossop, M., Bradley, B. The influence of psychological factors on opiate withdrawal syndrome. Brit. J. Psychiatry. 149:235–238, 1986.

17. Ruben, S. M., McLean, P. C., Melville, J. Cyclizine abuse among a group of opiate dependents receiving methadone. Br. J. Addict. 84:929–934, 1989.

18. De Wet, C.J., Reed, L.J., Glasper, A., Moran, P. Bearn, J., Gossop, M. Benzodiaz-epine co-dependence exacerbates the opiate withdrawal syndrome. SSA Sympo-sium Abstracts. Addict. Biol. 9:100, 2004.

19. Evans, J. V. Dihydrocodeine detox regime. HMP Manchester, personal communi-cation, 1998.

20. Washton, A. M., Resnick, R. B., Geyer, G. Opiate withdrawal using lofexidine, a clonidine analogue with few side effects. J. Clin. Psychiatry. 44, 335–337, 1983.

21. Ford, C., Morton, S., Lintzeris, N., Bury, J., Gerada C. Guidance for the Use of Buprenorphine for the Treatment of Opioid Dependence in Primary Care. Royal College of General Practitioners, London, 2003.

22. Stark, M. M. Substance misusers (drugs and alcohol) in custody. In: Stark M.M., Rogers D.J., and Norfolk G.A., eds., Good Practice Guidelines for Forensic Medi-cal Examiners—Metropolitan Police. GPG Editors, Oxford, 2004.

23a. Roth, B., Benowitz, N., Olson, K. Emergency management of drug-abuse-related disorders. In: Karch, S. B., ed., Drug Abuse Handbook, CRC Press, Boca Raton, FL, pp. 567–639, 1998.

23. Ghodse, H. Drugs of abuse and dependence. In: Ghodse, H. ed., Drugs and Addic-tive Behaviour—A Guide to Treatment. Cambridge University Press, Cambridge, 2002, p. 105.

24. Yealy, D. M., Paris, P. M., Kaplan, R. M., Heller, M. B., Marini, S. E. The safety of prehospital naloxone administration by paramedics. Ann. Emerg. Med. 19:902–905, 1990.

25. Jones, A. L. Initial management of poisoned patients in the out-of-hospital environ-ment. Pre-Hospital Immediate Care. 2:141–149, 1998.

26. Merigian, K. S. Cocaine-induced ventricular arrhythmias and rapid atrial fibrillation temporarily related to naloxone administration. Am. J. Emerg. Med. 11:96–97, 1993.

27. Ashton, H. Guidelines for the rational use of benzodiazepines. When and what to use. Drugs. 48:25–40, 1994.

28. Cowen, P. J. and Nutt, D. J. Abstinence symptoms after withdrawal of tranquillising drugs. Is there a common neurochemical mechanism? Lancet. 2:360–362, 1982.

29. Bezchlibnyk-Butler, K. Z., Jeffries, J. J. Clinical Handbook of Psychotropic Drugs. Hogrefe and Huber, Toronto, 1996.

30. Vgontzas, A. N., Kales, A., Bixler, E. O. Benzodiazepine side effects: role of pharmacokinetics and pharmacodynamics. Pharmacology. 51:205–223, 1995.

31. Editorial. Tranquillisers causing aggression. Br. Med. J. 1:113–114, 1975.

32. Gordon, E. B. Tranquillisers causing aggression. Br. Med. J. 2:36–37, 1975.

33. Zevin, S., and Benowitz, N. L. Drug-related syndromes. In: Karch, S. B., ed., Drug Abuse Handbook. CRC Press, Boca Raton, FL, pp. 559–560, 1998.

34. Ashton, H. Benzodiazepine withdrawal: an unfinished story. Br. Med. J. 288:1135–1140, 1984.
35. Petursson, H. The benzodiazepine withdrawal syndrome. Addiction. 89:1455–1459, 1994.
36. Roald, O. K., and Dahl, V. Flunitrazepam intoxication in a child successfully treated with the benzodiazepine antagonist flumazenil. Crit Care Med. 17:1355–1356, 1989.
37. Hojer, J., Baehrendtz, S., Matell, G., Gustafsson, L. L. Diagnostic utility of flumazenil in coma with suspected poisoning: a double blind randomised controlled study. Br. Med. J. 301:1308–1311, 1990.
38. Katz, Y., Boulos, M., Singer, P., Rosenberg, B. Cardiac arrest associated with Flumazenil. Br. Med. J. 304,:1415, 1992.
39. Ives, R. Drug Notes: 6 Solvents. Drugscope, London, 2002.
40. Al-Alousi, L. M. Pathology of volatile substance abuse: a case report and a literature review. Med Sci Law. 29:189–208, 1989.
41. Ron, M. A. Volatile substance abuse: a review of possible long-term neurological, intellectual and psychiatric sequelae. Br. J. Psychiatry. 148:235–246, 1986.
42. Shepherd, R. T. Mechanism of sudden death associated with volatile substance abuse. Hum Toxicol. 8:287–292, 1989.
43. Taylor, G. J. and Harris, W. S. Cardiac toxicity of aerosol propellants. JAMA. 214:81–85, 1970.
44. Merry, J. and Zachariadis, N. Addiction to glue sniffing. Br. Med. J. 2:1448, 1962.
45. Leikin, J. B., Krantz, A. J., Zell-Kanter, M., Barkin, R. L., Hryhorczuk, D. O. Clinical features and management of intoxication due to hallucinogenic drugs. Med. Toxicol. Adverse Drug Exp. 4:324–350, 1989.
46. Hollister, L. E. and Hartman, A. M. Mescaline, lysergic acid diethylamide and psilocybin: comparison of clinical syndromes, effects on color perception and biochemical measures. Comp. Psychiatry. 3:235–241, 1962.
47. Abraham, H. D. and Aldridge, A. M. Adverse consequences of lysergic acid diethylamide. Addiction. 88:1327–1334, 1993.
48. Schwartz, R. H. LSD. Its rise, fall and renewed popularity among high school students. Pediatric Clin. North Am. 42:403–413, 1995.
49. McCarron, M. M., Schulze, B. W., Thompson, G. A., Conder, M.C., Goetz, W. A. Acute phencyclidine intoxication: clinical patterns, complications and treatment. Ann. Emerg. Med. 10:290–297, 1981.
50. Brust, J. C. M. Other agents. Phencyclidine, marijuana, hallucinogens, inhalants and anticholinergics. Neurol. Clin. 11, 555–561, 1993.
51. Aniline, O. and Pitts Jr, F. N. Phencyclidine (PCP): a review and perspectives. Crit. Rev. Toxicol. 10:145–177, 1982.
52. Steele, T. D., McCann, U. D., Ricaurte, G. A. 3,4-Methylenedioxymethamphetamine (MDMA, "ecstasy"): pharmacology and toxicology in animals and humans. Addiction. 89:539–551, 1994.
53. Maxwell, D. L., Polkey, M. I., Henry, J. A. Hyponatraemia and catatonic stupor after taking "ecstasy." Br. Med. J. 307:1399, 1993.

54. Kessel, B. Hyponatraemia after ingestion of "ecstasy." Br. Med. J. 308:414, 1994.
55. Henry, J. A., Fallon, J. K., Kicman, A. T., Hutt, A. J., Cowan, D. A., Forsling, M. Low-dose MDMA ("ecstasy") induces vasopressin secretion. Lancet. 351:1784, 1998.
56. Redfearn, P. J., Agrawal, N., Mair, L. H. An association between the regular use of 3,4, methylenedioxy-methamphetamine (ecstasy) and excessive wear of the teeth. Addiction. 93:745–748, 1998.
57. Shearman, J. D., Chapman, R. W. G., Satsangi, J., Ryley, N. G. Misuse of ecstasy. Br. Med. J. 305:309, 1992.
58. Creighton, F. J., Black, D. L., Hyde, C. E. "Ecstasy" psychosis and flashbacks. Br. J. Psychiatry. 159:713–715, 1991.
59. Levine, A. J., Drew, S., Rees, G. M. "Ecstasy" induced pneumomediastinum. J. Royal Soc. Med. 86:232–233, 1993.
60. Bryden, A. A., Rothwell, P. J. N., O'Reilly, P. H. Urinary retention with misuse of "ecstasy". Br. Med. J. 310:504, 1995.
61. Chadwick, I. S., Curry, P. D., Linsley, A., Freemont, A. J., Doran, B. Ecstasy, 3-4 methylenedioxymethamphetamine (MDMA), a fatality associated with coagulopathy and hyperthermia. J. Royal Soc. Med. 84:371, 1991.
62. Brown, C., and Osterloh, J. Multiple severe complications from recreational ingestion of MDMA ("ecstasy"). JAMA. 258:780–781, 1987.
63. Dowling, G. P., McDonough, E. T., Bost, R. O. "Eve" and "ecstasy." A report of five deaths associated with the use of MDEA and MDMA. JAMA. 257:1615–1617, 1987.
64. Campkin, N. T. A. and Davies, U. M. Another death from Ecstasy. J. Royal Soc. Med. 85:61, 1992.
65. McGuire, P. and Fahy, T. Chronic paranoid psychosis after misuse of MDMA (ecstasy). Br. Med. J. 302:697, 1991.
66. Sternbach, H. The serotonin syndrome. Am. J. Psychiatry. 148:705–713, 1991.
67. Mueller, P. D. and Korey, W. S. Death by "ecstasy": the serotonin syndrome? Ann. Emerg. Med. 32:377–380, 1991.
68. McCann, U. D., Szabo, Z., Scheffel, U., Dannals, R. F., Ricaurte, G. A. Positron emission tomographic evidence of toxic effect of MDMA ("ecstasy") on brain serotonin neurons in human beings. Lancet. 352:1433–1437, 1998.
69. James, R. A. and Dinan, A. Hyperpyrexia associated with fatal paramethoxyamphetamine (PMA) abuse. Med Sci Law. 38:83–85, 1998.
70. Resnick, R. B., Kestenbaum, R. S., Schwartz, L. K. Acute systemic effects of cocaine in man—a controlled study by intranasal and intravenous routes. Science. 195:696–698, 1977.
71. Karch, S. B. Cocaine. In: Karch, S. B., ed., The Pathology of Drug Abuse. CRC Press, Boca Raton, FL, 2002, pp. 91-120.
72. Griffiths, P., Gossop, M., Wickenden, S., Dunworth, J., Harris, K., Lloyd, C. A transcultural pattern of drug use: qat (khat) in the UK. Br. J. Psychiatry. 170:281–284, 1997.
73. Ahmed, A. G., and Salib, E. The Khat users: a study of khat chewing in Liverpool's Somali men. Med Sci Law. 38:165–169, 1998.

74. Joyce, H. Khat. J. Forensic Psychiatry. 5:228–231, 1994.

75. Luqman, W., and Danowski, T. S. The use of khat (Catha edulis) in Yemen. Social and medical observations. Ann. Intern. Med. 85, 246–249, 1976.

76. Yousef, G., Huq, Z., Lambert, T. Khat chewing as a cause of psychosis. Br. J. Hosp. Med. 54:322–326, 1995.

77. Pantelis, C., Hindler, C. G., Taylor, J. C. Use and abuse of khat (Catha edulis): a review of the distribution, pharmacology, side effects, and a description of psychosis attributed to khat chewing. Psychol Med. 19:657–658, 1989.

78. Condon, J., and Smith, N. Prevalence of drug use: key findings from the 2002/2003 British Crime Survey. Home Office Research, Development and Statistics Directorate. London, 2003.

79. Cohen, J., and Hayes, G. Drug Notes: 3 Cannabis. Drugscope, London, 2002.

80. Wylie, A. S., Scott, R. T. A., Burnett, S. J. Psychosis due to "skunk." Br. Med. J. 311:125, 1995.

81. British Medical Association. Therapeutic Uses of Cannabis. Harwood Academic Publishers, Amsterdam, 1997, pp. 19–20.

82. Stephens, R. S., Roffman, R. A., Simpson, E. E. Adult marijuana users seeking treatment. J. Consult. Clin. Psychol. 61:1100–1104, 1993.

83. Bhasin, S., Storer, T. W., Berman, N., et al. The effects of superphysiologic doses of testosterone on muscle size and strength in normal men. N. Engl. J. Med. 335:1–7, 1996.

84. Kennedy, M. Athletes, drugs and adverse reactions. Adverse Drug Reaction Bull. 143, 536–539, 1990.

85. ISDD. Drug Notes 9: Anabolic Steroids. ISDD, London.

86. Haupt, H. A. and Rovere, G. D. Anabolic steroids: a review of the literature. Am. J. Sports Med. 12:469–484, 1984.

87. Stanley, A. and Ward, M. Anabolic steroids—the drugs that give and take away manhood. A case with an unusual physical sign. Med. Sci. Law. 34, 82–83, 1994.

88. Lloyd, F. H. Powell, P., Murdoch, A. P. Anabolic steroid abuse by body builders and male subfertility. Br. Med. J. 313:100–101, 1996.

89. Creagh, T. M., Rubin, A., Evans, D. J. Hepatic tumours induced by anabolic steroids in an athlete. J. Clin. Pathol. 41:441–443, 1988.

90. Su, T., Pagliaro M., Schmidt, P. J., Pickar, D., Wolkowitz, O., Rubinow D. R. Neuropsychiatric effects of anabolic steroids in male normal volunteers. JAMA. 269:2760–2764, 1993.

91. Pope, H. G. and Katz, D. L. Psychiatric and medical effects of anabolic-androgenic steroid use. Arch. Gen. Psychiatry. 51:375–382, 1994.

92. Corrigan, B. Anabolic steroids and the mind. Med. J. Aust. 165:222–226, 1996.

93. British Medical Association. Drugs in Sport. The Pressure to Perform. BMA, London, 2002.

94. Perry, H. M., Wright, D., Littlepage, B. N. C. Dying to be big: a review of anabolic steroid use. Br J Sports Med. 26:259–261, 1992.

95. Littlepage, B. N. C. and Perry, H. M. Misusing anabolic drugs: possibilities for future policies. Addiction. 88:1469–1471, 1993.

96. McBride, A. J., Williamson, K., Petersen, T. Three cases of nalbuphine hydrochloride dependence associated with anabolic steroid use. Br. J. Sports Med. 30:69–70, 1996.

97. Elkin, S. L., Brady, S., Williams, I. P. Bodybuilders find it easy to obtain insulin to help them in training. Br. Med. J. 314:1280, 1997.

98. FitzSimmons, C. R. and Kidner, N. Caffeine toxicty in a bodybuilder. J. Acid Emerg. Med. 15:196–1970, 1998.

99. Perry, H. M. and Littlepage, B. N. C. Misusing anabolic drugs. Br. Med. J. 305:1241–1242, 1992.

100. Roth, R. H. and Giarman, N. J. Natural occurrence of gamma-hydroxybutyrate in mammalian brain. Biochem. Pharmacol. 19:1087–1093, 1970.

101. Galloway, G. P., Frederick, S. L., Staggers Jr, F. E., Gonzales, M., Stalcup, S. A., and Smith, D. E. Gamma-hydroxybutyrate: an emerging drug of abuse that causes physical dependence. Addiction. 92:89–96, 1997.

102. Cohen, J. Drug Notes: 9 Poppers, Ketamine and GHB. London, Drugscope, 2002.

103. Ferrara, S. D., Zotti, S., Tedeshi, L., et al. Pharmacokinetics of gamma-hydroxybutyric acid in alcohol dependent patients after single and repeated oral doses. Br. J. Clin. Pharmacol. 34:231–235, 1992

104. Luby, S., Jones, J., and Zalewski, A. GHB use in South Carolina. Am. J. Public Health. 82:128, 1992.

105. Thomas, G., Bonner, S., and Gascoigne, A. Coma induced by abuse of gamma-hydroxybutyrate: a case report. Br. Med. J. 314, 35–36, 1997.

106. Dyer, J. E. ER admission cases discussed, in Getting the Scoop on GHB: The New Recreational Drug. Presented at the 49th Annual Meeting of the American Academy of Forensic Sciences, New York, 1997

107. Dyer, J. E., Kreutzer, R., Quatrrone, A., et al. Multistate outbreak of poisonings associated with the illicit use of gammahydroxybutyrate. JAMA. 265: 447–448, 1992.

108. McDonough, M. Glasper, A., Bearn, J. Managing gamma hydroxybutyrate or "liquid ecstasy" withdrawal – meta-analysis of published cases and reporting early experience in the UK. SSA Symposium Abstracts. Addiction Biology. 8:2, 241–242, 2003.

109. Cohen, J. Drug Notes: 9 Poppers, Ketamine and GHB. London, Drugscope, 2002

110. Jansen, K. L. R. Non-medical use of ketamine. BMJ. 306: 601–602, 1993.

111. Slogoff, S., Allen, G. W., Wessels, J. V. Clinical experience with subanaesthetic ketamine. Anesth Analg (Cleve). 53:354–358, 1974.

112. White, P. F., Way, W. L., Trevor, A. J. Ketamine: its pharmacology and therapeutic uses. Anaethesiology. 56:119–136, 1982.

113. Medicines Compendium. Ketalar. Datapharm Publications, London, 2002.

114. Moore, K. A., Kilbane, E. M., Jones, R., Kunsman, G. W., Levine, B., Smith, M. Tissue distribution of ketamine in a mixed drug fatality. J. Forensic Sci. 2:1183–1185, 1997.

115. Sigell, L. T., Kapp, F. T., Fusaro, G. A., Nelson E. D., Falck, R. S. Popping and snorting volatile nitrites: a current fad for getting high. Am J Psychiatry. 135:1216–1218, 1978.

116. Schwartz, R. H. and Peary, P. Abuse of isobutyl nitrite inhalation (rush) by adolescents. Clin Pediatr. 25:308–310, 1986.
117. Stambach, T., Haire, K., Soni, N., and Booth, J. Saturday night blue—a case of near fatal poisoning from the abuse of amyl nitrite. J. Accid. Emerg. Med. 14:339–340, 1997.
118. Virkkunen, M., and Linnoila, M. Brain serotonin, type II alcoholism and impulsive violence. J. Stud. Alcohol. 11(Suppl):163–169, 1993.
119. Magennis, P., Shepherd, J., Hutchison, I., Brown, A. Trends in facial injury. Br. Med. J. 316:325–326, 1998.
120. The All Party Group on Alcohol Abuse. Alcohol and Crime: Breaking the Link. Alcohol Concern, London, 1995.
121. Sumner, M., and Parker, H. Low in Alcohol. A Review of International Research into Alcohol's Role in Crime Causation. The Portman Group, London, 1995.
122. Moore, M. R. and Moore, S. R. The potential for the use of personal computers in clinical forensic medicine. J. Clin. Forensic Med. 1:139–143, 1994.
123. Robertson, G. The Role of Police Surgeons. The Royal Commission on Criminal Justice. Research Study No 6. Her Majesty's Stationery Office, London, 1992.
124. Payne-James, J. J., Keys, D. W., Wall, I., Jerreat, P. G., Dean, P. J. Alcohol misuse in clinical forensic medicine. J. Clin. Forensic Med. 4:17–19, 1997.
125. Best, D. Kefas, A. The role of alcohol in police-related deaths. Analysis of deaths in custody (Category 3) between 2000 and 2001. Police Complaints Authority, London, 2004.
126. Stockwell, T. and Stirling, L. Estimating alcohol content of drinks: common errors in applying the unit system. Br. Med. J. 298:571–572, 1989.
127. EEC Directive 766. 1976.
128. Ferner, R. E. Forensic Pharmacology. Medicines, Mayhem, and Malpractice. Oxford University Press, Oxford, 1996.
129. Baselt, R. C. Disposition of alcohol in man. In: Garriott, J, C., ed. Medicolegal Aspects of Alcohol, 3rd Ed. Lawyers and Judges Publishing Company, Tucson, AZ, 1996.
130. Stark, M. M. and Norfolk, G. A. Substance misuse. In: McLay, W. D. S. ed., Clinical Forensic Medicine. Greenwich Medical Media, London, 1996, pp. 173–179.
131. Holford, N. H. G. Clinical pharmacokinetics of ethanol. Clin. Pharmacokinet. 13:273–292, 1987.
132. Wilkinson, P. K., Sedman, A. J., Sakmar, E., Earhart, R. H., Kay, D. R., Wagner, J. G. Pharmacokinetics of ethanol after oral administration in the fasting state. J. Pharmacokinet. Biopharm. 5:207–224, 1977.
133. Jones, A. W. Biochemistry and physiology of alcohol: applications to forensic science and toxicology. In: Garriott, J. C., ed. Medicolegal Aspects of Alcohol, 3rd Ed. Lawyers and Judges, Tucson, AZ, 1996.
134. Drew, G. C., Colquhoun, W. P., Long, H. A. Effect of Small Doses of Alcohol on a Skill Resembling Driving. Medical Research Council Memorandum No. 38. Her Majesty's Stationery Office, London, 1959.

135. Jones, A. W. and Jonsson, K. A. Between-subject and within-subject variations in the pharmacokinetics of ethanol. Br. J. Clin. Pharmacol. 37:427–431, 1994.
136. Schultz, J., Weiner, H., Westcott, J. Retardation of ethanol absorption by food in the stomach. J. Stud. Alcohol. 41:861–870, 1980.
137. Jones, A. W., and Jonsson, K. A. Food-induced lowering of blood-ethanol profiles and increased rate of elimination immediately after a meal. J. Forensic Sci. 39:1084–1093, 1994.
138. Sedman, A. J., Wilkinson, P. K., Sakmar, E., Weidler, D. J., Wagner, J. G. Food effects on absorption and elimination of alcohol. J. Stud. Alcohol. 37:1197–1214, 1976.
139. Walls, H. and Brownlie, A. R. Drink, Drugs and Driving, 2nd Ed. Sweet and Maxwell, London, 1985.
140. Jones, A. W. and Sternebring, B. Kinetics of ethanol and methanol in alcoholics during detoxification. Alcohol Alcoholism. 27:641–647, 1992.
141. Manno, J. E. and Manno, B. R. Experimental basis of alcohol-induced psychomotor performance impairment. In: Garriott, J.C., ed., Medicolegal Aspects of Alcohol, 3rd Ed. Lawyers and Judges, Tucson, AZ, 1996.
142. Urso, T., Gavaler, J. S., Van Thiel, D. H. Blood ethanol levels in sober alcohol users seen in an emergency room. Life Sci. 28:1053–1056, 1981.
143. Sullivan, J. B., Hauptman, M., Bronstein, A. C. Lack of observable intoxication in humans with high plasma alcohol concentrations. J. Forensic Sci. 32:1660–1665, 1987.
144. Garriott, J. C. Pharmacology and toxicology of ethyl alcohol. In: Garriott, J.C., ed. Medicolegal Aspects of Alcohol, 3rd Ed. Lawyers and Judges, Tucson, AZ, 1996.
145. Money, K., and Myles, W. Heavy water nystagmus and effects of alcohol. Nature. 247:404–405, 1974.
146. Behrens, M. M. Nystagmus. J. Ophthalmol Clin. 18:57–82, 1978.
147. Aschan, G. Different types of alcohol nystagmus. Acta Otolaryngol. 140(Suppl):69–78, 1958.
148. Aschan, G., Bergstedt, M., Goldberg, L., Laurell, L. Positional nystagmus in man during and after alcohol intoxication. Q. J. Stud. Alcohol. 17:381–405, 1956.
149. Goding, G. S. and Dobie, R. A. Gaze nystagmus and blood alcohol. Laryngoscope. 96:713–717, 1986.
150. Belton, H. Lateral nystagmus: a specific diagnostic sign of ethyl alcohol intoxication. N. Z. Med. J. 100:534–535, 1987.
151. Eakins, W. A. Clinical signs and the level of blood alcohol. Police Surg. 11:8–15, 1977.
152. Willoughby, E. W. Nystagmus and alcohol intoxication. N. Z. Med. J. 100:640, 1987.
153. Moczula, B. Alcohol and the law: the legal framework of scientific evidence and expert testimony. In: Garriott, J. C., ed. Medicolegal Aspects of Alcohol, 3rd Ed. Lawyers and Judges, Tucson, AZ, 1996.
154. British Medical Association. The Recognition of Intoxication. Report of a Special Committee of the British Medical Association. BMA, London, 1954.
155. Tennant, F. The rapid eye test to detect drug abuse. Postgrad. Med. 84:108–114, 1988.
156. Fleming, P. and Stewart, D. Drugs and Driving: Training Implications for Police Officers and Police Surgeons. Home Office Police Policy Directorate, London, 1998.

157. Simpson-Crawford, T. and Slater, S. W. Eye signs in suspected drinking drivers: clinical examination and relation to blood alcohol. N. Z. Med. J. 74:92–96, 1971.

158. Johnson, K., Pisoni, D. B., Bernacki, R. H. Do voice recordings reveal whether a person is intoxicated? A case study. Phonetica. 47:215–237, 1990.

159. Martin, C. S. Measuring acute alcohol impairment. In: Karch, S. B., ed., Drug Abuse Handbook. CRC Press, Boca Raton, FL, 1998, pp. 309–326.

160. Potter, J. F., Watson, R. D. S., Skan, W., Beevers, D. G. The pressor and metabolic effects of alcohol in normotensive subjects. Hypertension. 8:625–631, 1986.

161. Kelbaek, H., Gjorup, T., Brynjolf, I., Christensen, N. J., Godtfredsen, J. Acute effects of alcohol on left ventricular function in healthy subjects at rest and during upright exercise. Am. J. Cardiol. 55:164–167, 1985.

162. Kaye, S. and Haag, H. B. Terminal blood alcohol concentrations in 94 fatal cases of alcoholism. JAMA. 165:451–452, 1957.

163. Johnson, R. A., Noll, E. C., MacMillan Rodney, W. Survival after a serum ethanol level of 1.5 per cent. Lancet. 2:1394, 1982.

164. Rix, K. J. B. "Alcohol intoxication" or "drunkenness": is there a difference? Med. Sci. Law. 29:100–106, 1989.

165. American Psychiatric Association. Diagnostic and Statistical Manual of Mental Disorders. 4th Ed. American Psychiatric Association, Washington, D.C., 1994.

166. Norfolk, G. A. Deaths in police custody during 1994: a retrospective analysis. J. Clin. Forensic Med. 5:49–54, 1998.

167. Royal College of Psychiatrists. Alcohol: Our Favourite Drug. Royal College of Psychiatrists, London, 1986.

168. Deehan, A., Stark, M. M., Marshall, E. J., Hanrahan, B., Strang, J. Drunken detainees in police custody: is brief intervention by the forensic medical examiner feasible? Crimin. Behav. Mental Health. 8:214–221, 1998.

169. Reilly, D., Van Beurden, E., Mitchell, E., Dight, R., Scott, C., Beard, J. Alcohol education in licensed premises using brief intervention strategies. Addiction. 93:385–398, 1998.

170. Midanik, L. The validity of self-reported alcohol consumption and alcohol problems: a literature review. Br. J. Addic. 77:357–382, 1982.

171. Babor, T. F., Ramon de la Fuente, J., Saunders, J., Grant, M. AUDIT, The Alcohol Use Disorders Identification Test: Guidelines for use in Primary Health Care. World Health Organization, Geneva, 1992.

172. Pokorny, A. D., Miller, B. A., Kaplan, H. B. The brief MAST: a shortened version of the Michigan alcoholism screening test. Am. J. Psychiatry. 129:342–345, 1972.

173. Hedlund, J. L., and Vieweg, B. W. The Michigan Alcoholism Screening Test (MAST): a comprehensive review. J. Operational Psychiatry. 15:55–65, 1984.

174. Mayfield, D., McLeod, G., Hall, P. The CAGE questionnaire: validation of a new alcoholism screening instrument. Am. J. Psychiatry. 131:1121–1123, 1974.

175. Ewing, J. A. Detecting alcoholism. The CAGE questionnaire. JAMA. 252:1905–1907, 1984.

176. Romach, M. K., and Sellers, E. M. Management of the alcohol withdrawal syndrome. Annu. Rev. Med. 42:323–340, 1991.

177. Naik, P., and Lawton, J. (1993) Pharmacological management of alcohol withdrawal. Br. J. Hosp. Med. 50:265–269, 1991.
178. Mayo-Smith, M. F. for the American Society of Addiction Medicine Working Group on Pharmacological Management of Alcohol Withdrawal. Pharmacological management of alcohol withdrawal. A meta-analysis and evidence-based practice guideline. JAMA. 278:144–151, 1997.
179. Naik, P. and Lawton, J. Assessment and management of individuals under the influence of alcohol in police custody. J. Clin. Forensic Med. 3:37–44, 1996.
180. Linnoila, M. I. Benzodiazepines and alcohol. J. Psychiatr Res. 24(Suppl 2):121–127, 1990.

Chapter 11

Deaths in Custody

Richard Shepherd

1. INTRODUCTION

The forensic physician will, in all probability, have to deal with a death in police custody at some point in his or her career. This chapter aims to provide a broad basis for the understanding of the disease processes and the mechanisms that may lead to death and also to provide some understanding of the current thinking behind deaths associated with restraint.

2. DEFINITION

In considering any death associated with detention by officials of any state, caused by whatever means, each state will define, according to its own legal system, the situations that are categorized as being "in custody" (1). The worldwide variations in these definitions have caused, and continue to cause, considerable confusion in any discussion of this subject. For the purposes of this chapter, "in custody" relates to any individual who is either under arrest or otherwise under police control and, although similar deaths may occur in prison, in psychiatric wards, or in other situations where people are detained against their will, the deaths specifically associated with police detention form the basis for this chapter.

It is important to distinguish between the different types of custodial deaths because deaths that are related to direct police actions (acts of commission) seem to cause the greatest concern to the family, public, and press. It is also important to remember that police involvement in the detention of individuals

From: *Clinical Forensic Medicine: A Physician's Guide, 2nd Edition*
Edited by: M. M. Stark © Humana Press Inc., Totowa, NJ

extends beyond direct physical contact and includes a "duty of care" to that individual, and "lack of care" may be termed "acts of omission." Lack of police action, or "care," has also been responsible for deaths in custody. These acts are considerably harder to define and perhaps sometimes result from the police being placed in, or assuming, a role of caring (e.g., in states of alcoholic intoxication or acute psychiatric conditions) that is beyond their competence or which they are not equipped or trained to fulfill.

Police involvement with an individual can also include those who are being pursued by the police either on foot or by vehicle, those who have been stopped and are being questioned outside the environment of a police station, and those who have become unwell through natural causes while in contact with or in the custody of the police.

The definitions of "death in custody" are therefore wide, and attempts at simple definitions are fraught with difficulty. Any definition will have to cover a multitude of variable factors, in various circumstances and with a variety of individuals. The crucial point is that the police owe a duty of care to each and every member of the public with whom they have contact, and it is essential that every police officer, whether acting or reacting to events, understands and is aware of the welfare of the individual or individuals with whom he or she is dealing.

3. STATISTICS

Because of the lack of a standard international definition of "death in custody," the simple comparison of the published raw data from different countries is of no value. The number of deaths recorded in police custody in England and Wales from 1990 to 2002 *(2)* shows considerable variation year to year but with an encouraging decline from the peak in 1998 (Fig. 1). In contrast, the data from Australia for much of the same period show little change *(3)* (Fig. 2). These raw data must be treated with considerable care because any changes in the death rates may not be the result of changes in the policy and practice of care for prisoners but of other undetermined factors, such as a decline in arrest rates during the period.

4. INVESTIGATION OF DEATHS IN CUSTODY

4.1. Legal Framework

In the United Kingdom, all deaths occurring in prison (or youth custody) *(4)* must be referred to the coroner who holds jurisdiction for that area. However, no such obligation exists concerning deaths in police custody, although the Home Office recommends *(5)* that all deaths falling into the widest defini-

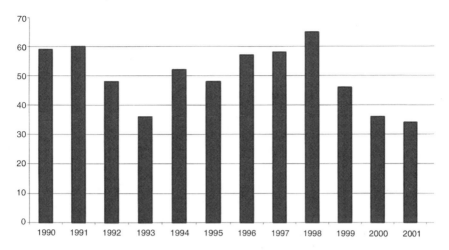

Fig. 1. Deaths in police custody in England and Wales.

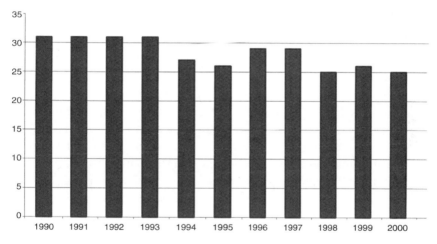

Fig. 2. Deaths in police custody in Australia.

tion of "in custody" should be subject to a coroner's inquest, and, hence, a full inquiry into the facts and a full postmortem examination should be performed. This acceptance that all deaths occurring in custody should be fully investigated and considered by the legal system must represent the ideal situation; however, not every country will follow this, and some local variations can and do occur, particularly in the United States.

4.2. Protocol

No standard or agreed protocol has been devised for the postmortem examination of these deaths, and, as a result, variation in the reported details of these examinations is expected. These differences in the procedures and the number and type of the specialist tests performed result in considerable variation in the pathological detail available as a basis for establishing the cause of death and, hence, available for presentation at any subsequent inquest. The absence of a defined protocol hinders the analysis of the results of these examinations and makes even the simplest comparisons unreliable. There is an urgent need for a properly established academic study of all of these deaths, such as that performed in Australia under the auspices of the Australian Institute of Criminology (6), to be instituted in the United Kingdom and the United States.

4.3. Terminology

In addition to the lack of reproducibility of the postmortem examinations, the terminology used by the pathologists to define the cause of death, particularly in the form required for the registration of the death, may often be idiosyncratic, and similar disease processes may be denoted by different pathologists using many different phrases. For example, damage to the heart muscle caused by narrowing of the coronary arteries by atheroma may be termed simply ischemic heart disease or it may be called myocardial ischemia resulting from coronary atheroma or even by the "lay" term, heart attack (7). This variation in terminology may lead to confusion, particularly among lay people attempting to understand the cause and the manner of death. A considerable amount of research (1,7) has been produced based on such lay assessments of the pathological features of a death, and this has, at times, resulted in increased confusion rather than clarification of the issues involved.

If the issues regarding the definition of "in custody," the variation in the postmortem examinations and the production of postmortem reports, and the use and analysis of subsequent specialist tests all raise problems within a single country, then the consideration of these deaths internationally produces almost insuperable conflicts of medical terminology and judicial systems.

5. DEATHS RELATED TO THE PHASES OF THE CUSTODIAL PROCESS

In an attempt to add some clarity to the situation, it is possible to state that whatever national definition of "in custody" is used, numerous phases of the custododial process can be identified, and the types of deaths that occur during these phases can be analyzed. Clearly, a death, whether sudden or delayed, may

Table 1
Expected Types of Deaths in Different Phases of Custody

	Natural	Accidental trauma	Alcohol	Drug	Self-inflicted	Deliberately inflicted
Prearrest	++	+++	++	++	±	±
Arrest	++	+++	++	++	±	+++
Detention	+	+	+++	+++	++	++
Interview	+	+	++	++	+++	++
Charge	+	+	−	−	+++	±

occur for many reasons even in the absence of police, but because it is the involvement of police that is the *sine qua non* of "in custody," deaths in the first phase must be considered to be the presence of police officers at the scene. Subsequently, an arrest may be made with or without the use of restraint techniques and the prisoner will then be transported to a police station. This transport will most commonly involve a period within a police vehicle, which may be a car, a van with seating, or some other vehicle. Many factors may determine the type of transport used and the position of the individual in that vehicle. Detention in the police station will be followed by an interview period interspersed with periods of time incarcerated, usually alone, within a cell. After the interview, the individual may be released directly, charged and then released, or he or she may be detained to appear before a court. It is at this point that custody moves from the police to other authorities, usually to the prison service.

When considering the types of death that can occur during each of these phases, six main groups can be identified based on the reported causes of death. The groups are composed of the following:

- Natural deaths.
- Deaths associated with accidental trauma.
- Deaths related directly to the use of alcohol.
- Deaths related to the use of other drugs.
- Deaths associated with self-inflicted injury.
- Deaths associated with injuries deliberately inflicted by a third party.

It is clear that different factors may lead directly to or play a major part in the death of an individual while in custody and that different factors will play their part at different phases in the period of custody (*see* Table 1).

Acute alcohol intoxication or the deleterious effects of drugs are, in most cases, likely to have a decreasing effect because they are metabolized or excreted from the individual's body. Therefore, they are most likely to cause death in the postarrest and early detention phases, and it is important to note that their effects will be least visible to those with the "duty of care" while the individual is out of sight, detained within a cell, particularly if he or she is alone within that cell. Similarly, the effects of trauma, whether accidentally or deliberately inflicted, are most likely to become apparent in the early phases of detention, and it would only be on rare occasions that the effects of such trauma would result in fatalities at a later stage, although this has occurred on several occasions, particularly with head injuries *(7)*. Conversely, death resulting from self-inflicted injuries is unlikely to occur in the prearrest and arrest phases of detention but it can and does occur when the individual is placed in a cell and is not under immediate and constant supervision.

On the other hand, deaths from natural causes can occur at almost any time during the arrest and detention period. It is possible that the stress (whether emotional, physical, or both) associated with the initial phases of arrest and with the subsequent, more emotionally stressful phases during detention are likely to precipitate the death of the susceptible individuals through the effects of sympathetic stimulation and adrenalin release. Deaths from natural causes should be reduced by the medical examination and supervision of detainees from the time of initial detention and throughout the period of detention (*see* Chapter 8).

However, it is quite clear that the deaths described in many reports are not "pure" (i.e., they are not attributable to any one single category). Individuals with heart disease may also be under the influence of alcohol; individuals under the influence of alcohol or drugs may also have suffered trauma, either accidental or deliberate, before or during their detention. In determining the cause of death, it can therefore be extremely difficult to weigh each of the factors that could be identified during the period of detention. There is great need for early assessment and accurate diagnosis of natural disease (physical or psychiatric),alcohol or drug intoxication, and for the identification, documentation, and treatment of all types of trauma.

The removal of an individual's freedom places on the police a duty of care to that individual, and it is only by the active assessment of each and every person entering police custody and the continuing care of that individual that the number of deaths in custody can be reduced.

6. Causes of Death

6.1. Natural Causes

Apart from a few unusual cases, deaths resulting from natural causes while in police custody fall into the groups of disease processes that are commonly associated with sudden natural death in the community.

6.1.1. Cardiovascular Disease

The most common cause of death in the community, and of sudden death particularly, is cardiac disease, and within this group, those deaths recorded as resulting from ischemic heart disease or coronary atheroma are the most common. The exact definitions and criteria for the pathological diagnosis of significant ischemic heart disease *(8)* are not within the scope of this chapter. Although there is a clear increase in the incidence of this cause of death with age *(9)*, it is important to remember that a small percentage of people in the younger age groups, most commonly those with hypercholesterolemia and hyperlipidemia, may also have significant coronary artery disease, and because the younger age groups are more likely to be arrested by the police, these few individuals may assume great significance.

The significance of coronary atheroma is that individuals with this disease are particularly prone to the development of dysrhythmias during periods of stress when their decreased ability to perfuse areas of the myocardium may result in the development of ectopic electrical foci. Deaths may be preceded by the development of classical cardiac chest pain, or it may present with sudden collapse and death without warning.

Individuals suffering from significant myocardial hypertrophy resulting from chronic hypertension are also at greater risk during periods of stress. Once again, it is the older age groups that are most commonly affected by essential hypertension, which may also render these individuals susceptible to focal lack of myocardial perfusion during periods of tachycardia. In addition to these two disease processes, there are also rarer diseases or syndromes that may cause sudden death, which are possibly more significant in the context of "deaths in custody" because some of them tend to affect younger age groups in particular. Congenital valvular disease (e.g., floppy mitral valve disease) and congenital myocardial disease (e.g., cardiomyopathies) may both render an individual more susceptible to sudden cardiac death and, as with ischemic or hypertensive heart disease, sudden death is more likely when the sympathetic stimulation that is associated with stress (emotional and/or physical) has resulted in tachycardia.

Current research is now focusing on a genetic basis for many other sudden cardiac deaths in the younger age groups. These genetically mediated disease processes (e.g., the prolonged QT intervals) can sometimes be diagnosed in life by electrocardiogram; however, after death, their presence—and hence their possible relationship to the sudden death—can only be inferred from the detection of specific gene defects *(10)*. The examination for these specific gene markers in any sudden death in police custody must now be considered in the absence of other causes of death.

Myocarditis and rheumatic heart disease are rare causes of death in young individuals, although such deaths may occur without any prior indication of a disease process in individuals in police custody and elsewhere.

Other cardiovascular causes of sudden death, for the most part, are also age related. The rupture of atheromatous aortic aneurysms is a disease almost entirely confined to late-middle and old age, whereas the rarer forms of aortitis and collagen diseases of the aorta *(11)*, which may also result in rupture, are more commonly seen in the younger age groups.

Pulmonary emboli can cause sudden death or may present as dyspnea and chest pain. It is most unusual for deep venous thrombosis of the leg veins to be present in a young active male; however, the association between some types of the combined oral contraceptive pill and the development of thromboses has been known for some time *(12)* and may render a small subgroup of the female population at greater risk of pulmonary emboli than the general population.

6.1.2. Central Nervous System

The stress associated with arrest and detention in custody may also have significant effects on the cerebrovascular system and may, in susceptible individuals, precipitate intracerebral hemorrhage by the rupture of congenital or acquired aneurysms or vascular malformations. Ruptured berry aneurysms will result in the development of acute subarachnoid hemorrhages. It is less likely that these intracranial hemorrhages will result in sudden death, but they may result in sudden unconsciousness, which ultimately leads to death. Clearly, the distinction between hemorrhage resulting from a natural disease process and death resulting from trauma will need to be established and a specialist neuropathological examination will be required should death occur.

As with the heart, the possibility that an infectious process within the central nervous system (CNS) is the cause of sudden collapse and death must be considered. However, it is unlikely that meningitis or encephalitis will present without any prodromal symptoms. Epilepsy is unlikely to develop *de novo* after arrest and detention, but epilepsy can and does lead to sudden collapse and death, and a pre-existing history of epilepsy is clearly important. Any individual known to suffer from epilepsy should be monitored with the utmost care and his or her prescribed medication continued.

Other forms of intracranial pathology that may lead to sudden death include tumors, both benign and malignant, and such rarities as the development of colloid cysts of the ventricular system.

6.1.3. Endocrine

Diabetes mellitus should raise similar concerns to those associated with epilepsy because poorly controlled diabetes occasionally may be the direct cause of sudden death and, through its association with an increased incidence of arterial disease, it is a major factor in the development of coronary artery disease in the younger age groups. At postmortem, consideration must be given in all cases of sudden death in a young individual, particularly when there is a history of diabetes mellitus, to the sampling of the vitreous humor to determine the blood glucose level at the time of death. The samples must be taken as soon after death as possible to avoid postmortem use of the intraocular glucose yielding erroneous results *(14)*.

6.1.4. Other Causes

There are many other natural disease processes that could theoretically lead to sudden collapse and death. Among them is asthma, a disease that is usually unlikely to lead to sudden death if adequately treated and supervised but that may, if untreated and unsupervised and in stressful circumstances, result in the individual being found dead in their cell. Other disease processes include the development of hemoptysis, from tuberculosis or pulmonary malignancy, or hematemesis, from peptic ulceration or esophageal varices, which can be life threatening and may, because of the bleeding, be considered to be the result of trauma rather than a natural disease process. These cases should present no problem to an experienced pathologist following a full postmortem examination.

6.1.5. Conclusion

The significant feature when considering possible natural causes of death of an individual in police custody is that some diseases can lead to rapid collapse and death with no warning in a young individual who is apparently fit and well immediately before the collapse. There is no method that the police can use to determine which of the individuals they encounter will be suffering from any of these diseases or from a genetic abnormality that may lead to electrical disturbances within the myocardium. Indeed, many of these disease processes can only be diagnosed after complex medical testing and after taking a full medical history.

That many of these diseases are rare in the age group that is most likely to be detained in custody places additional burdens on the police officers who are required to care for them and also on the doctors required to examine and treat them in the police station. The difficulties that these cases present to the pathologist lie in the need to have an awareness of all of the possible natural causes of sudden death and a careful determination and, if necessary, exclusion of all of these causes (cardiac, neurological, and endocrine) before forming the conclusion that some other factor has resulted in death.

6.2. Accidental Trauma

It is clear that determining whether trauma is the result of an accident may depend on the "eye of the beholder." For example, it is impossible at postmortem to determine if the injuries were caused by a fall from a window during arrest, were the result of an accidental fall, an intended jump, or a deliberate push from that window because the points of contact during the descent and the contact with the ground will result in the same injuries whatever the initial "cause." Pathologically, the only features of relevance in determining the exact cause of the initiation of the descent are the identification of specific gripping, holding, or other restraining injuries that could have occurred before the descent or the identification of marks or injuries that may or may not be present (for instance to the fingers) that could be ascribed to attempts to hold on to a window ledge. All of the injuries or marks found on the body will have to be correlated with witness statements from both the police and any other parties present at the time of the fall. Often the true interpretation of many of the injuries and marks found during the postmortem will only become clear when these statements are considered.

However, in general terms, accidental trauma can be caused by many events during the course of an arrest. Falls onto the ground may occur from a height or from standing. Gripping and restraining injuries are commonly present on many areas of the body. The site and significance of the injuries that are present will depend on the descriptions of the events before, during, and after the arrest.

It is essential that all injuries, no matter how apparently trivial, present on a detained individual are carefully documented by the forensic physician who examines the detainee whether at a police station or elsewhere. Contemporaneous photographs are always extremely helpful in these circumstances.

In terms of cause of death, few of the minor injuries will be relevant, but they may provide an indication of the extent and degree of the force that was applied to effect an arrest and, as such, they can be of immense value. Injuries present in high-risk sites (e.g., around the neck) must be examined, documented, and interpreted with particular care. All of the injuries must be interpreted in the light of witness statements and can provide useful corroborative evidence.

7. ALCOHOL- AND DRUG-RELATED DEATHS
7.1. Alcohol

Alcohol is one of the most commonly used drugs in the world. The small ethyl alcohol molecule can pass easily through the blood–brain barrier to the CNS where it has direct suppressant affects on the whole of the CNS. At low concentrations, the specialized cells of the cerebral cortex are affected, but as the concentration increases, the depressive effects involve the higher areas of the brain, resulting in increasingly disinhibited behavior. Still higher levels of alcohol result in the depressant effects involving the lower levels of brain function, including the vital cardiorespiratory centers in the midbrain and the medulla, predisposing the intoxicated individual to cardiorespiratory depression or arrest. Alcohol levels in excess of 300 mg/dL are considered to be potentially lethal, and although some individuals have survived, usually with medical attention, with higher levels, it should be remembered that some individuals have died with far lower levels of alcohol in their blood stream.

However, the effects of alcohol are not confined to the brain; there is also marked peripheral vasodilation, resulting in increased heat loss that may occasionally lead to hypothermia. The adverse effects of alcohol on the coronary circulation, particularly when associated with coronary atheroma, may lead to myocardial ischemia and the development of dysrhythmias and sudden death.

Alcohol also has marked diuretic effects and, when combined with the ingestion of large quantities of fluid (particularly in beer and lager drinking), it may result in electrolyte disturbances, particularly hyponatremia.

The chronic effects of alcohol involve many of the internal organs; alcoholic cardiomyopathy, hepatic steatosis, and cirrhosis are the most common, and all can lead to sudden death.

Alcohol may also be a major factor in causing death by predisposing the individual to accidental trauma and by obscuring the effects of that trauma. This is particularly the case in head injuries when the changes in the level of consciousness are attributed to the effects of alcohol rather than an identified or unidentified head injury.

Alcohol is also a gastric irritant and may precipitate vomiting when taken in excess. This, combined with the effects of decreased consciousness and the reduced laryngeal reflexes associated with intoxication may result in a significantly increased risk of aspiration of vomit into the airways and death. Such an event is unpredictable and, without constant supervision, unpreventable.

The anesthetic effects of alcohol may also result in deaths from asphyxiation. These deaths are the result of the intoxicated individual moving into or being placed or left in a position that impedes respiration either by occlusion of the external respiratory orifices or the internal airways (particularly the larynx) or restricts the free movement of the chest wall. These positions may result from lying face down on a bed, marked extension or flexion of the neck, or lying across an edge with the head down. Deaths resulting from impairment of respiration in this manner classically result in profound asphyxial changes involving the upper body, and these deaths are ascribed to postural asphyxia.

Given the speed with which an individual under the influence of alcohol can die from either the aspiration of vomit or postural asphyxia, it is doubtful if a police station cell is the correct environment for his or her recovery from intoxication.

7.2. Drugs

Drug use is now so ubiquitous in Western society that any examination of a potential detainee by a forensic physician must include a careful evaluation of drug use whether in the past or recently. The skill of the forensic physician will undoubtedly be stretched to the full in the evaluation of the history given, and this is discussed fully in Chapter 10. The failure to identify a drug abuser who then suffers from withdrawal while in custody is just as potentially life-threatening as the failure to continue a detainee's prescribed medication.

In terms of deaths in custody, all drug use, whether social, abusive, or therapeutic, is relevant *(13)*, and the possibility that a detainee may have abused just one drug or a combination of drugs with or without alcohol before death must be positively excluded. A full drug screen on blood and, if available, urine is imperative. Some laboratories will also examine samples of bile and/ or liver to detect evidence of previous drug abuse.

The management of acute drug intoxication is a matter of clinical judgment, but with adequate medical care, it is unlikely that, except in exceptional circumstances, drug intoxication alone will to lead to sudden death in custody.

8. DELIBERATE INJURIES
8.1. Baton Blows

Blows from a baton are usually easily identified because forceful blows produce the classic "tram line"-type injuries on the skin. "Tram line" injuries are typical of a blow from a linear blunt object; the areas of the skin that are most traumatized are not those at the middle of the site of contact where the skin is most evenly compressed but rather at the margins on the contact site where the stretching and distortion of the skin and, hence the damage to the underlying tissues, including the blood vessels, is most pronounced. A linear object will, almost by definition, have two such margins, which run parallel, and a blow from such an object results in two linear parallel bruises; hence, the terminology "tram line."

Blows from a baton may also result in deeper bruising, nerve damage, and fractured bones. The deeper injuries tend to reflect the use of greater force, but it is not possible to correlate with any degree of certainty the amount of force needed to cause a particular injury in any individual.

It is essential for both the forensic physician who examines a living victim of a baton blow to the head (or from any other cause) and the pathologist who performs a postmortem examination to remember that significant cerebral trauma can be caused in the absence of obvious external trauma or skull fractures, and it would be prudent to assess anyone who has received or complains of receiving a head injury from a baton or from any other cause and to consider carefully if referral to hospital for a full neurological assessment is advisable.

8.2. Neck Holds

Pressure on and around the neck is well-known to be a potentially lethal action *(14)*. Death can be caused after compression of the neck by any one of four mechanisms or by any combination of two or more of the following:

- Airway obstruction by direct compression of the larynx or trachea or by the pressure on the neck raising the larynx upward and causing the superior aspect of the pharynx to be occluded by the tongue base. This can be achieved by pressure of a forearm across the front of the neck, sometimes called the "choke hold."
- Occlusion of the veins in the neck. The low pressure in the venous system and the thin yielding nature of the vein walls make venous occlusion more easily achieved than arterial occlusion; however, the large reserve capacity of the venous system makes it unlikely that rapid death would result even if complete occlusion was achieved, unless some other factor supervened.
- Compression or occlusion of the carotid arteries. This is harder to achieve than venous occlusion because of the higher pressure in the arterial system and the thickness of the arterial walls; however, the effects of occlusion will become apparent much quicker. Saukko and Knight *(14)* record that occlusion of the carotid circulation for 4 min or more may result in brain damage, and Reay et al. *(15)* demonstrated significant changes in blood flow in the face of five individuals who were subjected to compression of the carotid arteries by the application of a "sleeper hold" in experimental conditions. A sleeper hold is applied when the upper arm compresses one side of the neck and the forearm the other and the larynx rests in the "V" formed by the elbow.
- The fourth mechanism by which death can occur during pressure to the neck results from stimulation of the vagus nerve by direct pressure in its course down the neck or as a result of stimulation of the carotid sinus. Vagal stimulation

results in bradycardia, which may progress to asystole or, in some cases, immediate asystole.

Mercy et al. *(16)* reviewed 20 deaths where neck holds had been applied and concluded that in 19 of these cases, the application of the neck hold was associated with the death. Conversely, Kowai *(17)* concluded that the use of the choke hold could take between 10 and 20 s to cause unconsciousness, and, therefore, it was safe. Clearly, they did not experience the vagal effects of this hold in their experiments.

Neck holds are commonly used in many forms of wrestling or martial arts, and in these situations, they are seldom associated with fatalities, possibly because of the ability of the person held to indicate his or her willingness to submit to a referee and so cause the hold to be released. No such authority is present during a restraint by police; perhaps this is why fatalities are recorded in this situation. In the United Kingdom, the use of neck holds by police during restraint is specifically prohibited and officers are warned during their training of the potentially fatal effects of applying any pressure to the neck. However, in the United States, neck holds are an approved method of restraint.

The pathological examination of deaths associated with compression of the neck requires a detailed and careful dissection of the neck structures *(18)*. The finding of injuries to the muscular, cartilaginous, vascular, or neural components of the neck must be interpreted in the light of the restraint events, the actions of the restrainers, and the subsequent resuscitation, if any. Pressure on the neck to maintain an airway after cardiac or respiratory arrest may result in bruising, which could be confused with pressure before or, indeed, causing that arrest. Therapeutic insertion of cannulae during active resuscitation by paramedics or in the hospital commonly leads to marked hemorrhage in the neck that, although it is unlikely to be confused with bruising caused by a neck hold, may mask any bruising that was present.

Pressure on the neck is not, of course, the only mechanism whereby an individual may suffer anoxia or asphyxiation. Any action that partially or completely occludes the mouth and/or the nose will result in difficulty in breathing and may result in asphyxiation. The features of these other causes of asphyxiation, traumatic or restraint asphyxia, are discussed in Subheading 11.

8.3. Homicide

There have been numerous cases where individuals have been murdered in the cell by another inmate. Such deaths are most commonly associated with blunt trauma, but strangulation, stabbing, and other methods may be employed if suitable weapons are available. It is also evident that individuals have been deliberately assaulted and killed by police officers during arrest and detention.

The forensic physician should always be aware of the possibility that police may have used excessive force or that deliberately homicidal injuries may have been inflicted. If injuries are present on any individual in their care, these injuries must be carefully documented and, if they are beyond that which the physician considers reasonable in the circumstances, their concerns should be expressed immediately to a senior officer, to a legal representative of the detainee, and an official complaints procedure. The physician also has the duty to ensure that no further harm comes to that person.

9. SELF-INFLICTED INJURIES

Suicidal deaths in custody are a cause for continuing public concern. The methods used are variable but reflect the materials available to the individual at that time.

9.1. Hanging

To effect a hanging suicide, the individual must have two things: an object that can be made into a noose and a point on which to tie it. In addition, the individual must be able to place his or her body so that his or her body weight can be used to apply pressure to the neck via the noose.

The materials and objects that can be made into a noose are many and vary from the obvious (ties, belts, shoelaces, etc) to the unusual (underwear, shirts, etc). To attempt to reduce the possibility of hanging suicides many police station cells have been redesigned and attachment points for the noose (pipes, bars, etc) have been removed or covered. However, the lack of these obvious points did not deter some individuals who placed the bed on end and used the upper end as the fixing point. Installation of fixed beds or benching should preclude the use of that method in future. It must be remembered that hanging can still be achieved, although is clearly more difficult, from a low suspension point, and any protrusion from a wall or fitment in a cell can potentially be used as the upper attachment for the noose.

In addition to removing the fixing points, attempts have been made to remove the items that have been used as nooses in the past and belts, shoelaces, etc. are sometimes taken from prisoners. Paper clothing has been used, although this has not been entirely successful because it entails removing all of the individual's clothing, which is clearly impractical in many cases and may raise problems with human rights. If made strong enough to withstand any degree of wear, the paper clothing would also be strong enough to act as a noose.

The key to preventing hanging suicides lies in the careful evaluation of all individuals who are to be detained and in the design of the cells in which they are held to preclude any possible point for the attachment of a noose.

Given the speed with which hanging can be effected, it is most unlikely that anything other than a permanent watch over the suicidal detainee would provide a foolproof method to prevent hanging in a cell. A cycle of 15-minutes checks will allow more than ample time for an individual to hang himself or herself and cannot be considered to be adequate protection against this type of suicide.

9.2. Ligature Strangulation

Because the possibility of suspension is reduced by the changes in the design of the cells, the possibility of other forms of self-asphyxiation are likely to increase. Self-strangulation by ligature is considered to be possible but difficult *(14)*; because the pressure has to be applied to the neck in these cases by the conscious muscular effort of the hands and arms, it follows that when consciousness is lost and the muscular tone lessens, the pressure on the ligature will decrease, the airway obstruction and/or the vascular occlusion will cease, and death will generally be averted. However, if the ligature is knotted or if the material is "non-slip" and looped around itself, then it is possible for the individual to apply the pressure to the neck and for that pressure to be maintained even after consciousness is lost and, as a result, death may follow.

As with hanging, the key to preventing these deaths lies in careful evaluation and, if necessary, the removal of clothing and observation.

9.3. Incised Injuries

All prisoners should be carefully searched before incarceration, and any sharp objects or objects that could be sharpened must be removed. The extent of the search will probably depend on the mental state of the individual, and the possibility of an intimate search to exclude weapons concealed in the vagina or rectum should be considered in those individuals who are considered most at risk. Death from deep incised wounds to the neck or arms can occur quickly. Even if the individual is found before death has occurred, the effects of profound blood loss may make death inevitable, despite resuscitation attempts.

9.4. Drugs

When considering the possibility of suicide using drugs while in police custody, the two key factors are, once again, evaluation and searching. Careful searching (possibly including intimate searches in some cases) will prevent the ingestion of drugs by an individual after he or she has been placed in the cell. The forensic physician must always be aware of the possibility that excessive quantities of a drug or drugs were taken before arrest and detention and may exert their effect when the individual is in the cell.

10. EXCITED DELIRIUM

10.1. Definition

The exact definition of this syndrome remains elusive, despite many publications apparently describing similar events *(19,20)*. Indeed, the many different names given to these apparently similar conditions (Bell's mania, agitated delirium, excited delirium, and acute exhaustive mania) throughout the years indicate that it is a syndrome that may have many different facets, not all of which may be present in any single case. However, all of these descriptions do comment on the high potential for sudden collapse and death while the individual is in the highly excited states that they all describe. It is now accepted that such syndromes do exist, and although it is now commonly associated with use and abuse of cocaine *(21)*, it is important to note that it was described in 1849 well before cocaine use and abuse became common *(19)*.

10.2. Features

The clinical features of excited delirium are generally accepted to be the following:

- A state of high mental and physiological arousal.
- Agitation.
- Hyperpyrexia associated with sweating.
- Violence, aggression, and hostility.
- Insensitivity to physical pain or to restraint sprays.

In addition to these clinical observable features, there will certainly also be significant physiological and biochemical sequelae, including dehydration, lactic acidosis, and increased catecholamine levels *(22)*. These biochemical and physiological features may be such that they will render the individual at considerable risk from sudden cardiac arrest, and the descriptions of cases of individuals suffering from excited delirium *(23)* indicates that the sudden death is not uncommon. Shulack *(23)* also records that: "the end may come so suddenly that the attending psychiatrist is left with a chagrined surprise," and continues: "the puzzlement is intensified after the autopsy generally fails to disclose any findings which could explain the death." More than 50 years after the publication of that paper, it is still true, but the site of the death may have moved from the psychiatric ward to a police station.

The findings noted in by Shulack in 1944 are also repeated today in many cases that have the features of excited delirium, the difference now being that toxicological examination not uncommonly reveals the presence of cocaine or, in a therapeutic environment, neuroleptic drugs and, as a result, it is tempting to relate the cause of death to the presence of the drug or drugs. In the context of restraint associated with death in cases of excited delirium, the presence of injuries to the neck may lead to the conclusion that death resulted from asphyxia, but this interpretation needs careful evaluation.

What is perhaps of greater importance is that in all of the cases described in the clinical literature *(19,20,23–25)*, there has been a prolonged period of increasingly bizarre and aggressive behavior, often lasting days or weeks before admission to hospital and subsequent death. The clinical evidence available for the deaths associated with police restraint indicates that although there may have been a period of disturbed behavior before restraint and death, the duration of the period will have been measured in hours and not days. This change in time scale may result from the different etiology of the cases of excited delirium now seen, and it is possible that the "natural" and the "cocaine-induced" types of excited delirium will have different time spans but a common final pathway. This feature also must be elucidated in the future.

The conclusion that can be reached concerning individuals displaying the symptoms of excited delirium is that they clearly constitute a medical emergency. The police need to be aware of the symptoms of excited delirium and to understand that attempts at restraint are potentially dangerous and that forceful restraint should only be undertaken in circumstances where the individual is a serious risk to himself or herself or to other members of the public.

Ideally, a person displaying these symptoms should be contained and a forensic physician should be called to examine him or her and to offer advice to the police at the scene. The possibility that the individual should be treated *in situ* by an emergency psychiatric team with resuscitation equipment and staff available needs to be discussed with the police, and, if such an emergency psychiatric team exists, this is probably the best and safest option. If such a team does not exist, then the individual will need to be restrained with as much care as possible and taken to the hospital emergency room for a full medical and psychiatric evaluation. These individuals should not be taken directly to a psychiatric unit where resuscitation skills and equipment may not be adequate.

11. RAPID UNEXPLAINED DEATHS DURING RESTRAINT

Deaths occurring while an individual is being restrained are extremely rare. In the UK Police Research Group Paper *(26)*, which covers the period

1990–1996, 16 cases are identified where police action "may have been associated with the death" amounting to 6% of the deaths that this group studied. From consideration of the medical aspects of these deaths recorded in their report, it would appear that six of the deaths resulted from natural disease and four were related to drug use or abuse. Of the remaining six cases, one was associated with a baton blow to the head, two to asphyxiation resulting from pressure to the neck, two to "restraint asphyxia," and one to a head injury. Therefore, in the deaths during the 7 years that this group considered, a total of four deaths (<1.5% of the 267 deaths in police custody reviewed by this group) were apparently directly associated with asphyxia during restraint.

However, the close association of these deaths with the actions of the police in restraining the individual raises questions about the pathologists' conclusions and their acceptance by the courts. It is common for several pathological opinions to be obtained in these cases; in a review of 12 in-custody deaths, an average of three opinions had been obtained (range 1–7) *(27)*. Indeed, in one of the cases cited as being associated with police actions, seven pathological opinions were sought, yet only one opinion is quoted. This points to the considerable difficulty in determining the relative significance of several different and, at times, conflicting areas of medical evidence that are commonly present in these cases.

The area of restraint that causes the most concern relates to asphyxiation during restraint. It has been known in forensic circles for many years that individuals may asphyxiate if their ability to breathe is reduced by the position in which they are placed or into which they fall (Subheading 7.1.; ref. *28*). This type of asphyxiation is commonly associated with alcohol or drug intoxication or, rarely, with neurological diseases that prevent the individual from extracting themselves from a position that either partially or completely occludes their mouth and nose or limits the freedom of movement of the chest wall. Death resulting from these events has been described as postural asphyxia to indicate that it was the posture of the individual that resulted in the airway obstruction rather than the action of a third party.

In 1988, research by Reay et al. *(29)* was published that was initially believed to show that in laboratory conditions, placing an individual in the hog-tie position significantly increased the time taken to return to resting blood oxygenation levels after moderate exercise. "Hog-tieing" is a form of restraint where the detainee is placed face down and the hands are tied together and then tied to the feet. Reay concluded that positional restraint (hog-tieing) had "measurable physiological effects." In 1992, Reay published an article *(30)* that recorded six cases where, in his opinion, individuals had died as a result of "hog-tieing" and being placed prone in police vehicles. This article raised the possibility that asphyxiation was occurring to individuals when they could not move themselves to safer positions because of the type of restraint used by the police. The concept of "restraint asphyxia," albeit in a specific set of circumstances, was born.

Since the description of deaths in the prone hog-tied position, Reay's original concepts have been extended to account for many deaths of individuals simply under restraint but not in the hog-tied position. The term *restraint asphyxia* has been widened to account for these sudden and unexpected deaths during restraint. Considerable pathological and physiological controversy exists regarding the exact effects of the prone position and hog-tieing in the normal effects upon respiration. Further experiments by Chan et al. *(31)* have cast considerable doubt on Reay's thesis, although other experiments by Roeggla et al. *(32)* support the original theory. Although the physiological controversy continues, it is clear to all those involved in the examination and investigation of these deaths that there is a small group of individuals who die suddenly and apparently without warning while being restrained.

Recent physiological research on simulated restraint *(33,34)* revealed that restraint did produce reductions in the ventilatory capacity of the experimental subjects but that this did not impair cardiorespiratory function. In two of the eight healthy subjects, breath holding after even moderate exercise induced hypoxia-related dysrhythmias, and it was noted that arterial oxygen saturation fell rapidly even with short breath hold times, especially if lung volume was reduced during exhalation.

The problem that currently faces the forensic pathologist is the determination of the cause or causes of these deaths. This is made harder because there are seldom any of the usual asphyxial signs to assist and, even if those signs are present, it is difficult to assign weight or significance to them because similar changes can be caused simply by resuscitation *(35,36)*.

The major features of asphyxiation are cyanosis, congestion, and petechial hemorrhages *(14)*. These features are seen to a greater or lesser extent in many, but not all, cases of asphyxiation. They often are completely absent in many plastic bag asphyxiations and in hanging, they have variable presence in manual strangulation, and they are most commonly seen in ligature strangulation. However, their most florid appearances are in deaths associated with postural asphyxia or crush asphyxia cases where death has occurred slowly and where it is associated with some form of pressure or force reducing the ability of the individual to maintain adequate respiratory movement, either from outside the body or from the abdominal contents splinting the diaphragm.

It is of interest then that these features, if present at all in these cases are, at most, scant and do not reflect their appearance in other cases of crush asphyxia, suggesting that different mechanisms are the cause of death in these two sets of circumstance.

The individuals who die during restraint are not infrequently under the influence of drugs (particularly cocaine) or alcohol; they may be suffering from some underlying natural disease (particularly of the cardiovascular system), or they may have suffered some trauma. These "additional" factors are sometimes seized by pathologists and courts to "explain" the death, sometimes even in the face of expert opinion that excludes the additional factor from playing a major part in the death. It would seem that there is a subgroup of the population that is either permanently or temporarily susceptible to the effects of restraint, whether those effects be mediated entirely or partially through decreased respiratory effort or some other factor.

There is a separate entity, the exact cause of which is not yet clear, where otherwise fit and healthy individuals die suddenly while being restrained and yet do not show significant features of asphyxiation. It is hoped that further research on the physiology of restraint will elucidate the mechanisms that cause death in these cases. Until these mechanisms are established, it is reasonable to propose that these deaths should be classified for what they are—rapid unexplained death during restraint—rather than to conclude that the cause of death cannot be determined or to ascribe a doubtful medical or toxicological cause of death that does not bear close scrutiny.

Deaths classified as rapid unexplained death during restraint must fulfill several of the following criteria:

1. The death must have occurred during restraint, and the individual must have collapsed suddenly and without warning.
2. A full external and internal postmortem examination must have been performed by a forensic pathologist, which did not reveal macroscopic evidence of significant natural disease, and subsequently a full histological examination of the tissues must have been performed, which did not reveal microscopic evidence of significant natural disease.
3. Studies must not reveal genetic markers of significant disease.
4. There must be no evidence of significant trauma or of the triad of asphyxial signs.
5. A full toxicological screen must have been performed that did not reveal evidence of drugs or alcohol that, alone or in combination, could have caused death.

The small numbers of these deaths in any single country or worldwide makes their analysis difficult; indeed, to search for a single answer that will explain all of these deaths may be futile. The bringing together of these deaths under a single classification would make the identification of cases and their analysis easier.

The problem for the police is that when approaching and restraining an individual, they cannot know the background or the medical history nor can they have any idea of the particular (or peculiar) physiological responses of that individual. The techniques that are designed for restraint and the care of the individual after restraint must allow for safe restraint of the most vulnerable sections of the community.

New research into the effects of restraint may possibly lead to a greater understanding of the deleterious effects of restraint and the development of safer restraint techniques. Although this experimental work is being performed, the only particular advice that can be offered to police officers is that the prone position should be maintained for the minimum amount of time only, no pressure should be applied to the back or the chest of a person restrained on the floor, and the individual should be placed in a kneeling, sitting, or standing position to allow for normal respiration as soon as practical.

It should be noted that an individual who is suffering from early or late asphyxiation may well struggle more in an attempt to breathe, and, during a restraint, this increased level of struggling may be perceived by police officers as a renewed attempt to escape, resulting in further restriction of movement and subsequent exacerbation of the asphyxial process. Officers must be taught that once restrained, these further episodes of struggling may signify imminent asphyxiation and not continued attempts to escape, that they may represent a struggle to survive, and that the police must be aware of this and respond with that in mind.

Since these matters were first brought to forensic and then public attention and training and advice to police officers concerning the potential dangers of face down or prone restraints, especially if associated with any pressure to the chest or back improved, there has been a decrease in the number of deaths during restraint. However, even one death in these circumstances is too many, and it is hoped that by medical research, improved police training, and increased awareness of the dangers of restraint that these tragic deaths can be prevented.

REFERENCES

1. Home Office. Consolidated Circular on Crime and Kindred Matters. 35/86, Her Majesty's Sationery Office, London, UK, 1996.
2. Inquest. Deaths in police custody (England & Wales). Available at Website: (http://inquest/gn/apc.org).
3. Australian Institute of Criminology. Deaths in custody in Australia. Available at Website: (http://www.aic.gov.au). Accessed November 18, 2002.

4. Matthews, P., Foreman, J. (eds.) Jervis on Coroners. Sweet & Maxwell, London, UK, 1993.

5. Home Office. Circular No 35 of 1969. Her Majesty's Stationery Office, London, UK, 1969.

6. Dalton,V. Australian deaths in custody & custody-related police operations 1997–98. Available at Website: (http://www.aic.gov. au). Accessed 1998.

7. Working Group of the Lambeth Community–Police Consultative Group. Lessons from Tragedies. Deaths in Custody in the Metropolitan Police District. 1986–1995, Furnival Press, London, UK, 1996.

8. Davies, M. J., Robertson, W. B., Pomerance, A., Davies, M. J. (eds.) Diseases of the coronary arteries. In: Pathology of the Heart. Blackwell Scientific Publications, Oxford, UK, pp. 81–126, 1975.

9. OPCS. Mortality Statistics (Cause). The Stationery Office, London, UK, 1997.

10. Burn, J., Camm, J., Davies, M. J., et al. The phenotype/genotype relation and the current status of genetic screening in hypertrophic cardiomyopathy, Marfan syndrome and long QT syndrome. Heart. 78:110–116, 1997.

11. Berry, C. L., McGee, J. O., Isaacson, P. G., Wright, N. A. (eds.) Arteritis. In: Oxford Textbook of Pathology. Oxford University Press, Oxford, UK, pp. 842–852, 1992.

12. Royal College of General Practitioners. Mortality among oral contraceptive users. Lancet. 1:727–731, 1977.

13. Havis, S., Best, D. Drug-Related Deaths in Police Custody. Police Complaints Authority, London, UK, 2003.

14. Saukko, P., Knight, B. Forensic Pathology. 3rd Ed. Arnold, London, UK, 2004.

15. Reay, D. T., Holloway, G. A. Changes in carotid blood flow produced by neck compression. Am. J. Forensic Med. Pathol. 3:199–202, 1982.

16. Mercy, J. A., Heath, C. W., Rosenberg, M. L. Mortality associated with the use of upper-body control holds by police. Violence Victims. 5:215–222, 1990.

17. Koiwai, E. K. Deaths allegedly caused by the use of "choke holds" (shime-waza). J. Forensic Sci. 32:419–432, 1987.

18. Vanezis, P. Techniques of examination. In: Pathology of Neck Injury. Butterworths, London, UK, pp. 22–27, 1989.

19. Bell, L. V. On a form of disease resembling mania and fever. Am. J. Insanity. 6:97, 1849.

20. Billig, O., Freeman, W. T. Fatal catatonia. Am. J. Psychiatry. 100:633, 1944.

21. Karch, S. B. Cocaine. In: Karch's Pathology of Drug Abuse, 2nd Ed. CRC Press, Boca Raton, FL, 2002, pp. 1–187.

22. Harries, M., Williams, C., Stanish, W.D., Micheli, L. J. Oxford Textbook of Sports Medicine. Oxford University Press, Oxford, UK, 1996.

23. Shulack, N. R. Sudden exhaustive death in excited patients. Psychiatric Q. 18:3, 1944.

24. Kraines, S. H. Bell's mania. Am. J. Psychiatry. 91:29, 1934.

25. O'Halloran, R. L., Lewman, L. V. Restraint asphyxiation in excited delirium [see comments]. Am. J. Forensic Med. Pathol. 14:289–295, 1993.

26. Leigh, A., Johnson, G., Ingram, A. Deaths in Police Custody—Learning the Lessons. Home Office, London, UK, 1998.

27. Morewood, T. C. G. In Custody Restraint Deaths [master's thesis]. University of London, UK, 1998.
28. Bell, M. D., Rao, V. J., Welti, C. V. Positional asphyxiation in adults: a series of 30 cases from the Dade and Broward County, Florida, medical examiners offices from 1982 to 1990. Am. J. Forensic Med. Pathol. 13:101–107, 1992.
29. Reay, D. T., Howard, J. D., Fligner, C. L., Ward, R. J. Effects of positional restraint on oxygen saturation and heart rate following exercise. Am. J. Forensic Med. Pathol. 9:16–18, 1998.
30. Reay, D. T., Fligner, C. L., Stilwell, A. D., Arnold, J. Positional asphyxia during law enforcement transport. Am. J. Forensic Med. Pathol. 13:90–97, 1992.
31. Chan, T. C., Vilka, G. M., Neuman, T., Clausen, J. L. Restraint position and positional asphyxia. Ann. Emerg. Med. 30:578–586.
32. Roeggla, M., Wagner, A., Muellner, M. Cardiorespiratory consequences to hobble restraint. Wiener Klinische Wochenschrift. 109:359–336, 1997.
33. Cary, N. R. B., Roberts, C. A., Cummin, A. R. C., Adams, L. The effect of simulated restraint in the prone position on cardiorespiratory function following exercise in humans. J. Physiol. 525P:31P, 2000.
34. Cummin, A. R. C., Roberts, C. A., Cary, N. R. B., Adams, L. The effect of breath holding on arterial oxygen saturation following exercise in man. J. Physiol. 525P:31P, 2000.
35. Hood, I. C., Ryan, D., Spitz, W. U. Resuscitation and petechiae. Am. J. Forensic Med. Pathol. 9:35–37, 1988.
36. Rao, V. J., Welti, C. V. The Forensic Significance of Conjunctival Petechiae. Am. J. Forensic Med. Pathol. 9:32–34, 1988.

Chapter 12

Traffic Medicine

Ian F. Wall and Steven B. Karch

1. INTRODUCTION

Driving a motor vehicle is a complex task requiring a reasonable level of physical fitness, accurate perception, and appropriate judgment. All these factors can be affected by drugs and alcohol, greatly increasing the risk of accidents. Many medical conditions (and their treatments) may impair fitness to drive and are considered first.

2. MEDICAL ASPECTS OF FITNESS TO DRIVE

Licensing requirements depend on the type of vehicle driven, with more stringent requirements for commercial purposes and multiaxle vehicles. In many jurisdictions, including Canada, Australia, and the United Kingdom, it is the motorist's responsibility to inform the licensing authority of any relevant medical conditions. Similar requirements generally apply in the United States, except that six states (California, Delaware, Nevada, New Jersey, Oregon, and Pennsylvania) require physicians to report patients with seizures (and other conditions that may alter levels of consciousness) to the department of motor vehicles *(1)*. Drivers have a legal responsibility to inform the licensing authority of any injury or medical condition that affects their driving ability, and physicians should take great pains to explain this obligation. Occasionally, especially when dealing with patients suffering from dementia, ethical responsibilities may require doctors to breach confidentiality and notify patients against their will or without their knowledge *(2)*; this situation is discussed in Subheading 2.5.

From: *Clinical Forensic Medicine: A Physician's Guide, 2nd Edition*
Edited by: M. M. Stark © Humana Press Inc., Totowa, NJ

Requirements vary in different countries and in different jurisdictions within the same country. When in doubt about the appropriate course of action, physicians should consult the appropriate guidelines. In the United Kingdom, the Driver and Vehicle Licensing Agency (DVLA) has made available the At-a-Glance Guide to the Current Medical Standards of Fitness to Drive *(3)*. In Australia, the Austroads Guidelines for Assessing Fitness to Drive provides similar information *(4)*. In the European Union, where European Community directives have developed basic standards but allow different countries to impose more stringent requirements, there is still variation from country to country. The situation is even more complicated in the United States, where each state sets its own rules and where federal regulations for commercial vehicles apply as well. Often, much of the required regulatory information can be acquired via the Internet or from organizations and foundations representing patients who have the particular disease in question.

It should be assumed that all adults drive; drivers with disabilities should be given special consideration and may require modification of their vehicle or have certain personal restrictions applied.

2.1. Cardiovascular Diseases

Several studies have demonstrated that natural deaths at the wheel are fairly uncommon and that the risk for other persons is not significant *(5,6)*. Even so, requirements for commercial drivers are generally much more rigid than for individuals, and in the United States, the Federal Highway Administration prohibits drivers with angina or recent infarction from driving. The length of prohibition varies from state to state. Restrictions for noncommercial car driving after first acute myocardial infarction are 4 weeks in United Kingdom but only 2 weeks in Australia. In the United States, they are entirely at the discretion of physicians. In general, ischemia itself is not considered an absolute disqualification, provided treadmill stress testing demonstrates that moderate reserves are present *(7)*. Similarly, individuals with controlled hypertension are usually considered fit to drive, although physicians, no matter what country they are in, must give serious thought to just what sort of medication is used to control hypertension; clonidine, methyldopa, reserpine, and prazosin can produce somnolence and/or impair reflex responses.

Patients with dysrhythmias treated with medication or with the implantation of a defibrillator/pacemaker present a special set of problems *(8)*. The tendency in the United States has been to treat such individuals as if they were epileptics (i.e., individuals with the potential to lose consciousness at the wheel). Most states set minimum requirements for seizure-free periods. Until recently, that period was 6 months in a majority of jurisdictions but is increasingly being shortened to 3 months in many locations. In the United Kingdom, patients with implantable cardioverter defibrillators are permanently barred from holding a group 2 license but may hold a group 1 license, providing the device has been implanted for 6 months and has not administered therapy (shock and/or symptomatic antitachycardia pacing) *(3)*.

2.2. Epilepsy

Epilepsy is the most common cause of collapse at the wheel, accounting for approx 30% of such incidents. In the United Kingdom, epilepsy is a prescribed disability (along with severe mental impairment, sudden attacks of disabling giddiness, and inability to meet eyesight requirements), and car driving is not allowed for at least 1 yr after a seizure. Restrictions vary from country to country. All 50 of the United States restrict the licenses of individuals with epilepsy if their seizures are not well controlled by medication. Most states require a 6-months seizure-free period and a physician's statement confirming that the individual's seizures have, in fact, been controlled and that the individual in question poses no risk to public safety. The letter from the physician is then reviewed by a medical advisory board, which may or may not issue a license. In the United States, even if the patient, at some later date, does have a seizure and cause an accident, the physician's act of writing to the board protects him or her from liability under American law, provided the letter was written in good faith.

Withdrawal of antiepileptic medication is associated with a risk of seizure recurrence. One study showed that 41% of patients who stopped treatment slowly developed a recurrence of seizures within 2 years, compared with only 22% of patients who continued treatment *(9)*. The legal consequences of discontinuing medication without a physician's order can be devastating. Patients who stop taking antiseizure medication and then cause an accident may face future civil liability and possibly even criminal charges if they cause physical injury *(10)*. Of course, rules vary from country to country but, in general, a patient with seizures who does not inform the appropriate regulatory agency may face dire consequences (including the legitimate refusal of the insurance carrier to pay for damages).

2.3. Diabetes

Diabetes may affect the ability to drive because of loss of consciousness from hypoglycemic attacks or from complications of the disease itself (e.g., retinopathy causing visual problems or peripheral vascular disease causing limb disabilities). In January 1998, the British government introduced new restrictions on licensing of people with insulin-dependent diabetes *(11)*. These restrictions were based on the second European Union driver-licensing directive (91/4389), and under most interpretations of the law, they prevent insulin-treated diabetics from driving light goods and small passenger-carrying vehicles. In response to concerns expressed by the diabetic community in Britain, the British Diabetic Association commissioned a report that found little evidence to support the new legislation. Regulations were therefore changed in April 2001 to allow "exceptional case" drivers to apply to retain their entitlement to drive class C1 vehicles (3500–7500 kg lorries) subject to annual medical examination.

In the United States, the situation varies from state to state, but in many states, individuals with diabetes are subject to restrictive licensing policies that bar them from driving certain types of motor vehicles *(12,13)*. However, the risk of hypoglycemia differs greatly among insulin-requiring diabetics, and today most insulin-dependent diabetics use self-monitoring devices to warn them when their blood glucose levels are becoming too low. Thus, several states have dropped blanket restrictions and allow for case-by-case evaluations to determine medical qualifications for diabetics. In some states, physicians are specifically required to notify authorities of the patient's diabetic conditions, but in all states, it is the patient's responsibility to do so. As with patients with seizure, failure to notify may expose the patient to both civil and criminal liability.

2.4. Vision and Eye Disorders

The two most important aspects of vision in relation to driving are visual acuity and visual fields. Visual acuity may simply be defined as the best obtainable vision with or without spectacles or contact lenses. Most countries require a binocular visual acuity greater than 6/12 for licensing purposes. In the United Kingdom, the eyesight requirements are to read a car number registration plate at 20.5 m, which corresponds to between 6/9 and 6/12 on the Snellen chart. The minimum field of vision for safe driving is generally regarded as at least 120° on the horizontal when measured with a Goldman IV4e target or its equivalent *(14)*.

2.5. Ethical Considerations

Although it is generally a patient's responsibility to inform the licensing authority of any injury or medical condition that affects his or her driving, occasionally ethical responsibilities may require a doctor to inform the licensing authorities of a particular problem. If a patient has a medical condition that renders him or her unfit to drive, the doctor should ensure that the patient understands that the condition may impair his or her ability to drive. If the patient is incapable of understanding this advice (e.g., because of dementia), the doctor should inform the licensing authority immediately *(15)*.

If patients continue to drive when they are not fit to do so, the doctor should make every reasonable effort to persuade them to stop, which may include informing their next of kin. If this still does not persuade the patient to stop driving, the doctor should disclose relevant medical information immediately, in confidence, to the medical adviser of the licensing authority. Before disclosing this information, the doctor should inform the patient of the decision to do so, and once the licensing authority has been informed, the doctor should also write to the patient to confirm that disclosure has been made *(15)*.

3. ALCOHOL AND DRIVING

3.1. Metabolism of Alcohol

Alcohol is absorbed through the stomach and duodenum. Absorption depends on many factors, including sex and weight of the individual, duration of drinking, nature of the drink, and presence of food in the stomach. Alcohol dehydrogenase in the gastric mucosa may contribute substantially to alcohol metabolism (gastric first-pass metabolism), but this effect is generally only evident with low doses and after eating. Studies of alcohol dehydrogenase activity in gastric biopsies of women suggest a significant decrease in activity in women compared with men, which could explain why women have higher peak blood alcohol levels and are more susceptible to liver damage after consumption of smaller quantities of alcohol when compared with men *(16)*. Further details of alcohol metabolism are given in Chapter 10.

Once absorbed, alcohol is eliminated at a fairly constant rate, with 90% being metabolized in the liver and the remainder excreted unchanged in urine, breath, and sweat. The rate of elimination in moderate drinkers may vary between 10 and 20 mg/100 mL blood/h, with a mean of 15 mg/100 mL blood/h. Chronic alcoholics undergoing detoxification have elimination rates of 19 mg/100 mL blood/h or even higher *(17)*. This increased rate of alcohol burnoff is believed to be a consequence of increased activity of hepatic microsomal enzymes (P450IIE).

3.2. Effects of Alcohol on Performance

Alcohol affects mood and behavior, causing euphoria (which is particularly significant in risk taking) but also depressing the central nervous system (CNS). Even at low doses, there is clear evidence that alcohol impairs performance, especially as the faculties that are most sensitive to alcohol are those most important to driving, namely complex perceptual mechanisms and states of divided attention. In a review of more than 200 articles (18), several behavioral aspects were examined, including reaction time, tracking, concentrated attention, divided attention, information processing, visual function, perception, psychomotor performance, and driver performance. Most of the studies showed impairment at 70 mg/100 mL of blood, but approx 20% showed impairment at concentrations between 10 and 40 mg/100 mL of blood.

The definitive study on the relationship between risk of accident and blood alcohol concentration is that conducted in the 1960s in Grand Rapids, Mich., by Borkenstein and Dale (19); data were collected on 5895 drivers involved in accidents and on 7590 drivers not involved in accidents. Comparison of the two groups disclosed that an accident was statistically more likely at blood alcohol levels greater than 80 mg/100 mL of blood, with accidents occurring more frequently as follows:

Blood alcohol (mg/100 mL)	Accident occurrence
50–100	1.5 times as frequently
100–150	4 times as frequently
Over 150	18 times as frequently

Further analysis of the data by Allsop (20) quantified the risks for different ages and different drinking habits. On average, the risk doubles at 80 mg/100 mL, increasing sharply to a 10 times risk multiplier at 150 mg/100 mL and a 20 times risk multiplier at 200 mg/100 mL of blood. For inexperienced and infrequent drinkers, the sharp increase occurs at much lower levels, whereas for the more experienced drinking driver it may not occur until 100 mg/100 mL (Fig. 1).

Therefore, this research has encouraged some countries to have a lower blood alcohol level for legal driving; in Australia, Canada, and some states of the United States, different levels and rules are applied for younger and/or inexperienced drivers (see Subheading 3.3.). Further evidence of the relationship between crash risk and blood alcohol levels has been shown by Compton and colleagues (21), who studied drivers in California and Florida. This recent research studying a total of 14,985 drivers was in agreement with previous studies in showing increasing relative risk as blood alcohol levels increase, with an accelerated rise at levels in excess of 100 mg/100 mL of blood. However, after adjustments for missing data (hit-and-run drivers, refusals, etc.), the result was an even more dramatic rise in risk, with the relative risk of crash involvement being significantly elevated at blood alcohol levels of 40 mg/100 mL.

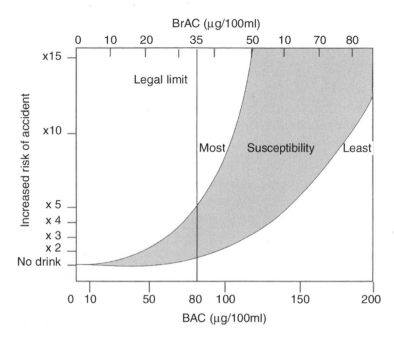

Fig. 1. Risk of road traffic accidents related to level of alcohol in the blood and breath. BAC, blood alcohol concentration; BrAC, breath alcohol concentration. Permission by Greenwich Medical Media.

3.3. Road Traffic Legislation

In the United Kingdom, this research led to the introduction of the Road Safety Act 1967, which set a legal driving limit of 80 mg/100 mL of blood (or 35 µg/100 mL of breath or 107 mg/100 mL of urine). This law also allows mandatory roadside screening tests and requires the provision of blood or urine tests at police stations. The Transport Act 1981 provided that quantitative breath tests, performed with approved devices, could be used as the sole evidence of drunk driving. Although the level for UK drivers is set at 80 mg/100 mL of blood, in practice, drivers are not usually prosecuted at blood levels below 87 mg/100 mL of blood because during the analysis, a series of results by gas chromatography, which must fall within 3 standard deviations (or 6%) of each other, is averaged, and then 6% (or 6 mg below 100 g/100 mL) is deducted from the result, which is then reported as not less than X mg/100 mL of blood.

In the United States, permissible blood levels vary from state to state and also by age. Many states have enacted "zero tolerance" laws, and the detection of any alcohol in an individual younger than 21 years old is grounds for license revocation. Some states permit levels as high as 100 mg/100 mL, but most enforce the same limit as in the United Kingdom, and legislation to reduce the 80 mg/100 mL level further is under consideration. Repeated attempts to introduce one nationwide level have been rebuffed by the US Congress.

3.4. Equivalent Limits in Other Body Fluids

Statutes have been used to establish blood alcohol concentration equivalents in other tissues and breath. Not infrequently, alcohol concentrations will be measured in accident victims taken for treatment at trauma centers. However, there are two important differences between alcohol measurements made in hospitals and those made in forensic laboratories; first, in hospitals, standard international units are the norm, the mole is the unit of mass, the liter is the unit of volume, and alcohol concentrations are reported in mmol/L. In forensic laboratories, results are expressed as gram/deciliter or liter, or even milligrams per milliliter, and measurements are made in whole blood, not serum or plasma. Because 1 mL of whole blood weighs, on average, 1.055 g, a blood alcohol concentration of 100 mg/dL is actually the same as 95 mg/ 100 g or 21.7 mmol/L *(17)*.

There is another, even more important, difference between serum/plasma and whole blood. The former contains 91.8% water, whereas the latter contains only 80.1% water. Because alcohol has a large volume of distribution, this difference in water content means that alcohol concentrations measured in serum/plasma will be higher than concentrations measured in whole blood by approx 14%. In practice, if plasma alcohol concentrations are to be introduced as evidence, they should be related back to whole blood concentrations using an even higher ratio (1.22:1), which corresponds to the mean value, ± 2 standard deviations. As mentioned, if whole blood is tested, drivers are not usually prosecuted at blood levels below 87 mg/100 mL of blood *(17)*.

Breath testing is equally problematic. The instruments used are calibrated to estimate the concentrations of alcohol in whole blood, not plasma or serum. To estimate the serum or plasma alcohol concentration from breath measurements, a plasma/breath ratio of 2600:1 must be used (because, as explained, whole blood contains 14% less alcohol). In Europe, but not necessarily in the United States, two specimens of breath are taken for analysis, and the specimen with the lower proportion of alcohol should be used as evidence.

Bladder urine, because it contains alcohol (or other drugs) that may have accumulated over a long period, is generally not considered a suitable specimen for forensic testing, especially because the presence of alcohol in the

Table 1
Prescribed Blood Alcohol Levels in Various Jurisdictions

Country	Level	Country	Level	Country	Level
Australia	50	France	50	Poland	20
Austria	80	Germany	80	Romania	0
Belgium	80	Greece	50	Russia	0
Bulgaria	0	Hungary	0	Sweden	20
Canada	80	Italy	80	Spain	80
Czechoslovakia	80	Luxembourg	80	Turkey	0
Denmark	80	Netherlands	50	United States	100[a]
Ireland	80	Norway	50	Yugoslavia	50
Finland	50				

[a] Some states in the United States have reduced the legal level to 80 mg/100 mL of blood.

urine only proves that alcohol is present in the body. Alcohol concentrations in bladder urine cannot be used to infer the blood levels reliably. Even so, UK legislation and most US states still allow drivers the option of providing breath, blood, or urine specimens, but, as of 1999, the State of California has dropped the option of providing urine samples, and other states are considering similar actions. Under the new California provisions, police can still request a urine test if a suspect's breath test is negative *(22)*.

Other options are available in the case of alcohol-related fatalities. Comparison of alcohol concentrations in vitreous and blood can provide a good indication of whether concentrations were rising or falling at the time of death (alcohol is distributed mainly in water and the water content of vitreous is lower than that of blood). Urine obtained from the kidney pelvis can also be used, because its alcohol content can be precisely related to blood concentration *(23)*.

3.5. Legal Limits in Other Jurisdictions

Table 1 shows permissible alcohol limits for various countries. All figures are the maximum permissible amount in milligrams per 100 mL of blood (in the United States, referred to as deciliters [dL]). Although legislation has been introduced to enforce uniform standards, these standards have not been enacted, and in the United States, permissible alcohol levels vary from state to state.

3.6. Countermeasures

Numerous measures have already been taken to discourage drivers from drinking, and they have had a considerable degree of success.

3.6.1. Lowering the Legal Limit

When the legal limit was reduced in Sweden from 50 to 20 mg, there was a fall in casualties *(24)*. It has been estimated that a similar reduction in the United Kingdom would save 50 lives, prevent 250 serious injuries, and eliminate another 1200 slight injuries each year. A cost/benefit analysis suggests that this would save £75 million a year *(25)*. However, the UK government ultimately decided against reducing the legal limit.

3.6.2. Widening Police Breath-Testing Powers

Currently in the United Kingdom, a police officer may stop any person driving a motor vehicle on the road, but that does not necessarily mean that the officer can administer a breath test. As is the case in the United States, police officers can require a breath test only if there is reasonable cause to suspect that the person detained has alcohol in his or her body, has committed a moving traffic offense, or has been involved in an accident.

In Finland, random breath testing, along with a legal limit of 50 mg/ 100 mL of blood, was introduced in 1977; highly visible check points are established where typically 8–12 police officers with breath alcohol screening devices are placed along the center of the road, the sites being chosen so that it is impossible for a driver to avoid being tested. All drivers are tested, except those of emergency vehicles. The procedure takes only seconds to perform, the system receives general public support *(26)*, and it has resulted in a marked reduction in the number of accidents and injuries.

In the state of Victoria, Australia, "booze buses" are set up along with a roadblock—any driver who fails a roadside breath test is taken into the bus and given an evidentiary breath test (Drager 7100 machine). Every driver in Victoria is said to be tested on average at least once a year *(27)*.

3.6.3. Ignition Interlocks for Repeat Drunk-Driving Offenders

These devices prevent the car ignition from being started unless the concentration of breath alcohol blown into the device is below a predetermined level, often well below the legal limit. Thereafter, during the journey, the driver is required to undertake random rolling retests. A failure of these tests activates the vehicle's lights and horn. These devices have been used in several states of the United States and also in Alberta, Canada. They are generally applied to repeat offenders, either as an alternative to disqualification or in succession to a period of disqualification. Results in the United States have shown that repeat offenses occur rapidly once the restriction is removed *(28)*. However, in Alberta, where there is closer supervision of the program, supplemented by counseling, more long-term improvements have been experienced.

3.6.4. High-Risk Offender Scheme

A special program in England, Wales, and Scotland was introduced in 1983, and the criteria widened in 1990 to cover drivers who were convicted of having a blood alcohol concentration (BAC) in excess of 200 mg/100 mL of blood, or refusing to provide an evidential specimen, or two offenses involving BACs in excess of 80 mg/100 mL of blood within a 10-yr period. This group accounts for approx 30–40% of drunk drivers in Britain. To regain their licenses at the end of a period of disqualification, the drivers must undergo a medical examination (including blood tests to discover biochemical evidence of excessive alcohol consumption) to demonstrate with reasonable certainty that they are not alcohol abusers *(3)*. Similar statues apply in the United States. In California, drivers with a BAC higher than 200 mg/100 mL, in addition to whatever other sanctions are imposed, are required to attend a 6-months educational program *(22)*. In the United States, penalties for drunk driving may be "enhanced" under special circumstances, such as a second conviction for drunk driving, speeding at the time of arrest, the presence of a child in the car, or the causation of property damage or injury.

3.7. Procedural Issues

Although the procedures involved may seem simple, numerous technical defenses have been raised in most countries throughout the world. Not surprisingly, many of these challenges are similar, no matter the country in which they are offered. Challenges to the UK Road Traffic Act are illustrative of the problem.

3.7.1. Definitions

Section 5(1) of the Road Traffic Act 1988 (RTA) states that if a person drives or attempts to drive a motor vehicle on a road or other public place, or is in charge of a motor vehicle on a road or other public place, after consuming so much alcohol that the proportion of it in his or her breath, blood, or urine exceeds the prescribed limit, he or she is guilty of an offense. Unfortunately, the word "drive" is not defined, but in fact, three points need to be proved: first, that the person is in the driving seat or has control of the steering; second, that the person charged must have something to do with the propulsion of the vehicle; and finally, that what the individual was doing must fall within the normal meaning of driving.

Attempting to drive has produced an abundance of case law, but it has been held that acts of mere preparation (e.g., checking the engine, finding keys, or opening the car door) do not amount to attempting to drive but steps on the way to what would have been driving, if not interrupted, may amount to an attempt (e.g., putting the key in the ignition). However, in a recent test case in the United Kingdom, when police found a man asleep in his van with the doors locked with a BAC over the legal limit, judges ruled by a majority decision that the laws that led to his conviction were disproportionate and violated the presumption of innocence to which he was entitled under Article 6(2) of the European Convention on Human Rights (29).

In Section 185(1) of the RTA, a motor vehicle is defined as a "mechanically propelled vehicle intended or adapted for use on a road"—the words "mechanically propelled" are intended to have a wide meaning and will cover any transmission of power from the engine to the wheels by mechanical means. Similar regulations are to be found throughout the European Union, and if further evidence is needed regarding just how vague the definition of "mechanically propelled" may be, one needs only to consider the arrest in 1997 of a paraplegic Scandinavian who was arrested (and tried) for unsafe driving of his wheelchair.

In Section 192(1) of the RTA, the word "road" is defined as any highway and any other road to which the public has access and includes bridges over which a road passes. Public place is a question of fact for the court to determine. In English law, a car park attached to a public house was held, during opening hours, to be a public place because it was attached to a tavern that offered its services to all members of the public, whereas the same car park would not be regarded as a public place if it were attached to a private club (30).

"In charge" is a question of fact, not law. As a general rule, the person remains in charge until he or she takes the vehicle off the road unless some intervening act occurs (e.g., handing keys to another person prevents him or her from retaining control). There is a statutory defense in that a person shall be deemed not to be in charge if he or she can prove that at the time, the circumstances were such that there was no likelihood of his or her driving the vehicle while the proportion of alcohol in the blood was over the prescribed limit. That the driver was injured or that the vehicle was damaged may be disregarded by the court if it is put forward as a defense. Therefore, the court is entitled to consider what the position would have been had the defendant not been prevented from driving by damage or injury. Of course, the state must always prove that the defendant was actually driving the car. That may prove difficult if, as is the case in many accidents, there are no witnesses.

3.7.2. Breath Testing

Section 6(1) of the RTA conferred the power to require a breath test only to officers in uniform. The courts have already ruled against a challenge where the officer was not wearing his helmet *(31)*. In the United Kingdom, the breath test may be taken either at or near the place where the officer makes a request for one. Normally, that would be at the roadside but not necessarily at the scene of the offense. If an accident occurs owing to the presence of a motor vehicle on a road or other public place, a police officer may require any person who he or she has reasonable cause to believe was driving or attempting to drive or in charge of the vehicle at the time of the accident to provide a specimen of breath for a breath test. The test may be taken at or near the place where the requirement was made or, if the police officer thinks fit, at a police station specified by the officer. In the United States, roadside breath testing, with nonevidentiary screening devices, is permitted only in "zero tolerance" states, with drivers under the age of 21 years.

In the United Kingdom, a person failing to provide a specimen of breath without reasonable excuse is guilty of an offense. A reasonable excuse would include someone who is physically or mentally unable to provide a sample, or if the act of providing the sample would, in some way entail risk to health. In most US states, refusal to submit to a breath (or blood or urine) test is admissible as evidence in criminal proceedings and, as a rule, leads to license suspension, even if guilt is not proved in court. In some states, refusal is actually considered a separate crime. This somewhat strange situation comes about because most US states and most other countries have *per se* laws for alcohol: an alcohol level above some preset limit is, by law, proof of intoxication *(32,33)*.

Section 6 of the RTA allows police officers to arrest a driver without a warrant if the breath test is positive or if the driver fails or refuses to provide a specimen of breath and the officer has reasonable cause to suspect alcohol in his or her body. Additionally, if an accident occurs owing to the presence of a motor vehicle on a road or public place and a police officer reasonably suspects that the accident involved injury to another person, then for the purpose of requiring a breath test or arresting a person, the officer may enter (by force if need be) any place where that person is or where the officer reasonably suspects the person to be.

3.7.3. Hospital Procedure

In the United Kingdom, patients at a hospital do not have to produce a breath test or provide a specimen for a laboratory testing unless the practitioner in immediate charge of their case has been notified and does not object on the grounds that the requirement would be prejudicial to the proper care and treatment of the person. In the United States, forensic blood samples can be taken from unconscious patients who are not able to give informed consent. Recent legislative changes in the United Kingdom in the Police Reform Act 2002 give doctors similar powers with a few subtle differences in that blood can be taken providing the person has been involved in an accident, the doctor is satisfied that the person is not able to give valid consent (for whatever reason, which could include mental health problems) and the person does not object to or resist the specimen being taken *(34)*. After death, a coroner can order that the blood alcohol level be measured (remembering always that the value measured will be 14% lower than if serum or plasma had been measured at a clinical laboratory). In the United States, medical examiners and coroners do not require special permission to measure ethanol (or any drug for that matter), and they do so routinely. Ethanol concentrations in vitreous humor are made and may be introduced in court. However, no fixed relationship between postmortem blood and vitreous concentrations is recognized in law. Additionally, when bodily harm has resulted, or when there is evidence of criminal activity (such as leaving the scene of an accident), then it is within the power of the officer to order that blood be drawn, even if the suspect is unwilling or unconscious.

3.7.4. Police Station Procedure

Police may require a suspect to provide either two breath samples for analysis by means of an approved device or a sample of blood or urine for laboratory testing. This is usually done at a police station, because it is almost unheard of for a hospital in the United Kingdom or the United States to be equipped with an evidentiary breath testing device. Blood or urine samples can only be collected at a police station or hospital. In the United Kingdom, such a request cannot be made at a police station, unless the constable making the requirement has reasonable cause to believe that, for medical reasons, a specimen of breath cannot be provided, or at the time the requirement is made, an approved breath analysis device is not available, or not practical to use, or that the suspected offense is one under Section 3A or 4 of the RTA, and the constable making the requirement has been advised by a doctor that the condition of the person may result from some drug. This situation does not occur in the United States where, if appropriate staff are available, both blood and urine may be obtained at the police station.

In the United Kingdom, if a specimen other than breath is required, police may demand either a urine or blood test. If blood cannot be obtained as, for example, might well be the case in a chronic intravenous drug abuser, then a urine sample must be provided within 1 hour of the request for its provision being made and after the provision of a previous specimen of urine. In the United States, urine specimens are generally not considered admissible proof of intoxication. A large number of studies have shown that the ratio between blood alcohol and pooled urine is highly unreliable and unpredictable *(35,36)*. Ureteral urine, on the other hand, has an alcohol concentration 1.3 times greater than blood *(23)*. Collection of ureteral urine is often attempted at autopsy, but for obvious reasons, is not an option with living patients.

Breath samples can only be analyzed with approved devices. Those currently in use include the Intoximeter EC/IR, Camic Datamaster, Lion Intoxilyzer 6000, and Drager Alcotest 7100 (Australia). Only officers who are trained to use the machine are allowed to conduct the intoximeter procedure, and the lower of two readings is taken. The subject must not have smoked for 10 minutes or have consumed alcohol or used a mouth spray or mouthwash, taken any medication, or consumed any food for 20 minutes before the breath test.

If the reading is below the prescribed limit of 35 µg of alcohol per 100 mL of breath, no action is taken unless impairment through drugs is suspected. If that is the case, a forensic physician should be called. If the level is between 36 and 39, no prosecution can occur unless there is impairment. If the level is between 40 and 50, the person is given the option of having the breath sample reading replaced by a specimen of blood or urine, but it is for the police officer to decide which, in accordance with Section 7. At levels over 51, the person is charged with an offense. Different rules and regulations, but with much the same intent, apply in other countries.

3.7.5. Blood Samples

It is wise to have a standardized routine for this procedure, if only to help prevent some of the technical defenses that are frequently raised in court. RTA blood alcohol kits are available with all the necessary equipment, and similar kits are sold in the United States, although their use is not mandatory. Regardless of whether or not a kit is used, appropriate chain of custody forms must be completed, and the record must reflect that alcohol-containing swabs were not used to cleanse the skin (actually, studies have shown that alcohol swabs contribute negligibly to the final result, but the issue is routinely raised in court) *(37)*.

The police officer should identify the doctor to the person, and the doctor should obtain witnessed informed consent. The physician must then determine whether there are any medical reasons why a sample of blood cannot be taken. It is for the doctor to decide from where the sample of blood is taken. The sample should be divided equally between the two bottles and shaken to disperse the preservative (an additional needle through the rubber membrane helps to equalize the pressure). The bottles should be labeled and placed in the secure containers and caps applied. The driver is allowed to retain one sample, which is placed in an envelope and sealed. The driver is then given a list of analysts.

Under US law, blood may be taken even if the driver objects, providing the driver has been involved in an accident leading to injury or a crime has been committed. Most US states have statutes that excuse individuals with hemophilia and patients taking anticoagulants from blood testing (22). Under British law, a forensic physician may make up to three unsuccessful attempts at taking blood before the driver can reasonably refuse to give blood on grounds that the defendant has lost confidence in the doctor. No such protection exists in US law.

3.7.6. Section 4, RTA

The medical examination and procedure to be adopted when it is suspected that a person is unfit through drink or drugs will be discussed later in Heading 4., Drugs and Driving.

3.8. Complex Defenses

Numerous technical defenses have been advocated over the years, and doctors should be aware of the most common. Failure to provide a sample of breath or blood will be considered separately.

3.8.1. Failure to Provide a Sample of Breath

Unless there is a reasonable excuse, failure to provide a specimen of breath, blood, or urine is an offense under Section 7 of the RTA. In the United States, refusal leads to automatic license suspension and, in some states, may actually constitute a separate crime; police are under an obligation to ensure that drivers are made aware of that. The motorist must understand the mandatory warning of prosecution if a specimen is not produced. Failure to understand, at least in the United Kingdom, is a reasonable excuse for the nonprovision of a sample (38). The decision regarding whether there is a medical reason not to supply a sample of breath is left to the police officer and is summarized in case law. There is no provision or requirement at that stage for a doctor to be summoned or to give an opinion.

Examples of medically acceptable reasons include mouth, lip, or facial injury; tracheotomy; rib injury; and neurological problems. Case law has stated that fear of acquired immune deficiency syndrome (AIDS) not amounting to phobia (39), shock (40), and even intoxication (41) can, in certain circumstances, be regarded as reasonable excuses.

Many cases have been challenged on the basis that the person was unable to blow into the intoximeter because of respiratory problems. Research has now clarified some of these situations. Spirometry has shown that if a person has a forced expiratory volume in 1 s (FEV1) of less than 2 L and a forced vital capacity (FVC) of less than 2.6 L, then that person would generally be unable to use a breath alcohol testing device *(42)*. A further study of healthy people of small stature (less than 166 cm tall) showed that if their FEV1, FVC, and peak expiratory flow rate were greater than 2.31, 2.61, and 330 L/min, respectively, then they should be capable of supplying a suitable breath sample *(43)*. This article was particularly useful because most forensic physicians do not have access to spirometry but do have access to a simple peak flow reading in the custody situation.

A study in Victoria, Australia, showed that persons with an FEV1 greater than 1.51 could provide an adequate screening sample on the Lion Alcolmeter SD2 roadside screening device *(44)* and that with an FEV1 greater than 1.0 and FVC greater than 1.75, individuals were able to provide adequate samples on the Drager Alcotest 7110 (as used in Victoria) evidentiary breath testing machine.

A more recent study *(45)* on the new Lion Intoxilyzer 6000 concluded that some subjects with lung diseases may have difficulty in providing evidential breath samples. However, these were subjects who would generally have been considered to have severe lung diseases.

A recent fashionable defense is that the presence of a metal stud through a hole pierced in the tongue invalidates the breath alcohol test because of the prohibition against foreign substances in the mouth and because of the potential for the jewelery to retain alcohol and interfere with the breath test. However, experimental work has shown that the rates of elimination of mouth alcohol were no different in subjects with a tongue stud as opposed to controls and that for the purposes of breath alcohol testing, oral jewelery should be treated the same as metallic dental work and left in place without affecting the outcome of the breath test *(46)*.

3.8.2. *Failure to Provide a Sample of Blood*

First, there must be a definite request to provide a sample of blood. In *Kuldip Singh Gill v DPP (47)*, it was held that a driver could not be convicted of failing to supply a specimen of blood or urine if he or she was not requested to do so. Where the sample of blood is taken from is solely the choice of the forensic physician (or, in the United States, the emergency room physician). In *Solesbury v Pugh (48)*, the defendant was found guilty of failing to supply a specimen as he would only allow a sample to be taken from his big toe, which the doctor was not prepared to do.

It is reasonable for the person to request that his or her own doctor take the sample of blood, providing this does not delay the sample being taken *(49)*. In the United Kingdom, if the patient's own doctor and forensic physician are both present, the person can choose which doctor takes the sample. Similar rules apply in the United States, where statutes generally spell out that financial responsibility for such services rests with the driver and not the state. In the United Kingdom, if a blood sample is provided but the doctor spills the sample, then the law has been complied with on the basis that removal of the syringe from the vein by the doctor completes the provision of the specimen by the defendant *(50)*. In the United Kingdom, a minimum of 2 mL of blood is required (the laboratory requires a minimum of 1 mL for analysis) for an adequate sample *(51)*. If less than this is obtained, the sample should be discarded and another one attempted or the police officer advised that there is a medical reason why a sample of blood should not be provided and the urine option can then be selected. In the United States, minimum quantities are generally not written into statute. As indicated, alcohol swabs should not be used. In the early 1980s, one police force purchased and used swabs containing alcohol with the result that numerous convictions were later overturned *(52)*.

Probably the most common defense for failure to provide a sample of blood is that of needle phobia. If this is alleged, a full medical history should be obtained and enquiry made of whether the person has had blood tests before, whether ears or other parts of the body have been pierced, or whether there have been foreign travel immunizations or any other medical or dental procedure undertaken in which an injection may have been administered. Specific inquiry about the phobia should be made. British appellate judges *(53)* have stated that "no fear short of phobia recognized by medical science to be as strong and as inhibiting as, for instance, claustrophobia can be allowed to excuse failure to provide a specimen for a laboratory test, and in most if not all cases where the fear of providing it is claimed to be invincible, the claim will have to be supported by medical evidence." Stark and Brener *(54)* stress the importance of having a standardized approach for assessing needle phobia using diagnostic guidelines for a definite diagnosis of a specific phobia and wisely conclude that the best way to ensure a successful prosecution is to obtain a sample, any sample, for analysis. Rix also gives some practical advice to police surgeons: be able to distinguish between repugnance and phobia, be able to distinguish between unwillingness and inability, document the history and examination with emphasis on the presence or absence of signs of anxiety, and ensure that the decision is based on firm medical evidence. Finally, record all this information, specifically note in the police record whether a medical condition has been identified, and then verbally communicate this opinion to the police officers *(55)*.

Another common defense is that of consuming alcohol after the offense–the hip flask defense *(56)*. It is used almost universally and is based on the fact that although it is unlawful to have an excessive BAC at the time of driving, it is not unlawful to have an elevated blood alcohol at the time of being tested. In the United Kingdom, Section 15(3) of the RTA allows for a driver to prove that he or she had imbibed alcohol after ceasing to drive and that the amount of such consumption was the sole reason for being over the legal limit or unfit to drive, at the time he or she gave a sample for analysis. It will be necessary for a scientist to prove that it was only the postdriving consumption that caused the analysis to reveal an alcohol level above the prescribed limit. The quantity of alcohol in the after-drink, the time of intake, and the age, sex, height, and body weight of the driver can all be used to calculate the theoretical expected BAC *(57)*. Back calculations can only be approximate because they are based on average values, and although they are reasonable estimates for most people, they may occasionally fail to reflect accurately the situation of a particular individual, regardless of whether the calculation is for preincident or postincident drinking.

3.8.3. Failure to Provide a Urine Sample

If a woman is requested to provide a urine sample, it is important to have a female officer present because it has been held that because of the embarrassment that it could involve, the refusal to supply a sample of urine could be regarded as a reasonable excuse *(58)*. However, any embarrassment at having to urinate in front of an officer of the same sex is not regarded as a reasonable excuse for not having supplied a specimen. Similar statutes apply in the United States. Methadone and other opiates have an effect on the bladder sphincter and can thus cause delayed bladder emptying; this effect could be considered a reasonable excuse for failing to provide a urine sample *(59)*. In Sweden, Jones *(56)* reported the top 10 defense challenges for driving under the influence of alcohol (Table 2). This situation may be subject to some change, because medications, such as tolterodine (Detrusitol) and other muscarinic receptor antagonists, are being increasingly prescribed for treatment of patients with symptoms of an unstable bladder. This may explain why California has already dropped urine from its list of testing options.

3.9. Postmortem Alcohol Measurements

This topic has recently been reviewed in depth by Pounder and Jones *(23)*. High postmortem alcohol concentrations do not imply that impairment

Table 2
Top 10 Defense Challenges For Driving Under the Influence of Alcohol

1. Drinking after the offense—the hip flask defense.
2. Laced drinks.
3. Inhalation of ethanol vapors from the work environment.
4. Pathological condition or trauma.
5. Use of skin antiseptics containing ethanol.
6. Alleged mix-up of blood specimens.
7. Postsampling formation of alcohols.
8. Drug–alcohol interactions.
9. Consumption of elixirs or health tonics containing alcohol.
10. Infusion of blood or other liquids during surgical emergency treatment.

was evident during life. Of 32 alcoholics presented at an emergency room for medical treatment, only 23 had apparent behavioral abnormalities, six were confused, and three were drowsy, even though the mean alcohol concentration was 313 mg/100 mL (range 180–450 mg/100 mL) *(60)*. Alcohol can be measured in numerous tissues, but the most accurate picture is usually obtained when multiple sites are sampled (e.g., vitreous, gastric contents, blood, and urine) particularly if ureteral urine is available and the alcohol concentrations compared.

Because the eye is anatomically isolated, putrefaction is delayed, and there is little problem with postmortem redistribution, vitreous measurements can be used to confirm values obtained from whole blood and urine, to distinguish postmortem alcohol production from antemortem ingestion, and to determine whether blood alcohol concentrations were rising or falling at the time of death. Vitreous contains more water than blood so that the blood/vitreous alcohol ratio is less than 1. Ratios greater than 1 suggest that death occurred before equilibrium had been reached (i.e., blood alcohol was still rising) *(61)*. Vitreous alcohol concentrations can be related to blood concentrations; however, there is so much intraindividual variation that extrapolation in an individual case is probably unwise and unsound scientifically.

As mentioned, serum and plasma contain more water than whole blood, and it follows that the alcohol content of the former will be 10–15% higher than the latter. Because postmortem measurements are made with whole blood and the water content of the cadaver begins to decrease almost immediately after death, estimating antemortem values with any precision is difficult, especially if only blood has been sampled. However, if samples from multiple sites are obtained, and vitreous, blood, and urine (urine as it is being formed contains 1.3 times as much alcohol as whole blood) are all analyzed, it may be possible to make a reasonable estimate of what the alcohol concentration was at the time of death *(23)*.

4. DRUGS AND DRIVING

4.1. The Problem

Increasing alcohol levels are associated with increased risk of accidents, but fatigue, drug abuse, and even the use of prescription medication can also increase risk *(62)*. The danger associated with sedatives and hypnotics is readily appreciated, but other drugs, such as anticholinergics, antidepressants, antihistamines, and antihypertensive medications, may occasionally cause drowsiness. Patients should be warned about this, and after starting therapy or after a significant change in dose, they should avoid driving until it is known that unwanted effects do not occur *(63,64)*.

4.2. The Scale of the Problem

The size of the problem is not really known. In the United Kingdom in 1997, more than 860,000 breath tests for alcohol were conducted, with a refusal (presumed positive) rate of 12% (103,000) (D. Rowe, DETR, personal communication, 1999). During the same period, the Forensic Science Service (FSS) dealt with only 1850 drugs/driving submissions. In a 2-weeks period in August 1996, the FSS received 270 blood specimens for testing for driving with excess alcohol. Further examination revealed that 18% contained one or more drugs, and of those that fell below the legal alcohol limit, a further 18% were positive for drugs. If this 18% figure were applied to those 103,000 cases in 1997, more than 18,000 cases would have been identified in which drivers had drugs in their body *(65)*.

In October 1999, the UK Department of Environment, Transport and the Regions completed a 3-years study into the incidence of drugs in road accident fatalities *(66)*. There were a total of 1138 road user fatalities, including drivers, riders of two-wheeled vehicles (34 of them cyclists), passengers in vehicles, and pedestrians; more than 6% tested positive for medicinal drugs, 18% for illicit drugs (mainly cannabis), and 12% for alcohol.

In this study, urine was tested by immunoassay for the following drugs: alcohol, amphetamines, methyl amphetamines (including ecstasy), cannabis, cocaine, opiates, methadone, lysergic acid diethylamide, benzodiazepines, and tricyclic antidepressants. The incidence of medicinal drugs likely to affect driving had not significantly changed from the 1985–1987 study *(67)*. However, illicit drug taking in drivers had increased sixfold in percentage terms, and there was a comparable increase among passengers. In addition, an in-

Table 3
Type of Drug Detected in Samples
Submitted to the FSS in 1997

Amphetamine	13%	Methylamphetamine	3%
Cannabis	28%	Cocaine	6%
Opiates	16%	Methadone	7%
Benzodiazepines	24%	Others	3%

creasing number had taken more than one illicit drug. In 1997, drugs were detected in approx 90% of samples submitted to the UK FSS for analysis (Table 3).

4.3. Effects of Different Drugs

The effects on driving of different drugs are now considered.

4.3.1. Cannabis

Numerous studies have been undertaken to examine the effects of cannabis on driving. One large meta-analysis of more than 150 studies showed that cannabis impairs the skills important for driving, including tracking, psychomotor skills, reaction time, and performance, with the effects most marked in the first 2 h after smoking and with attention, tracking, and psychomotor skills being affected the most (68). The study also showed that impairment is most marked in the absorption phase as opposed to the elimination phase and that frequent cannabis users become less impaired than infrequent users. These are, for the most part, older studies, done during the 1970s. Impairment is dosage dependent, and externally observable symptoms (e.g., impairment of psychomotor skills or the impression of absent-mindedness), disappear quickly during the early elimination phase. More recent studies (69) conducted with volunteer marijuana smokers who were actually driving found that the main effect of marijuana was to increase lateral movement of the vehicle moderately within the driving lane on a highway (70,71). A UK study (72) offered further support for the view that when under the influence of cannabis, users are acutely aware of their impairment but attempted to compensate for their impairment by driving more cautiously.

4.3.2. Opiates

Single doses of narcotics can have marked effects on performance, such as reaction time. However, most studies of opiates among regular users suggest that they do not present a hazard or exist as a significant factor in driving.

One study compared the effects of alcohol, diazepam, and methadone on clients commencing or stabilized on a methadone program. The battery of tests showed no evidence for an effect of the acute dose of methadone; thus, clients on a methadone program should not be considered impaired in their ability to perform complex tasks, such as driving a motor vehicle. Thus, in the United Kingdom, persons on a stable methadone program who have not abused other drugs for 1 yr and who have clear urine drug screening tests regularly are allowed a driving license subject to annual review. However, it should be remembered that users of heroin are also prone to heavy use of other psychoactive drugs, such as cocaine, alcohol, and tranquilizers, which are all dangerous when it comes to driving.

This problem is illustrated by a more recent study from Germany *(73)*. Thirty-four methadone substitution patients, all of them volunteers, were subjected to a battery of psychological tests. Twenty-one of these patients had to be excluded from the study because the toxicological analysis of repeated blood and urine samples revealed the presence (or possibly chronic use) of substances other than methadone. Of the remaining 13 (age range 26 to 42 years, 8 males and 5 females) 6 were selected who, based on the impression of the physicians, could be described as optimal methadone patients. Although some personality scales and psychopathological findings revealed shortcomings for a few of these patients, they could not be regarded as factors ruling out driver fitness, and the authors concluded that under certain conditions, long-term methadone maintenance patients under strict medical supervision do not suffer significant driving impairment, providing that no other drugs have been taken.

4.3.3. Cocaine and Methamphetamine

Although the argument often goes unchallenged in court, all drugs do not, by definition, produce impairment. Even though some US states define "being under the influence" as synonymous with the presence of any drug, some drugs do improve performance. In fact, low to moderate acute doses of cocaine and amphetamine can be expected to increase positive mood, energy, and alertness, especially in nontolerant individuals *(74)*. It has been known since World War II that use of D-amphetamine can increase the ability to sustain attention for prolonged periods when performing monotonous tasks. For that reason, radar operators and pilots of both Allied and Japanese armies were issued supplies of amphetamine. Many of the performance tasks related to driving can be improved, at least in the laboratory, by treatment with stimulants *(75)*. Although the results of one retrospective autopsy study suggest that methamphetamine users seem more likely to be involved in traffic accidents *(76)*, a driving simulator study *(77)* of young people who had taken ecstasy (3,4-methylenedioxymethamphetamine) showed that basic vehicle control is only moderately affected but risk taking is increased. It seems likely that abrupt discontinuation of either drug in a chronic user could result in driving impairment, but that situation has never been tested *(70)*. Large doses can result in toxic psychosis with symptoms indistinguishable from paranoid schizophrenia, a condition that is extremely unlikely to improve driving performance.

4.3.4. Sedative Hypnotics

Benzodiazepines impair psychomotor performance in nontolerant individuals, generally in a dose-dependent manner. Most of the widely prescribed benzodiazepines increase lateral lane movement and slow response time to a lead car's change in speed. Several of the benzodiazepines (50 mg of oxazepam, 30 mg of flurazepam, and 2 mg of lormetazepam) predictably impair driving the morning after. Diazepam (15 mg) impaired performance on a clinical test for drunkenness, which comprised 13 tests assessing motor, vestibular, mental, and behavioral functioning *(78,79)*. A recent study *(80)* showed a clear relationship between dose of benzodiazepines and risk of impairment, which the authors believed probably supported a limit for benzodiazepines and driving as low as within the therapeutic range.

Acute doses of many benzodiazepines slow response time in simple or choice visual reaction time tests and impair attentional performance and cause deficits that do not result from sedation. In fact, the impairment of sustained attention and vigilance in benzodiazepine users is the direct result of some as yet uncharacterized direct action on perceptual sensitivity *(70)*.

4.3.5. Multiple Drug Use

Polydrug use is common and can result in complex interactions, with the drugs having additive, antagonistic, or overlapping effects. Alcohol is commonly consumed in addition to abused drugs. In a study on alcohol and cannabis *(81)*, it has been shown that when they are administered together, the result was one of additive impairment. This finding was confirmed in a recent UK study *(82)*. However, in the laboratory setting, simultaneous administration of alcohol and cocaine seems to minimize alcohol-related deficits *(75)*.

4.3.6. Antidepressants

There are many side effects associated with the use of the tricyclic antidepressants (TCAs) (e.g., amitriptyline), that are relevant to the ability to drive, such as blurred vision, slow visual accommodation, disorientation, and eye–hand coordination; the most important are the induction of drowsiness, lethargy, and sedation. An analysis of 500 road traffic accidents showed that victims who had taken TCAs had a relative accident risk 2.2 times greater than non-TCA users and that patients using TCAs with a daily dose greater than or equivalent to 125 mg of amitriptyline had a sixfold increase in road traffic crash risk *(83)*. The newer antidepressant drugs of the serotonin reuptake inhibitor class (e.g., fluoxetine, paroxetine, or the selective serotonin and no-radrenaline re-uptake inhibitors [venlafaxine]) do not generally affect driving performance and are safe for use by patients who drive *(84)*.

4.3.7. Over-the-Counter Preparations

An increasing number of drugs can now be bought over the counter from pharmacies. Many of these preparations (e.g., cough mixtures and deconges-tants), contain drugs that can cause sedation, particularly the older antihista-mines (e.g., chlorpheniramine). The newer nonsedating antihistamines, such as terfenadine and astemizole, generally do not impair driving. However, one study that measured driving performance across differing doses of terfenadine found that performance was impaired at very high doses (240 mg), stressing the need to establish the behavioral effects of drugs over a range of doses *(85)*. The second-generation group of antihistamines is less lipophilic than the pre-vious generation and thus cross the blood–brain barrier less readily, which accounts for the lower levels of sedation observed with the newer drugs. Thus, although the second-generation antihistamines generally produce less seda-tion than first-generation compounds, if therapeutic doses are exceeded, the so-called nonsedating antihistamines become sedating and can impair driving.

4.4. Assessment in the Field by Police

In the United Kingdom, if a police officer stops a driver, for whatever reason, and believes the driver is unfit to drive, it is highly likely that a road-side breath test will be conducted. That is not the case in the United States, where field breath testing is only permitted in some states, and then only for drivers under the age of 21 years *(22)*. The laws of the United States also prevent random breath testing. Under the Fourth Amendment, searches and seizures must be reasonable. Stopping a vehicle is a seizure, but it may be reasonable if the police officer has a justifiable suspicion that an offense is being committed. The procedures American officers follow in driving under the influence cases are surprisingly similar to the procedures under the United Kingdom Section 4 RTA. To gain powers to conduct further tests, officers in most US states first have to be satisfied that the driver is impaired. This then gives them the probable cause to carry out subsequent tests similar to the Sec-tion 4 procedure to prove impairment.

If breath testing is negative, impairment resulting from drugs or medical illness must be considered. Until recently in the United Kingdom, police traffic officers received little or no training in the recognition of signs and symptoms of drug effects. However, a pilot study *(86)* was carried out in England, Wales, and Scotland in 1999, whereby police officers were trained to perform roadside impairment tests; this study showed that forensic analysis confirmed the presence of a drug in 92% of the drivers who were suspected of taking a drug, who had failed the field impairment tests (FIT) and who had provided a sample. As a consequence, FIT is now slowly being introduced across the United Kingdom. This contrasts dramatically with the United States, where in 1979, the Drug Recognition Expert (DRE) Program was introduced. Police officers were trained to observe and document known indicators of drug use and impairment.

Instead of breath testing, a series of standardized field sobriety tests, which include psychomotor and divided attention tests, is conducted. If alcohol is suspected, the following tests are carried out: walk and turn test, one-leg stand, and the horizontal gaze nystagmus test. In addition, if drugs are suspected, a Romberg balance test is also carried out. Unlike chemical tests (with refusal to submit possibly resulting in immediate license suspension), drivers in the United States are not legally required to take any field sobriety tests; however, if the driver submits, the results can be introduced as additional evidence of impairment.

These tests are all divided attention tests, which assess the individual's balance and coordination, as well as the ability to follow simple instructions (i.e., to divide attention between multiple tasks). They are as follows:

- Horizontal gaze nystagmus: nystagmus may be caused by any number of conditions, but its presence could indicate drugs or alcohol.
- Walk and turn: nine steps heel to toe are taken in one direction, and then the individual turns and repeats the process in the other direction. Eight impairment indicators are measured; if two of the eight are present, impairment would be indicated.
- One-leg stand: the subject has to stand on alternate feet for 30 s while counting aloud. Failing two of the four recognized indicators would indicate impairment.
- Romberg balance test: the subject stands with eyes closed and estimates a period of 30 s during which body sway is estimated. Some drugs alter the body's internal clock and make the person act faster or slower than normal. The test allows for a tolerance of ±10 s.

If impairment is identified and alcohol is suspected, the driver performs a breathalyzer test and a similar procedure to the United Kingdom Section 5 RTA procedure is conducted. However, if drugs are suspected, the police officer would call on a DRE to carry out a more detailed examination.

The DRE will use a 12-step procedure as follows:

1. Breath alcohol test: this is carried out by the arresting officer; if the reading is not consistent with the degree of impairment, the DRE is called in.
2. Interview with the arresting officer: the purpose is to ascertain baseline information, including the circumstances of the arrest, whether an accident occurred, whether drugs were found, and if so, what they looked like.
3. Preliminary examination: the purpose of the preliminary examination is to determine whether if there is sufficient reason to suspect a drug offense and to try to exclude any underlying medical problems. General observations and details of any current medical problems are ascertained, and the first measurement of the pulse is taken. If no signs of drug influence are found, the procedure is terminated; if any medical problems are found, a medical assessment is obtained, and if drugs are still suspected, a full assessment is carried out. If at any time during the assessment a serious medical condition is suspected, a medical opinion will be obtained.
4. Eye examination: the driver is assessed for horizontal gaze nystagmus, vertical gaze nystagmus, and convergence.
5. Divided attention tests: once at a police station, the Romberg balance test, walk and turn test, one-leg stand test, and the finger-to-nose test are carried out. These are all examples of divided attention tests whereby balance and movement tests are performed in addition to remembering instructions.
6. Vital signs examination: blood pressure, temperature, and a second recording of the pulse are carried out.
7. Darkroom examination: pupil size is measured in room light and then in near total darkness, using both indirect artificial light and direct light. The mouth and nose are also examined for evidence of drug use.
8. Muscle tone: limb tone is assessed as some drugs cause rigidity, whereas others, for example, alcohol, cause flaccidity.
9. Injection sites examination: the purpose is to seek evidence of intravenous or injection drug abuse. A third pulse reading is taken.
10. Interrogation: a structured interview about the use of drugs is carried out.
11. Opinion: based on all the previous assessments, the DRE forms an opinion as to drug impairment and also the type of drug causing the problem, the legal standard being a reasonable degree of certainty.
12. Toxicology testing: at the same time, samples arc obtained for toxicological examination, either a blood or urine sample being taken for analysis of common drugs.

Initial studies, suggesting high sensitivity and specificity for DRE examination *(87)*, have not been confirmed in controlled laboratory studies. The results of the few studies that have been performed suggest that the accuracy of DRE assessment in general may not be sufficiently good to provide evidence in court fairly *(70,71)*. Several field studies have indicated that a DRE's opinions were confirmed by toxicological analysis in 74–92% of cases when DREs concluded that suspects were impaired. However, published controlled trials, in which blood levels were measured before and during DRE examination, have shown that except in the case of alcohol, DRE assessment agreed with toxicology findings only 32–44% of the time.

There are other options for roadside screening tests. Both sweat and saliva have been used *(88)*. Devices are already available, and some have been approved by the US Department of Transportation for the testing of commercial drivers. The mere detection of a drug does not prove impairment unless, of course, the jurisdiction has *per se* laws whereby the detection of drugs at some predetermined level is ruled, by law, to be proof of impairment. Roadside drug screening tests are acceptable to the public; a UK study *(89)* found that 98% of drivers were in favor of the principle of road side drug screening and found the test methods of saliva or forehead perspiration generally acceptable. The UK Home Office Police Scientific Development Branch are currently researching the use of computer program for detecting impairment and Surface Enhanced Raman Spectroscopy as a means of quantitative analysis of saliva for drugs.

4.5. Medical Examination Under Section 4 of the RTA

In the United Kingdom, it is not necessary to prove impairment, as Section 7(3)(c) of the RTA states that: "the suspected offence is one under Section 3A or 4 of this Act and the constable has been advised by a medical practitioner that the condition of the person required to provide the specimen *might* [author's emphasis] be due to some drug." It is for the court to decide whether the driver is unfit to drive on the evidence before it.

Whether the examination is carried out by a forensic physician in London or an emergency room physician in San Francisco, the aim of the examination is to exclude any medical condition other than alcohol or drugs as the cause of the driver's behavior. The differential diagnosis is wide and includes head injury, neurological problems (e.g., epilepsy, stroke, cerebral tumour, and multiple sclerosis), metabolic problems (e.g., hypoglycemia), hepatic or renal failure, and mental illness. The procedure should include introductory details, full medical history, and clinical examination. In Scotland, forensic physicians use form F97. Appendix 6 contains a form that has been found useful. Similar forms are not available in the United States, but there is nothing to prevent any emergency department in the United States from drafting and providing a similar document. Even if no special form is provided, most of the relevant material will have been (or at least should be) recorded in the emergency department record.

4.5.1. Introductory Details

These should include the name, address, and date of birth of the driver and the name and number of the police officer, as well as the place and date the examination took place, and various times, including time doctor contacted, time of arrival at police station/hospital, and time the examination commenced and ended.

The doctor will need to know brief details of the circumstances leading to arrest and the results of any field impairment tests that may have been carried out by the police officer. Informed consent should be obtained.

4.5.2. Full Medical History

Details of any current medical problems and details of recent events, particularly whether there was a road traffic accident that led to the event, should be recorded. Past medical history (with specific reference to diabetes, epilepsy, asthma, and visual and hearing problems), past psychiatric history, and alcohol and drug consumption (prescribed, over the counter, and illicit) should be noted.

4.5.3. Clinical Examination

This should include general observations on demeanor and behavior, a note of any injuries, speech, condition of the mouth, hiccoughs, and any smell on the breath. The cardiovascular system should be examined and pulse, blood pressure, and temperature recorded. Signs of drug abuse should be looked for (e.g., needle marks). Examination of the eyes should include state of the sclera, state of the pupils (including size, reaction to light, convergence, and the presence of both horizontal or vertical nystagmus).

A series of divided attention tests should be performed including the Romberg test, finger–nose test, one-leg-stand test, and walk and turn test. A survey of forensic physicians' opinions within Strathclyde police demonstrated concerns regarding the introduction of standardized field sobriety tests with the walk and turn test and the one-leg-stand test, causing the highest levels of concern *(90)*. The mental state should be assessed and consideration given to obtaining a sample of handwriting. Fitness for detention is of paramount importance, and any person who is not fit to be detained because of illness or injury should be transferred to hospital and not subjected to a Section 4 assessment. If the person refuses to consent to an examination, it is prudent to make observations on his or her manner, possible unsteadiness, etc. and make written note of these.

At the end of the examination, the doctor should decide whether there is a condition present that may result from some drug. In the case of short-acting drugs, the observations of the police officer or other witnesses can be of crucial importance. In a recent case, a person was found guilty of driving while unfit resulting from drug use on the basis of the officer's observations and the results and opinion of the toxicologist; the forensic physician was not called to give evidence *(91)*. Similarly, if the police officer reports that the person was swerving all over the road but the doctor later finds only minimal physical signs, this may be sufficient to indicate that a condition may be present because of some drug (e.g., cannabis) and that it is appropriate to proceed to the next part of the procedure.

The doctor should inform the police officer whether there is a condition present that may be the result of a drug, and if so, the police officer will then continue with the blood/urine option. Consent will need to be obtained for a blood specimen. On this occasion, 10 mL of blood should be taken and divided equally into two septum-capped vials because the laboratory requires a greater volume of blood for analysis because of the large number of drugs potentially affecting driving performance and their limited concentration in body fluids; indeed, if the driver declines the offer of a specimen, both samples should be sent.

As a means of further validating FIT as an effective means of detecting drivers who are impaired because of drugs, the University of Glasgow is carrying out further research *(92)*. Those drivers stopped under suspicion of impairment who are under the legal alcohol limit but still considered impaired will be offered a FIT test. If they fail, they will be considered as a suspect drug driver and examined by a forensic physician and a forensic sample obtained and analyzed if appropriate. Those who pass a FIT assessment will be asked to voluntarily supply a sample of saliva, which will be analyzed for drugs. The drug incidence in the two groups will then be compared, as will the police officers' and doctors' assessments using standardized proformas. The results are awaited with interest.

In Victoria, Australia *(93)*, forensic physicians with relevant qualifications and experience act as experts for the court by reviewing all the evidence of impaired driving, the police Preliminary Impairment Test, the forensic physician's assessment, and toxicological results and provide an opinion. So far, no expert opinions have been challenged in court. However, there were several inconsistencies in the physical examination with the drugs eventually found on toxicological examination, cases where the individual were barely conscious, where a formal assessment should not even have been considered, and missed medical and psychiatric conditions.

REFERENCES

1. Finucane, A. K. Legal aspects of epilepsy. Neurol. Clin. 17:235–243, 1999.
2. Fitten, L. J. The demented driver: the doctor's dilemma. Alzheimer Dis. Assoc. Disord. 11 (Suppl 1):57–61, 1997.
3. Driver and Vehicle Licensing Agency. For Medical Practitioners: At a Glance Guide to the Current Medical Standards of Fitness to Drive. Drivers Medical Unit. DVLA, Swansea, Wales, 2003.

4. Austroads Assessing Fitness to Drive: Austroads Guidelines for Health Professionals and Their Legal Obligations. Austroads, Sydney, 1998.
5. Osawa, M., Nagasawa, T., Yukawa, N., et al. Sudden natural death in driving: case studies in the western area of Kanagawa. Nippon Hoigaku Zasshi. 52:315–318, 1998.
6. Cheng, L. H., Whittington, R. M. Natural deaths while driving: would screening for risk be ethically justified? J. Med. Ethics. 24:248–251, 1998.
7. Belkic, K., Emdad, R., Theorell, T. Occupational profile and cardiac risk: possible mechanisms and implications for professional drivers. Int. J. Occup. Med. Environ. Health. 11:37–57, 1998.
8. Conti, J. B., Woodard, D. A., Tucker, K. J., Bryant, B., King, L. C., Curtis, A. B. Modification of patient driving behavior after implantation of a cardioverter defibrillator. Pacing Clin. Electrophysiol. 20(9 Pt. 1):2200–2204, 1997.
9. Medical Research Council Antiepileptic Drug Withdrawal Study Group. Prognostic index for recurrence of seizures after remission of epilepsy. Br. Med. J. 306:1374–1378, 1993.
10. Krumholz, A. Driving and epilepsy: a historical perspective and review of current regulations. Epilepsia. 35:668–674, 1994.
11. MacLeod, K. M. Diabetes and driving: towards equitable, evidence-based decision-making. Diabetes Med. 16:282–290, 1999.
12. Ehrlich, E. N. Diabetes and the license to drive. Wis. Med. J. 90:115–118, 1991.
13. Distiller, L. A., Kramer, B. D. Driving and diabetics on insulin therapy. S. Afr. Med. J. 86 (Suppl 8):1018–1020, 1996.
14. Charman, W. N. Vision and driving–a literature review and commentary. Ophthalmic Physiol. Opt. 17:371–391, 1997.
15. General Medical Council. Duties of a Doctor–Confidentiality. Guidance from the General Medical Council. GMC, London, UK, 1995.
16. Ellenhorn, M. J., Schonwald, S., Ordog, G., Wasserberger, J. Ellenhorn's Medical Toxicology: Diagnosis and Treatment of Human Poisoning. Williams & Wilkins, Baltimore, MD, 1997.
17. Jones, A., Pounder, D. Measuring blood-alcohol concentration for clinical and forensic purposes. In: Karch, S., ed., Drug Abuse Handbook. CRC Press, Boca Raton, FL, pp. 327–356, 1998.
18. Noordzij, P. C., Roszbach, R. Alcohol, drugs, and traffic safety. In: T86: Proceedings of the 10th International Conference on Alcohol, Drugs, and Traffic Safety, Amsterdam, September 9–12, 1986. Excerpta Medica, New York, NY, 1987.
19. Borkenstein, R. F., Dale, A. The role of the drinking driver in traffic accidents. Department of Police Administration, Indiana University, Bloomington, IN, 1964.
20. Allsop, R. Alcohol and road accidents: a discussion of the Grand Rapids study: RRL 6. Transport and Road Research Laboratory, Crowthorne, UK, 1996.
21. Compton, R.P., Blomberg, R.D., Moskowitz, H., Burns, M., Peck, R.C., Fiorentino, D. Crash Risk of Alcohol Impaired Driving in T2002 Proceedings of the 16th International Conference on Alcohol, Drugs and Traffic Safety. Montreal, Canada, 2002.
22. California Code of Regulations. Title 13. Motor Vehicles and Traffic Regulations, CA, 1999.

23. Pounder, D., Jones, G. Measuring alcohol post-mortem. In: Karch, S., ed., Drug Abuse Handbook, CRC Press, Boca Raton, FL, pp. 356–374, 1998.
24. Aberg, L. Utzelmann, H. D., Berghaus, G., eds. Behaviours and opinions of Swedish drivers before and after the 0.02% legal BAC limit of 1990, in T9. Proceedings of the 12th International Conference on Alcohol, Drugs, and Traffic Safety, Cologne, Germany, 1992.
25. Department of Environment, Transport and the Regions. Combating Drunk-Driving—Next Steps. A Consultation Document. DETR, UK, 1998.
26. Dunbar, J. A., Penttila, A., Pikkarainen, J. Drinking and driving: success of random breath testing in Finland. Br. Med. J. 295:101–103. 1987.
27. Marsden, A. Accidental injury and traffic medicine. In: McLay, W. D. S., ed., Clinical Forensic Medicine, Greenwich Medical Media, London, UK, p. 231, 1996.
28. Coben, J. H., Larkin, G. L. Effectiveness of ignition interlock devices in reducing drunk driving recidivism. Am. J. Prev. Med. 16 (Suppl 1):81–87, 1999.
29. *Sheldrake v Director of Public Prosecutions* [2003] EWHC 273 (Admin).
30. *Pugh v Knipe.* R.T.R. 286. 1972.
31. *Wallwork v Giles.* 114 S.J. 36. 1969.
32. Krause, K. R., Howells, G. A., Bair, H. A., Bendick, P. J., Glover, J. L. Prosecution and conviction of the injured intoxicated driver. J. Trauma. 45:1069–1073, 1998.
33. McArthur, D. L., Kraus, J. F. The specific deterrence of administrative per se laws in reducing drunk driving recidivism. Am. J. Prev. Med. 16 (Suppl 1):68–75, 1999.
34. Association of Police Surgeons/British Medical Association. Taking blood from incapacitated drivers. Guidance for doctors on the provisions of the Police Reform Act 2002. Available at Website: (http://www.afpweb.org.uk/Pages/Publications-Guidelines&Advice.htm). Accessed on October 2002.
35. Kaye, S., Cardona, E. Errors of converting a urine alcohol value into a blood alcohol level. Am. J. Clin. Pathol. 52:577–584, 1969.
36. Winek, C. L., Esposito, F. M. Comparative study of ethanol levels in blood versus bone marrow, vitreous humor, bile and urine. Forensic Sci. Int. 17:27–36, 1981.
37. Carter, P. G., McConnell, A. A. Alcohol in drink driving swabs: does it make any difference? [letter]. Med. Sci. Law. 30:90, 1990.
38. *Chief Constable of Avon and Somerset v Singh.* R.T.R. 107. 1988.
39. *D.P.P. v Kinnersley.* The Times, December 29 D.C. 1992.
40. *D.P.P. v Pearman.* R.T.R. 407. 1992.
41. *Young v D.P.P.* R.T.R. 328. 1992.
42. Gomm, P. J., Osselton, M. D., Broster, C. G., Johnson, N. M., Upton, K. Study into the ability of patients with impaired lung function to use breath alcohol testing devices. Med. Sci. Law. 31:221–225, 1991.
43. Gomm, P. J., Broster, C. G., Johnson, N. M., Hammond, K. Study into the ability of healthy people of small stature to satisfy the sampling requirements of breath alcohol testing instruments. Med. Sci. Law. 33:311–314, 1993.
44. Odell, M., McDonald, C., Farrar, J., Natsis, J. S., Pretto, J. F. Breath testing in patients with respiratory disability. J. Clin. Forensic Med. 5:45–48, 1998.
45. Honeybourne, D., Moore, A. J., Butterfield, A. K., Azzan, L. A study to investigate the ability of subjects with chronic lung diseases to provide evidential breath samples

using the Lion Intoxilyzer ® 6000 UK breath alcohol testing device. Respiratory Med. 94:684–688, 2000.
46. Logan, B. K., Gullberg, R. G. Lack of effect of tongue piercing on an evidential breath alcohol test. J. Forensic Sci. 43:239–240, 1998.
47. *Kuldip Singh Gill v D.P.P.* January 16, 1995.
48. *Solesbury v Pugh.* 1 W.L.R. 1114. 1969.
49. *Bayliss v Thames Valley Police Chief Constable.* R.T.R. 328, 1978.
50. *Beck v Watson.* R.T.R. 91. 1980.
51. Robinson, S. P. Road traffic offences. In Robinson, S. P., ed., Principles of Forensic Medicine, Greenwich Medical Media, London. Distributed worldwide by Oxford University Press, Oxford, UK, pp. 139–147, 1996.
52. *R v Bolton JJ. Ex p. Scally* 1 Q.B. 537. 1991.
53. *R v Harding.* R.T.R. 325. 1974.
54. Stark, M.M., Brener, N. Needle Phobia. J. Clin. Forensic Med. 7:35–38, 2000.
55. Rix, K. Blood or needle phobia as a defence under the Road Traffic Act of 1988. J. Clin. Forensic Med. 3:173–177, 1996.
56. Jones, A. W. Top ten defence challenges among drinking drivers in Sweden. Med. Sci. Law. 31:229–238, 1991.
57. Jones, A., Logan, B. DUI defenses. In: Karch, S., ed., Drug Abuse Handbook , CRC Press, Boca Raton, FL, pp. 1006–1046, 1998.
58. *Rowland v. Thorpe.* 3 All E.R. 195. 1970.
59. Acevedo, C. G., Tamayo, L., Contreras, E. Effects of morphine in the isolated mouse urinary bladder. Gen. Pharmacol. 17:449–452, 1986.
60. Davis, A. R., Lipson, A. H. Central nervous system tolerance to high blood alcohol levels. Med. J. Aust. 144:9–12, 1986.
61. Felby, S., Olsen, J. Comparative studies of postmortem ethyl alcohol in vitreous humor, blood, and muscle. J. Forensic Sci. 14:93–101, 1969.
62. Seppala, T., Linnoila, M., Mattila, M. J. Drugs, alcohol and driving. Drugs. 17:389–408, 1979.
63. Mattila, M. J., Vanakoski, J., Kalska, H., Seppala, T. Effects of alcohol, zolpidem and some other sedatives and hypnotics on human performance and memory. Pharmacol. Biochem. Behav. 59:917–923, 1998.
64. Ramaekers, J. G. Behavioural toxicity of medicinal drugs. Practical consequences, incidence, management and avoidance. Drug Saf. 18:189–208, 1998.
65. Osselton, M. D., Owen, P., Fysh, R. Drugs and Driving, Forensic Science Service Report No. TN816. Forensic Science Service, London, UK, p. 3, 1996.
66. Tunbridge, R. J., Keigan, M., James, F. J. The Incidence of Drugs in Road Accident Fatalities. TRL report 495. TRL Ltd, Crowthorne, UK, 2001.
67. Everest J, T,, Tunbridge, R J , B Widdop. The Incidence of Drugs in Road Accident Fatalities. TRL Report RR202. Transport and Road Research Laboratory, Crowthorne, UK, 1989.
68. Berghaus, G., Scheer, N., Schmidt, P. Effects of cannabis on psychomotor skills and driving performance–a meta-analysis of experimental studies, in T95 Proceedings of the 13th International Conference on Alcohol, Drugs, and Traffic Safety, Adelaide, 1994.

69. Chait, L., Pierri, J. Effects of smoked marijuana on human performance: a critical review. In: Murphy, L., Bartke, A., eds., Marijuana/Cannabinoids: Neurobiology and Neurophysiology. CRC Press, Boca Raton, FL, 1992.
70. Heishman, S., Karch, S. Drugs and driving. In: Siegel, J., Saukko, P., Knupfer, G., eds., Encyclopaedia of Forensic Sciences. Academic Press, London, UK, 2000.
71. Heishman, S. J., Singleton, E. G., Crouch, D. J. Laboratory validation study of drug evaluation and classification program: alprazolam, δ-amphetamine, codeine, and marijuana. J. Anal. Toxicol. 22:503–514, 1998.
72. Sexton, B.F., Tunbridge, R.J., Brook-Carter, N., et al. The influence of cannabis on driving. TRL Report 477. TRL Limited, Crowthorne, UK, 2000.
73. Friedel, B., Berghaus, S. Methadone and Driving. In: T95 Proceedings of the 13th International Conference on Alcohol, Drugs, and Traffic Safety, Adelaide, Australia, 1995.
74. Koelega, H. S. Stimulant drugs and vigilance performance: a review. Psychopharmacology. 111:1–16, 1993.
75. Farre, M., Llorente, M., Ugena, B., Lamas, X., Cami, J. Interaction of cocaine with ethanol. NIDA Res Monogr. 105:570–571, 1991.
76. Logan, B. K. Methamphetamine and driving impairment. J. Forensic Sci. 41:457–464, 1996.
77. De Waard, D., Brookhuis, K. A., Pernot, L. M. C. A driving simulator study on the effects of MDMA (Ecstasy) on driving performance and traffic safety. In: T2000 Proceedings of the International Conference on Alcohol, Drugs, and Traffic Safety, Stockholm, Sweden, May 26, 2000.
78. O'Hanlon, J. F., Vermeeren, A., Uiterwijk, M. M., van Veggel, L. M., Swijgman, H. F. Anxiolytics' effects on the actual driving performance of patients and healthy volunteers in a standardized test. An integration of three studies. Neuropsychobiology. 31:81–88, 1995.
79. Barbone, F., McMahon, A. D., Davey, P. G., et al. Association of road-traffic accidents with benzodiazepine use [see comments]. Lancet. 352:1331–1336, 1998.
80. Bramness, J. G., Skurtveit, S., Mørland. J. Clinical Impairment of Benzodiazepines–Relation between Benzodiazepine Concentrations and Impairment in Apprehended Drivers. Pompidou Group, Strasbourg, France, 2003.
81. Chesher, G. B., Dauncey, H., Crawford, J., Horn, K. The Interaction Between Alcohol and Marijuana. Report to the Australian Federal Office of Road Safety. Department of Pharmacology, University of Sydney, Sydney, Australia, 1996.
82. Sexton, B. F., Tunbridge, R. J., Brook-Carter, N., et al. The influence of cannabis and alcohol on driving. TRL Report 543. TRL Limited, Crowthorne, UK, 2002.
83. Hindmarch, I. Psychiatry in practice. Winter:23–25, 1993.
84. O'Hanlon, J. F., Robbe, H. W., Vermeeren, A., van Leeuwen, C., and Danjou, P. E. Venlafaxine's effects on healthy volunteers' driving, psychomotor, and vigilance performance during 15-day fixed and incremental dosing regimens. J. Clin. Psychopharmacol. 18:212–221, 1998.
85. Bhatti, J. Z., Hindmarch, I. The effects of terfenadine with and without alcohol on an aspect of car driving performance. Clin. Exp. Allergy. 19:609–611, 1989.

86. Tunbridge, R. J., Keigan, M., James, F. J. Recognising drug use and drug related impairment in drivers at the roadside. TRL report 464. TRL Ltd, Crowthorne, UK, 2001.
87. Burns, M., Adler, E. Study of a Drug Recognition Expert (DRE) program, in T95. Proceedings of the 13th International Conference on Alcohol, Drugs, Traffic Safety, Adelaide, Australia, 1995.
88. Kidwell, D. A., Holland, J. C., Athanaselis, S. Testing for drugs of abuse in saliva and sweat. J. Chromatogr. B Biomed. Sci. Appl. 713:111–135, 1998.
89. Tunbridge, R. J., Rowe, D. J. Roadside identification of drug impaired drivers in Great Britain. 10th International Conference on Road safety in Europe, Malmo, 1999.
90. O'Keefe, M. Drugs driving—standardized field sobriety tests: a survey of police surgeons in Strathclyde. J. Clin. Forensic Med. 8:57–65, 2001.
91. *Leetham v. D.P.P.* Q.B. 488. 1998.
92. Stark, M. M., Tunbridge, R. J., Rowe, D., Fleming, D., Stewart, D. Drugs, driving and sobriety tests–a review of recent developments. J. Clin. Forensic Med. 9:126–132, 2002.
93. Odell, M.S. Expert Opinion in DUID Cases Based on Interpretation and Observation and Toxicology in T2002. Proceedings of the 16th International Conference on Alcohol, Drugs and Traffic Safety. Montreal, Canada, 2002.

Appendices

CONTENTS

1. Ethical Documents
2. Guidance Notes on UK Statutory Provisions Governing Access to Health Records
3. Management of Head-Injured Detainees
4. The Mini-Mental State Examination
5. Alcohol Assessment Questionnaires
6. Drink/Drugs Driving Impairment Assessment Form
7. Useful Web Site Addresses

PREFACE

The attached appendices include international ethical documents and samples of forms used in clinical forensic practice, as well as guidance notes on key topics.

The appendices contain useful information for a worldwide audience of physicians working in the field of clinical forensic medicine. They provide comparative data and are not meant to be exhaustive.

From: *Clinical Forensic Medicine: A Physician's Guide, 2nd Edition*
Edited by: M. M. Stark © Humana Press Inc., Totowa, NJ

Appendix 1

Ethical Documents

DOCUMENT 1

Code of Conduct for Law Enforcement Officials (Adopted by the United Nations General Assembly, 17 December 1979).

G.A. res. 34/169, annex, 34 U.N. GAOR Supp. (No. 46) at 186, U.N. Doc. A/34/46 (1979).

Article 1

Law enforcement officials shall at all times fulfill the duty imposed upon them by law, by serving the community and by protecting all persons against illegal acts, consistent with the high degree of responsibility required by their profession.

Commentary:

a. The term "law enforcement officials" includes all officers of the law, whether appointed or elected, who exercise police powers, especially the powers of arrest or detention.

b. In countries where police powers are exercised by military authorities, whether uniformed or not, or by State security forces, the definition of law enforcement officials shall be regarded as including officers of such services.

c. Service to the community is intended to include particularly the rendition of services of assistance to those members of the community who by reason of personal, economic, social or other emergencies are in need of immediate aid.

d. This provision is intended to cover not only all violent, predatory, and harmful acts, but extends to the full range of prohibitions under penal statutes. It extends to conduct by persons not capable of incurring criminal liability.

From: *Clinical Forensic Medicine: A Physician's Guide, 2nd Edition*
Edited by: M. M. Stark © Humana Press Inc., Totowa, NJ

Article 2

In the performance of their duty, law enforcement officials shall respect and protect human dignity and maintain and uphold the human rights of all persons.

Commentary:

a. The human rights in question are identified and protected by national and international law.

Among the relevant international instruments are the Universal Declaration of Human Rights; the International Covenant on Civil and Political Rights; the Declaration on the Protection of All Persons from Being Subjected to Torture and Other Cruel, Inhuman or Degrading Treatment or Punishment; the United Nations Declaration on the Elimination of All Forms of Racial Discrimination; the International Convention on the Elimination of All Forms of Racial Discrimination; the International Convention on the Suppression and Punishment of the Crime of Apartheid; the Convention on the Prevention and Punishment of the Crime of Genocide; and the Standard Minimum Rules for the Treatment of Prisoners and the Vienna Convention on Consular Relations.

b. National commentaries to this provision should indicate regional or national provisions identifying and protecting these rights.

Article 3

Law enforcement officials may use force only when strictly necessary and to the extent required for the performance of their duty.

Commentary:

a. This provision emphasizes that the use of force by law enforcement officials should be exceptional; although it implies that law enforcement officials may be authorized to use force as is reasonably necessary under the circumstances for the prevention of crime or in effecting or assisting in the lawful arrest of offenders or suspected offenders, no force going beyond that may be used.

b. National law ordinarily restricts the use of force by law enforcement officials in accordance with a principle of proportionality. It is to be understood that such national principles of proportionality are to be respected in the interpretation of this provision. In no case should this provision be interpreted to authorize the use of force that is disproportionate to the legitimate objective to be achieved.

c. The use of firearms is considered an extreme measure. Every effort should be made to exclude the use of firearms, especially against children. In general, firearms should not be used except when a suspected offender offers armed resistance or otherwise jeopardizes the lives of others and less extreme measures are not sufficient to restrain or apprehend the suspected offender. In every instance in which a firearm is discharged, a report should be made promptly to the competent authorities.

Article 4

Matters of a confidential nature in the possession of law enforcement officials shall be kept confidential, unless the performance of duty or the needs of justice strictly require otherwise.

Commentary:

By the nature of their duties, law enforcement officials obtain information that may relate to private lives or be potentially harmful to the interests, especially the reputation of others. Great care should be exercised in safe-guarding and using such information, which should be disclosed only in the performance of duty or to serve the needs of justice. Any disclosure of such information for other purposes is wholly improper.

Article 5

No law enforcement official may inflict, instigate, or tolerate any act of torture or other cruel, inhuman, or degrading treatment or punishment, nor may any law enforcement official invoke superior orders or exceptional circumstances, such as a state of war or a threat of war, a threat to national security, internal political instability, or any other public emergency as a justification of torture or other cruel, inhuman, or degrading treatment or punishment.

Commentary:

a. This prohibition derives from the Declaration on the Protection of All Persons from Being Subjected to Torture and Other Cruel, Inhuman or Degrading Treatment or Punishment, adopted by the General Assembly, according to which: "[Such an act is] an offense to human dignity and shall be condemned as a denial of the purposes of the Charter of the United Nations and as a violation of the human rights and fundamental freedoms proclaimed in the Universal Declaration of Human Rights [and other international human rights instruments]."

b. The Declaration defines torture as follows: torture means any act by which se-vere pain or suffering, whether physical or mental, is intentionally inflicted by or at the instigation of a public official on a person for such purposes as obtaining from him or a third person information or confession, punishing him for an act he has committed or is suspected of having committed, or intimidating him or other persons. It does not include pain or suffering arising only from, inherent in or incidental to, lawful sanctions to the extent consistent with the Standard Mini-mum Rules for the Treatment of Prisoners."

c. The term "cruel, inhuman, or degrading treatment or punishment" has not been defined by the General Assembly but should be interpreted to extend the widest possible protection against abuses, whether physical or mental.

Article 6

Law enforcement officials shall ensure the full protection of the health of persons in their custody and, in particular, shall take immediate action to secure medical attention whenever required.

Commentary:

a. "Medical attention," which refers to services rendered by any medical personnel, including certified medical practitioners and paramedics, shall be secured when needed or requested.
b. Although the medical personnel are likely to be attached to the law enforcement operation, law enforcement officials must take into account the judgment of such personnel when they recommend providing the person in custody with appropriate treatment through, or in consultation with, medical personnel from outside the law enforcement operation.
c. It is understood that law enforcement officials shall also secure medical attention for victims of violations of law or of accidents occurring in the course of violations of law.

Article 7

Law enforcement officials shall not commit any act of corruption. They shall also rigorously oppose and combat all such acts.

Commentary:

a. Any act of corruption, in the same way as any other abuse of authority, is incompatible with the profession of law enforcement officials. The law must be enforced fully with respect to any law enforcement official who commits an act of corruption, because governments cannot expect to enforce the law among their citizens if they cannot, or will not, enforce the law against their own agents and within their agencies.
b. Although the definition of corruption must be subject to national law, it should be understood to encompass the commission or omission of an act in the performance of or in connection with one's duties; in response to gifts, promises, or incentives demanded or accepted; or the wrongful receipt of these once the act has been committed or omitted.
c. The expression "act of corruption" referred to should be understood to encompass attempted corruption.

Article 8

Law enforcement officials shall respect the law and the present Code. They shall also, to the best of their capability, prevent and rigorously oppose any violations of them. Law enforcement officials who have reason to believe that a violation of the present Code has occurred or is about to occur shall report the matter to their superior authorities and, where necessary, to other appropriate authorities or organs vested with reviewing or remedial power.

Commentary:

a. This Code shall be observed whenever it has been incorporated into national legislation or practice. If legislation or practice contains stricter provisions than those of the present Code, those stricter provisions shall be observed.

b. The article seeks to preserve the balance between the need for internal discipline of the agency on which public safety is largely dependent, on the one hand, and the need for dealing with violations of basic human rights, on the other. Law enforcement officials shall report violations within the chain of command and take other lawful action outside the chain of command only when no other remedies are available or effective. It is understood that law enforcement officials shall not suffer administrative or other penalties because they have reported that a violation of this Code has occurred or is about to occur.

c. The term "appropriate authorities or organs vested with reviewing or remedial power" refers to any authority or organ existing under national law, whether internal to the law enforcement agency or independent thereof, with statutory, customary, or other power to review grievances and complaints arising out of violations within the purview of this Code.

d. In some countries, the mass media may be regarded as performing complaint review functions similar to those described in the paragraph above. Law enforcement officials may, therefore, be justified if, as a last resort and in accordance with the laws and customs of their own countries and with the provisions of article 4 of the present Code, they bring violations to the attention of public opinion through the mass media.

e. Law enforcement officials who comply with the provisions of this Code deserve the respect, the full support, and the cooperation of the community and of the law enforcement agency in which they serve, as well as the law enforcement profession.

DOCUMENT 2

Declaration on the Police (extract from Resolution 690 of the Parliamentary Assembly of the Council of Europe, 1979).

The Assembly

1. Considering that the full exercise of human rights and fundamental freedoms, guaranteed by the European Convention on Human Rights and other national and international instruments, has as a necessary basis the existence of a peaceful society that enjoys the advantages of order and public safety;

2. Considering that, in this respect, police play a vital role in all the member states, that they are frequently called on to intervene in conditions which are dangerous for their members, and that their duties are made yet more difficult if the rules of conduct of their members are not sufficiently precisely defined;

3. Being of the opinion that it is inappropriate for those who have committed violations of human rights while members of police forces, or those who have belonged to any police force that has been disbanded on account of inhumane practices, to be employed as policemen;

4. Being of the opinion that the European system for the protection of human rights would be improved if there were generally accepted rules concerning the professional ethics of the police that take account of the principles of human rights and fundamental freedoms;

5. Considering that it is desirable that police officers have the active moral and physical support of the community they are serving;

6. Considering that police officers should enjoy status and rights comparable to those of members of the civil service;

7. Believing that it may be desirable to lay down guidelines for the behavior of police officers in case of war and other emergency situations and in the event of occupation by a foreign power;

8. Adopts the following Declaration on the Police, which forms an integral part of this resolution;

9. Instructs its Committee on Parliamentary and Public Relations and its Legal Affairs Committee and the Secretary General of the Council of Europe to give maximum publicity to the declaration.

Appendix Declaration on the Police

Ethics

1. A police officer shall fulfill the duties the law imposes upon him by protecting his fellow citizens and the community against violent, predatory, and other harmful acts, as defined by law.

2. A police officer shall act with integrity, impartiality, and dignity. In particular, he shall refrain from and vigorously oppose all acts of corruption.

3. Summary executions, torture, and other forms of inhuman or degrading treatment or punishment remain prohibited in all circumstances. A police officer is under an obligation to disobey or disregard any order or instruction involving such measures.

4. A police officer shall carry out orders properly issued by his hierarchical superior, but he shall refrain from carrying out any order he knows, or ought to know, is unlawful.

5. A police officer must oppose violations of the law. If immediate or irreparable and serious harm should result from permitting the violation to take place he shall take immediate action, to the best of his ability.

6. If no immediate or irreparable and serious harm is threatened, he must endeavor to avert the consequences of this violation, or its repetition, by reporting the matter to his superiors. If no results are obtained in that way he may report to higher authority.
7. No criminal or disciplinary action shall be taken against a police officer who has refused to carry out an unlawful order.
8. A police officer shall not cooperate in the tracing, arresting, guarding, or conveying of persons who, while not being suspected of having committed an illegal act, are searched for, detained, or prosecuted because of their race, religion or political belief.
9. A police officer shall be personally liable for his own acts and for acts of commission or omission he has ordered and that are unlawful.
10. There shall be a clear chain of command. It should always be possible to determine which superior may be ultimately responsible for acts or omissions of a police officer.
11. Legislation must provide for a system of legal guarantees and remedies against any damage resulting from police activities.
12. In performing his duties, a police officer shall use all necessary determination to achieve an aim that is legally required or allowed, but he may never use more force than is reasonable.
13. Police officers shall receive clear and precise instructions as to the manner and circumstances in which they should make use of arms.
14. A police officer having the custody of a person needing medical attention shall secure such attention by medical personnel and, if necessary, take measures for the preservation of the life and health of this person. He shall follow the instructions of doctors and other competent medical workers when they place a detainee under medical care.
15. A police officer shall keep secret all matters of a confidential nature coming to his attention, unless the performance of duty or legal provisions require otherwise.
16. A police officer who complies with the provisions of this declaration is entitled to the active moral and physical support of the community he is serving.

Document 3

Declaration of Tokyo

Guidelines for Medical Doctors concerning Torture and Other Cruel, Inhuman or Degrading Treatment or Punishment in relation to Detention and Imprisonment. (Adopted by the 29th World Medical Assembly, Tokyo, Japan, October 1975.)

Preamble

It is the privilege of the medical doctor to practice medicine in the service of humanity, to preserve and restore bodily and mental health without distinction as to persons, and to comfort and ease the suffering of his or her patients. The utmost respect for human life is to be maintained even under threat, and no use made of any medical knowledge contrary to the laws of humanity.

For the purpose of this Declaration, torture is defined as the deliberate, systematic, or wanton infliction of physical or mental suffering by one or more persons acting alone or on the orders of any authority to force another person to yield information, to make a confession, or for any other reason.

Declaration

The doctor shall not countenance, condone, or participate in the practice of torture or other forms of cruel, inhuman, or degrading procedures, whatever the offence of which the victim of such procedure is suspected, accused, or guilty, and whatever the victim's belief or motives, and in all situations, including armed conflict and civil strife.

The doctor shall not provide any premises, instruments, substances, or knowledge to facilitate the practice of torture or other forms of cruel, inhuman, or degrading treatment or to diminish the ability of the victim to resist such treatment.

The doctor shall not be present during any procedure during which torture or other forms of cruel, inhuman, or degrading treatment are used or threatened.

A doctor must have complete clinical independence in deciding on the care of a person for whom he or she is medically responsible. The doctor's fundamental role is to alleviate the distress of his or her fellow men, and no motive, whether personal, collective, or political, shall prevail against this higher purpose.

Where a prisoner refuses nourishment and is considered by the doctor as capable of forming an unimpaired and rational judgment concerning the consequences of such voluntary refusal of nourishment, he or she shall not be fed artificially. The decision regarding the capacity of the prisoner to form such a judgment should be confirmed by at least one other independent doctor. The consequences of the refusal of nourishment shall be explained by the doctor to the prisoner.

The World Medical Association will support and should encourage the international community the national medical associations and fellow doctors to support the doctor and his or her family in the face of threats or reprisals resulting from a refusal to condone the use of torture or other forms of cruel, inhuman, or degrading treatment.

DOCUMENT 4

Principles of Medical Ethics Relevant to the Role of Health Personnel, Particularly Physicians, in the Protection of Prisoners and Detainees against Torture and Other Cruel, Inhuman or Degrading Treatment or Punishment.

G.A. res. 37/194, annex, 37 U.N. GAOR Supp. (No. 51) at 211, U.N. Doc. A/37/51 (1982).

Principle 1

Health personnel, particularly physicians, charged with the medical care of prisoners and detainees have a duty to provide them with protection of their physical and mental health and treatment of disease of the same quality and standard as is afforded to those who are not imprisoned or detained.

Principle 2

It is a gross contravention of medical ethics, as well as an offense under applicable international instruments, for health personnel, particularly physicians, to engage, actively, or passively, in acts that constitute participation in, complicity in, incitement to or attempts to commit torture or other cruel, inhuman or degrading treatment or punishment.

Principle 3

It is a contravention of medical ethics for health personnel, particularly physicians, to be involved in any professional relationship with prisoners or detainees the purpose of which is not solely to evaluate, protect or improve their physical and mental health.

Principle 4

It is a contravention of medical ethics for health personnel, particularly physicians:

a. To apply their knowledge and skills in order to assist in the interrogation of prisoners and detainees in a manner that may adversely affect the physical or mental health or condition of such prisoners or detainees and which is not in accordance with the relevant international instruments;
b. To certify or to participate in the certification of the fitness of prisoners or detainees for any form of treatment or punishment that may adversely affect their physical or mental health and which is not in accordance with the relevant international instruments or to participate in any way in the infliction of any such treatment or punishment that is not in accordance with the relevant international instruments.

Principle 5

It is a contravention of medical ethics for health personnel, particularly physicians, to participate in any procedure for restraining a prisoner or detainee unless such a procedure is determined in accordance with purely medical criteria as being necessary for the protection of the physical or mental health or the safety of the prisoner or detainee himself, of his fellow prisoners or detainees, or of his guardians and presents no hazard to his physical or mental health.

Principle 6

There may be no derogation from the foregoing principles on any ground whatsoever, including public emergency.

DOCUMENT 5

The Nurse's Role in the Care of Detainees and Prisoners (International Council of Nurses, 1975).

At the meeting of the Council of National Representatives of the International Council of Nurses in Singapore in August 1975, a statement on the role of the nurse in the care of detainees and prisoners was adopted. The text, last reviewed in 1991, is as follows:

The International Council of Nurses (ICN) Code for Nurses[1] states that:

1. The fundamental responsibility of the nurse is fourfold: to promote health, to prevent illness, to restore health, and to alleviate suffering.
2. The nurse's primary responsibility is to those people who require nursing care.
3. The nurse, when acting in a professional capacity, should at all times maintain standards of personal conduct that reflect credit on the profession.
4. The nurse takes appropriate action to safeguard the individual when his or her care is endangered by a coworker or any other person.

ICN has reaffirmed its support of the Geneva Conventions of 1949[2], and the additional protocols, which state that, in case of armed conflict of international, as well as national character (i.e., internal disorders, civil wars, armed rebellions):

---

[1]International Council of Nurses, Code for Nurses, Geneva, ICN, Adopted 1973, Reaffirmed in 1989.

[2]International Committee of the Red Cross, Rights and Duties of Nurses under the Geneva Convention of August 12, 1949, Geneva, ICRC, 1970.

1. Members of the armed forces, prisoners and persons taking no active part in the hostilities
   a. shall be entitled to protection and care if wounded or sick,
   b. shall be treated humanely, that is:
      • they may not be subjected to physical mutilation or to medical or scientific experiments of any kind which are not justified by the medical, dental or hospital treatment of the prisoner concerned and carried out in his interest;
      • they shall not be willfully left without medical assistance and care, nor shall conditions exposing them to contagion or infection be created;
      • they shall be treated humanely and cared for by the party in conflict in whose power they may be, without adverse distinction founded on sex, race, nationality, religion, political opinion or any other similar criteria.
2. The following acts are and shall remain prohibited at any time and in any place whatsoever with respect to the above-mentioned persons:
   a. violence to life and person, in particular murder of all kinds, mutilation, cruel treatment, and torture;
   b. outrages on personal dignity, in particular humiliating and degrading treatment.

ICN has endorsed the United Nations Universal Declaration of Human Rights[1] and, hence, accepted that:

   a. Everyone is entitled to all the rights and freedoms, set forth in this Declaration, without distinction of any kind, such as race, color, sex, language, religion, political or other opinion, national or social origin, property, birth or other status (Article 2),
   b. No one shall be subjected to torture or to cruel, inhuman, or degrading treatment or punishment (Article 5).

In relation to detainees and prisoners of conscience, interrogation procedures are increasingly being employed resulting in ill effects, often permanent, on the person's mental and physical health. ICN condemns the use of all such procedures harmful to the mental and physical health of prisoners and detainees.

Nurses having knowledge of physical or mental ill-treatment of detainees and prisoners must take appropriate action, including reporting the matter to appropriate national and/or international bodies.

---

[1]United Nations Universal Declaration of Human Rights, United Nations, Adopted 10 December 1948.

Nurses employed in prison health services do not assume functions of prison security personnel, such as body search for prison security reasons.

Nurses participate in clinical research carried out on prisoners only if the freely given consent of the patient has been secured after a complete explanation and understanding by the patient of the nature and risk of the research.

The nurse's first responsibility is to the patients, notwithstanding considerations of national security and interest.

DOCUMENT 6

Human Rights Act 1998

This Act, which received royal assent in November 1998, will have a most profound effect on the rights of the individual in European Community member states and on the interpretation of UK statute law (*see* Appendix 1 for relevant Articles). It will come into effect at some future date (unknown at the time of writing), and the Act will give effect to rights and freedoms guaranteed under the European Convention on Human Rights. U.K. primary and subordinate legislation "so far as it is possible to do so...must be read and given effect in a way which is compatible with the Convention rights." When the Act is in force, by section 19, "A Minister of the Crown in charge of a Bill in either House of Parliament must, before second reading of the Bill—(a) make a statement to the effect that in his view the provisions of the Bill are compatible with the Convention Rights" or must make clear that he or she cannot make such a statement but wishes in any event to proceed with the Bill. It will assuredly have a far-reaching and wide-ranging impact on UK law and practice.

Document 7

Relevant Articles of the European Convention on Human Rights.

Article 2

1. Everyone's right to life shall be protected by law. No one shall be deprived of his life intentionally save in the execution of a sentence of a court following his conviction of a crime for which this penalty is provided by law.
2. Deprivation of life shall not be regarded as inflicted in contravention of this article when it results from the use of force that is no more than absolutely necessary:
   a. in defense of any person from unlawful violence;
   b. in order to effect a lawful arrest or to prevent the escape of a person lawfully detained;
   c. in action lawfully taken for the purpose of quelling a riot or insurrection.

Article 3

No one shall be subjected to torture or to inhuman or degrading treatment or punishment.

Article 5

1. Everyone has the right to liberty and security of person. No one shall be deprived of his liberty save in the following cases and in accordance with a procedure prescribed by law:
    a. the lawful detention of a person after conviction by a competent court;
    b. the lawful arrest or detention of a person for noncompliance with the lawful order of a court or in order to secure the fulfillment of any obligation prescribed by law;
    c. the lawful arrest or detention of a person effected for the purpose of bringing him before the competent legal authority on reasonable suspicion of having committed an offence or when it is reasonably considered necessary to prevent his committing an offence or fleeing after having done so;
    d. the detention of a minor by lawful order for the purpose of educational supervision or his lawful detention for the purpose of bringing him before the competent legal authority;
    e. the lawful detention of persons for the prevention of the spreading of infectious diseases, of persons of unsound mind, alcoholics or drug addicts, or vagrants;
    f. the lawful arrest or detention of a person to prevent his effecting an unauthorized entry into the country or of a person against whom action is being taken with a view to deportation or extradition.
2. Everyone who is arrested shall be informed promptly, in a language that he understands, of the reasons for his arrest and of any charge against him.
3. Everyone arrested or detained in accordance with the provisions of paragraph 1(c) of this article shall be brought promptly before a judge or other officer authorized by law to exercise judicial power and shall be entitled to trial within a reasonable time or to release pending trial. Release may be conditioned by guarantees to appear for trial.
4. Everyone who is deprived of his liberty by arrest or detention shall be entitled to take proceedings by which the lawfulness of his detention shall be decided speedily by a court and his release ordered if the detention is not lawful.
5. Everyone who has been the victim of arrest or detention in contravention of the provisions of this article shall have an enforceable right to compensation.

Article 6

1. In the determination of his civil rights and obligations or of any criminal charge against him, everyone is entitled to a fair and public hearing within a reasonable time by an independent and impartial tribunal established by law. Judgment shall

be pronounced publicly but the press and public may be excluded from all or part of the trial in the interests of morals, public order or national security in a democratic society, where the interests of juveniles or the protection of the private life of the parties so require, or to the extent strictly necessary in the opinion of the court in special circumstances where publicity would prejudice the interests of justice.

2. Everyone charged with a criminal offence shall be presumed innocent until proved guilty according to law.
3. Everyone charged with a criminal offence has the following minimum rights:
   a. to be informed promptly, in a language which he understands and in detail, of the nature and cause of the accusation against him;
   b. to have adequate time and facilities for the preparation of his defense;
   c. to defend himself in person or through legal assistance of his own choosing or, if he has not sufficient means to pay for legal assistance, to be given it free when the interests of justice so require;
   d. to examine or have examined witnesses against him and to obtain the attendance and examination of witnesses on his behalf under the same conditions as witnesses against him;
   e. to have the free assistance of an interpreter if he cannot understand or speak the language used in court.

Article 7

1. No one shall be held guilty of any criminal offence on account of any act or omission that did not constitute a criminal offence under national or international law at the time when it was committed. Nor shall a heavier penalty be imposed than the one that was applicable at the time the criminal offence was committed.
2. This article shall not prejudice the trial and punishment of any person for any act or omission which, at the time when it was committed, was criminal according to the general principles of law recognized by civilized nations.

Article 8

1. Everyone has the right to respect for his private and family life, his home and his correspondence.
2. There shall be no interference by a public authority with the exercise of this right except such as in accordance with the law and is necessary in a democratic society in the interests of national security, public safety or the economic well-being of the country, for the prevention of health or morals, or for the protection of the right and freedoms of others.

Appendix 2

Guidance Notes on UK Statutory Provisions Governing Access to Health Records

DATA PROTECTION ACT 1998

The 1998 Act replaced the 1984 Act, making some important changes including extending the provisions of the Act to "relevant filing systems," whether manual (paper-based) or computerized. It also replaced the Access to Health Records Act 1990, with the exception of those sections of the latter Act dealing with requests for access to information about deceased patients, and enacted new provisions about access to health records, both computerized and paper-based, in respect of living persons.

The 1998 Act introduced sweeping changes to the UK law governing all aspects of processing information about identifiable individuals. Much of the Act is already in force but some provisions are not yet operative. The Act applies to all personal and sensitive data held within 'a relevant filing system,' whether or not the system is computerized. It regulates the processing, use, and storage of information relating to individuals including the obtaining, holding, use, or disclosure of such information, which is "being processed by means of equipment operating automatically in response to instructions given for that purpose" (that is, data held on computers). It gives individuals rights of access to personal data and to know how they are stored and processed. All those who control data (that is, determine the purposes for which data are stored and the manner in which data are processed) must comply with the provisions of the Act. Comparable provisions extend throughout the European Union, giving effect to the Data Protection Principles[1].

---

[1]Schedule 1, Part 1 of the Data Protection Act 1998.

From: *Clinical Forensic Medicine: A Physician's Guide, 2nd Edition*
Edited by: M. M. Stark © Humana Press Inc., Totowa, NJ

The individual whose data is stored has rights of access to check what is held and to require correction of inaccurate information. Those who suffer financial loss as a consequence of inaccurate information can seek compensation. Those who operate the data systems (and this may include doctors who use computers to record information about patients) must ensure that they comply with the provisions of the legislation, including the rights of data subjects to have access to personal data.

There are exceptions for the processing of sensitive personal data (as defined in section 2 of the Act) for medical purposes by a health professional (as defined in section 69). Medical purposes include the provision of preventative medicine, medical diagnosis, medical research, the provision of care and treatment, and the management of health care services. Readers are referred to texts on the provisions of the Act for a more detailed exposition of its provisions and ramifications.

ACCESS TO MEDICAL REPORTS ACT 1988

This Act gives individuals a right of access to any medical report prepared for insurance or employment purposes by a doctor "who is or has been responsible for the patient's care" provided that allowing the individual to see the report will not endanger his or her health or disclose information about another person who is not a health professional. If access is denied on this ground the individual has a right of challenge in the county court (England and Wales) or Sheriff's court (Scotland).

Individuals who exercise their right of access but dispute the content of the report may request amendments. If these are not agreed to by the doctor, the individual may either refuse to allow the report to be dispatched or may request that it be accompanied by a statement prepared by the individual.

The statute applies only to reports prepared by a doctor who is or has been responsible for the care of the patient and not to an independent occupational physician who has not provided care. Where the doctor occupies a dual role (e.g., as both general practitioner and as part-time occupational physician or insurance medical examiner), the provisions of the Act do apply.

Appendix 3

Management of Head Injured Detainees

Table 1
Glasgow Coma Scale

	Score
Eye opening	
• Spontaneous	4
• To speech	3
• To painful stimulus	2
• None	1
Best motor response	
• Obeys commands	6
• Localises painful stimulus	5
• Withdraws (normal flexion)	4
• Flexes abnormally (spastic flexion)	3
• Extension	2
• No response	1
Best verbal response	
• Orientated	5
• Confused	4
• Says inappropriate words	3
• Makes incomprehensible sounds	2
• No verbal response	1
Maximum	15

From Jennett, B., Teasdale, G. Aspects of coma after severe head injury. Lancet. 1:878–881,

From: *Clinical Forensic Medicine: A Physician's Guide, 2nd Edition*
Edited by: M. M. Stark © Humana Press Inc., Totowa, NJ

1997.

Table 2
Detained Person: Observation List

If any detainee fails to meet any of the following criteria, an appropriate health care professional or ambulance must be called.

When assessing the level of rousability consider:

Rousability—can they be woken?

- Go into the cell
- Call their name
- Shake gently

Response to questions—can they give appropriate answers to questions such as:

- What's your name?
- Where do you live?
- Where do you think you are?

Response to commands—can they respond appropriately to commands such as:

- Open your eyes!
- Lift one arm, now the other arm!

Remember—take into account the possibility or presence of other illnesses, injury, or mental condition. A person who is drowsy and smells of alcohol may also have the following:

- Diabetes
- Epilepsy
- Head injury
- Drug intoxication or overdose
- Stroke

From Home Office. Annex H. Police and Criminal Evidence Act 1984 (s.60[1][a] and s.66[1]). Codes of Practice A–E revised edition. Effective 1 April 2003. Her Majesty's Stationery Office, Norwich, UK, 2003.

Appendix 4

The Mini-Mental State Examination

	Score
Orientation	
What is the (year) (season) (date) (day) (month)?	.... /5
Where are we: (country) (state) (county) (town) (police station)?	.... /5
Registration	
Examiner names three objects (e.g., orange, key, ball). Patient asked to repeat the three names. Score one for each correct answer. Then ask the patient to repeat all three names three times.	.... /3
Attention	
Serial 7's. Stop after 5 correct answers. Alternatively, if patient makes errors on serial subtraction: spell 'world' backwards: D L R O W. Score best performance on either task.	.... /5
Recall	
Ask for the names of the objects learned earlier.	.... /3
Language	
Show and ask the patient to name a pencil and a watch.	.... /2
Repeat the phrase 'No ifs, and, or buts.'	.... /1
Give a three-stage command. Score one for each stage (e.g., 'Take this piece of paper in your right hand, fold it in half, and place it on the chair next to you).	.... /3

From: *Clinical Forensic Medicine: A Physician's Guide, 2nd Edition*
Edited by: M. M. Stark © Humana Press Inc., Totowa, NJ

Ask patient to read and obey a written command on a piece
    of paper stating: "Close your eyes."   .... /1
Ask the patient to write a sentence. Score correct if it has a
    subject and a verb.   .... /1

Copying
    Ask the patient to copy intersecting pentagons. Score as correct
        if they overlap and if each has five sides.   .... /1

Total Score   .... /30

From: Folstein, M. F., Folstein, S. E., McHugh, P. R. "Mini-Mental State." A practical method for grading the cognitive state of patients for the clinician. J. Psychiat. Res. 12:189–198, 1975.

Appendix 5

Alcohol Assessment Questionnaires

The Brief MAST

	Score	
Questions	Yes	No
1. Do you feel you are a normal drinker?	0	2
2. Do friends or relatives think you're a normal drinker?	0	2
3. Have you ever attended a meeting of Alcoholics Anonymous?	5	0
4. Have you ever lost boyfriends/girlfriends because of drinking?	2	0
5. Have you ever got into trouble at work because of drinking?	2	0
6. Have you ever neglected your obligations, your family or your work for more than 2 days in a row because you were drinking?	2	0
7. Have you ever had DTs, sever shaking, heard voices or seen things that weren't there after heavy drinking?	2	0
8. Have you ever gone to anyone for help about your drinking?	5	0
9. Have you ever been in a hospital because of drinking?	5	0
10. Have you ever been arrested for drunk driving or driving after drinking?	2	0
Total	___	___

The brief MAST is useful as a quick screening instrument to distinguish between alcohol dependent (a score of 6 or above) and non-alcohol dependent individuals.

From Pokorny, A., D., Miller, B. A., Kaplan, H. B. The Brief MAST: a shorten version of the Michigan Alcoholism Screening Test. Am. J. Psychiat. 131:1121–1123, 1971.

From: *Clinical Forensic Medicine: A Physician's Guide, 2nd Edition*
Edited by: M. M. Stark © Humana Press Inc., Totowa, NJ

The CAGE Questionnaire

	Score	
Questions	Yes	No
1. Have you ever felt you should **C**ut down on your drinking?	___	___
2. Have people **A**nnoyed you by criticizing your drinking?	___	___
3. Have you ever felt bad or **G**uilty about your drinking?	___	___
4. Have you ever had a drink first thing in the morning to steady your nerves, or to get rid of a hang over (**E**ye-opener)?	___	___

Two or more positive responses sensitive indicator of alcohol dependence.

From Mayfield, D., McLeod, G. and Hall, P. The CAGE Questionnaire: Validation of a New Alcoholism Screening Instrument. Am. J. Psychiatry. 131:1121–1123, 1974.

The AUDIT Questionnaire

Circle the number that comes closest to the patient's answer.

1. How often do you have a drink containing alcohol?
    (0) NEVER (1) MONTHLY OR (2) TWO TO FOUR (3) TWO TO THREE 4) FOUR OR MORE
    LESS TIMES A MONTH TIMES A WEEK TIMES A WEEK

2. How many drinks containing alcohol do you have on a typical day when you are drinking?
    (CODE NUMBER OF STANDARD DRINKS)
    (0) 1 OR 2 (1) 3 OR 4 (2) 5 OR 6 (3) 7 OR 8 (4) 10 OR MORE

3. How often do you have six or more drinks on one occasion?
    (0) NEVER (1) LESS THAN (2) MONTHLY (3) WEEKLY (4) DAILY OR
    MONTHLY ALMOST DAILY

4. How often during the last year have you found that you were not able to stop drinking once you had started?
    (0) NEVER (1) LESS THAN (2) MONTHLY (3) WEEKLY (4) DAILY OR
    MONTHLY ALMOST DAILY

5. How often during the last year have you failed to do what was normally expected from you because of drinking?
    (0) NEVER (1) LESS THAN (2) MONTHLY (3) WEEKLY (4) DAILY OR
    MONTHLY ALMOST DAILY

6. How often during the last year have you needed a first drink in the morning to get yourself going after a heavy drinking session?
    (0) NEVER (1) LESS THAN (2) MONTHLY (3) WEEKLY (4) DAILY OR
    MONTHLY ALMOST DAILY

7. How often during the last year have you had a feeling of guilt or remorse after drinking?
    (0) NEVER (1) LESS THAN (2) MONTHLY (3) WEEKLY (4) DAILY OR
    MONTHLY ALMOST DAILY

8. How often during the last year have you been unable to remember what happened the night before because you had been drinking?
    (0) NEVER (1) LESS THAN (2) MONTHLY (3) WEEKLY (4) DAILY OR
    MONTHLY ALMOST DAILY

9. Have you or someone else been injured as a result of your drinking?
    (0) NO (2) YES, BUT NOT IN THE LAST YEAR(4) YES, DURING THE LAST YEAR

10. Has a relative or friend or a doctor or other health worker, been concerned about your drinking or suggested you cut down?
    (0) NO (2) YES, BUT NOT IN THE LAST YEAR(4) YES, DURING THE LAST YEAR

*   In determining the response categories it has been assumed that one "drink" contains 10g alcohol. In countries where the alcohol content of a standard drink differs by more than 25% from 10g, the response category should be modified accordingly.

Record sum of individual item scores here _____

A score of 8 produces the highest sensitivity; a score of ten or more results in higher specificity. In general high scores on the first three items in the absence of elevated scores on the remaining items suggest hazardous alcohol use. Elevated scores on items 4 through 6 imply the emergence of alcohol dependence. High scores on the remaining items suggest harmful alcohol use.

For details see: Babor, T. F., Ramon de la Fuente, J., Saunders, J., Grant, M. (1992) *AUDIT The Alcohol Use Disorders Identification Test: Guidelines for use in Primary Health Care*. World Health Organisation.

Appendix 6

Drink/Drugs Driving Impairment Assessment Form

From: *Clinical Forensic Medicine: A Physician's Guide, 2nd Edition*
Edited by: M. M. Stark © Humana Press Inc., Totowa, NJ

ASSOCIATION OF FORENSIC PHYSICIANS
SECTION 4 RTA ASSESSMENT FORM (Version 6.1 1/04)

1 | INTRODUCTION AND GENERAL GUIDANCE

> **Note**:   This form has been designed by Dr Ian F Wall on behalf of the Education and
> Research Committee of the Association of Police Surgeons for use by Police Surgeons (also
> known as Forensic Medical Examiners or Forensic Physicians) who have been trained in the
> use of Standardised Impairment Tests. The form is provided to assist Police Surgeons in
> determining whether a person has a condition, which may be due to drink or drugs and not
> necessarily due to impairment . It is to be regarded as an aide-memoire and it is therefore not
> necessary for all parts of the form to be completed. Some details are included so as to aid
> possible subsequent assessment of fitness for detention in custody. Where a test is abandoned
> the reasons should be recorded in Additional Particulars at 12. If the questions are read from a
> card, the wording should be identical to those used in this form and the card must remain
> available for production at court. On completion this form is the personal property of the
> examining doctor.
>   Whilst this form is designed to provide for the recording of findings following the
> examination of a subject to determine both the persons general medical condition and the
> degree of any impairment present, it is important to stress that the primary question police
> require to be answered is Has the person a condition which might be due to some drug?   It
> is not necessary to determine impairment or unfitness to drive.

2 | GENERAL DETAILS

Name:	Police station:
Address:	Custody record No:
	Date of birth:
	Occupation:
Arrest date:	Arrest time:
PNC warnings:	
Time Called:	Time Arrived:
Time examination started:	Time examination completed:

3 | BACKGROUND INFORMATION

Road side breath test:	Intoximeter readings:

Information from arresting officer (PC......................)............................

....

....

Field impairment test results...

....

....

Information from Custody Officer

(PS...................).....................

....

Dr's name........................Date................   * Delete as Applicable   Page 1

ASSOCIATION OF FORENSIC PHYSICIANS
SECTION 4 RTA ASSESSMENT FORM (Version 6.1 1/04)

....

4   <u>**CONSENT**</u>

Consent witnessed by:

"My name is Dr. .... and I have been asked to examine you to ascertain whether in my opinion, you have a condition which might be due to drink or drugs. You should be aware that any conversation with me might not be treated confidentially"

"Do you agree to a medical examination?" ***YES/NO**

If **NO** make observations of accused's behaviour:...............................
....
....
....

If **YES**, consider written consent:

I consent to a medical examination as explained to me above:

Signed...

5   <u>**MEDICAL CONSULTATION**</u>

Consultation commenced at: hours

History of recent events:...
....
....

Current medical problems..
....
....

Past medical history:...
....
....
....

Dr's name......................Date................   * Delete as Applicable   Page 2

ASSOCIATION OF FORENSIC PHYSICIANS
SECTION 4 RTA ASSESSMENT FORM (Version 6.1 1/04)

HEARING PROBLEMS		**BALANCE PROBLEMS**	
VISUAL PROBLEMS		**ASTHMA**	
DIABETES RENAL IMPAIRMENT		**EPILEPSY HEPATIC IMPAIRMENT**	

Alcohol intake and times in last 24 hours:…...………………….………

…………………………………………………………………………………

WEEKLY ALCOHOL INTAKE [   ] Units per week

TIME LAST ATE [   ]   **TIME LAST SLEPT** [   ]

Past psychiatric history:…...………..………………………………………

…………………………………………………………………………………

…………………………………………………………………………………

Previous self harm attempts:………………………………………..………

…………………………………………………………………………………

Social history:………………………………………………………………...

…………………………………………………………………………………

Relevant educational history (to assess if learning disability etc):……………

…………………………………………………………………………………

MEDICATION	DOSE	DURATION	ROUTE	LAST TAKEN
Prescribed				
OTC medicines				
Non-prescribed				

Dr's name………………..Date…………….   * Delete as Applicable   Page 3

ASSOCIATION OF FORENSIC PHYSICIANS
SECTION 4 RTA ASSESSMENT FORM (Version 6.1 1/04)

6	**MEDICAL EXAMINATION**

EXAMINED IN PRESENCE OF:

General demeanour:...

....

State of clothing:...

....

Mental state:..

....

....

....

Specimen of handwriting:...

....

....

Areas of body examined:...

....

SPEECH		**MOUTH**	
BREATH		**BLOOD SUGAR**	

DRUG MISUSE	**CVS**	**RS**	**GIT**
Needle marks:	Initial pulse:	PN:	Soft:
Shivering:	BP:	BS:	Tender:
Yawning:	Temp:	Added sounds:	LKKS:
Rhinorrhoea:	Heart sounds:	VR:	BS:
Gooseflesh:		PEFR:	
Lachrymation:			

Other abnormal findings:...

....

....

ASSOCIATION OF FORENSIC PHYSICIANS
SECTION 4 RTA ASSESSMENT FORM (Version 6.1 1/04)

EYE EXAMINATION

Use the gauge below or a printed laminated card to assess pupil size:

1.0 1.5 2.0 2.5   3.0   3.5   4.0   4.5 5.0 5.5   6.0   6.5   7.0   7.5   8.0   8.5   9.0

EYE SIGNS	RIGHT	LEFT
Conjunctiva		
Pupil Size		
Direct reflex		
Indirect reflex		
Visual acuity:		
Visual fields:		
Horizontal gaze nystagmus		
Lack of smooth pursuit		

Vertical gaze nystagmus: *YES/NO   Convergence: *YES/NO

Spectacles: *YES/NO   Contact lens: *YES/NO

Other abnormal eye findings:………………………………………………....

……………………………………………………………………………………...

7 | ## IMPAIRMENT TESTS

"I would like you to perform a series of tests to enable me to ascertain whether you have a condition which might be due to drink or drugs, or whether your ability to drive is impaired by drink or drugs. The tests are simple and part of my evaluation will be based on your ability to follow instructions. If you do not understand any of the instructions, please tell me so that I can clarify them."

ASSOCIATION OF FORENSIC PHYSICIANS
SECTION 4 RTA ASSESSMENT FORM (Version 6.1 1/04)

8	**ROMBERG TEST**

*"Stand up straight with your feet together and your arms down by your sides. Maintain that position while I give you the remaining instructions. Do not begin until I tell you to do so. When I tell you to start, you must tilt your head back slightly and close your eyes **(demonstrate but do not close your eyes)**. Keep your head tilted backwards with your eyes closed until you think that 30 seconds have passed, then bring your head forward and say 'Stop'".*

"Do you understand?" **YES/NO***

ABLE TO STAND STILL DURING INSTRUCTIONS: *****YES/NO**

EXCESSIVE BODY SWAY SEEN: *****YES/NO**

INTERNAL BODY CLOCK: 30SECONDS AT ....SECS

  "How long was that?"...............................

ABLE TO COMPLETE TEST: *****YES/NO**

COMMENTS:

| **Front/Back view**
(Indicate direction
& degree of sway) | | **Side view**
(Indicate direction
& degree of sway) | |

9	**WALK AND TURN TEST**

Identify a real or imaginary line.
*"Place your left foot on the line. Place your right foot on the line in front of your left touching heel to toe **(demonstrate)**. Put your arms down by your sides and keep them there throughout the entire test. Maintain that position whilst I give you the remaining instructions".*

"Do you understand?" **YES/NO***

*"When I say start, you must take nine heel to toe steps along the line. On each step the heel of the foot must be placed against the toe of the other foot **(demonstrate)**. When the ninth step has been taken, you must leave the front foot on the line and turn around using a series of small steps with the other foot. After turning you must take another nine heel to toe steps along the line. You must watch your feet at all times and count each step out loud. Once you start walking do not stop until you have completed the test".*

"Do you understand?" **YES/NO***

Dr's name.......................Date................ * Delete as Applicable Page 6

ASSOCIATION OF FORENSIC PHYSICIANS
SECTION 4 RTA ASSESSMENT FORM (Version 6.1 1/04)

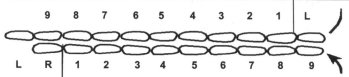

Any deviation from the instructions and any observations should be indicated below and on the diagram above

Able to stand still during instructions: *YES/NO

Start too soon: *YES/NO   Stops walking: *YES/NO

Turn: *Correct/Incorrect

Misses heel/toe: *YES/NO   Steps off line: *YES/NO

Raises arms: *YES/NO   Correct step count: *YES/NO

Notes:

10   **ONE LEG STAND TEST**

"Stand with your feet together with your arms by your sides. Maintain that position while I give you the remaining instructions. Do not begin until I tell you to start."

"Do you understand?"   *YES/NO

"When I tell you to start you must raise your right foot six to eight inches off the ground, keeping your leg straight and your toes pointing forward, with your foot parallel to the ground (demonstrate). You must keep your arms by your sides and keep looking at your elevated foot while counting out loud in the following manner, 'one thousand and one, one thousand and two' and so on until I tell you to stop."

"Do you understand?"   *YES/NO

Repeat procedure with each foot

	LEFT	RIGHT			LEFT	RIGHT
SWAYS	YES/NO	YES/NO	**HOPS**		YES/NO	YES/NO
	*	*			*	*

	LEFT	RIGHT			LEFT	RIGHT
PUTS FOOT DOWN	YES/NO	YES/NO	**RAISES ARMS**		YES/NO	YES/NO
	*	*			*	*

- If YES –
record at what point(s) in the count that it occurred i.e. one thousand and six (1006)

ASSOCIATION OF FORENSIC PHYSICIANS
SECTION 4 RTA ASSESSMENT FORM (Version 6.1 1/04)

| 11 | **FINGER AND NOSE TEST** |

"Stand with your feet together and your arms in this position. **(Demonstrate extending both hands out in front, palms side up and closed with the index finger of both hands extended).** *Maintain that position while I give you the remaining instructions. Do not begin until I tell you to start. When I tell you to start you must tilt your head back slightly* **(demonstrate)** *and close your eyes. When I tell you which hand to move, you must touch the tip of your nose with the tip of that finger and lower your hand once you have done so* **(demonstrate).**
"Do you understand?"   ***YES/NO**

Call out the hands in the following order, left, right, left, right, right, left.

EXCESSIVE BODY SWAY:	**YES/NO**
CORRECT HAND USE:	**YES/NO**
ADDITIONAL COMMENTS:	

2   1
4   3
5   6

Draw lines to spots touched

| 12 | **ADDITIONAL PARTICULARS** (see notes at 1). |

....
....
....
....
....
....
....
....
....
....
....
....

| **FINAL PULSE:** | | **CONSULTATION ENDED AT:** | **hours** |

ASSOCIATION OF FORENSIC PHYSICIANS
SECTION 4 RTA ASSESSMENT FORM (Version 6.1 1/04)

13	**CONCLUSIONS**

Is the person fit to be detained?   ***YES/NO**

If **NO** make note of reasons and subsequent action.................................
....

Is there a condition present which might be due to a drug?"   ***YES/NO**

If **YES** make note of conditions:...
....
....

**POLICE OFFICER ADVISED THAT A CONDITION
PRESENT THAT MIGHT BE DUE TO A DRUG AT:**

hours

Is there impairment present?"   ***YES/NO**

If **YES** make note of reasons:..
....
....

**If there is a condition present which might be due to a drug the police
officer will proceed as on Form MG DD/B at B18.**

14	**SUBSEQUENT PROCEDURES**

Blood or Urine decision

Are there medical reasons for the sample not to be of blood?   ***YES/NO**

If **YES** make note of reasons (Officer will then proceed to require Urine)
....

15	**CONSENT FOR BLOOD SAMPLE**

Consent witnessed by:

*"My name is Dr. .... and I have been asked to take a sample of blood
from you which will be tested for alcohol and/or drugs"*

"Do you agree to a blood test?"   ***YES/NO**

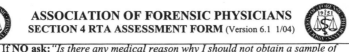

ASSOCIATION OF FORENSIC PHYSICIANS
SECTION 4 RTA ASSESSMENT FORM (Version 6.1 1/04)

If **NO** ask: *"Is there any medical reason why I should not obtain a sample of blood from you?"*

Make notes of accused's reasons:...

....

....

....

If **YES,** details as below:

Blood specimen successfully taken at...........................hours

Site............................... Venting needle used?   ***YES/NO**

Blood specimen given to .... at.................hours

If venepuncture unsuccessful, reasons:..

....

...........(Police can still proceed with a urine requirement on form MG DD/B).

It is also useful to assist the Police Officer in completion of Form MG DD/E Drugs Sample Information Form.

Appendix 7

Useful Website Addresses

Arrestee Drug Abuse Monitoring Program	http://www.adam-nij.net
Association of Forensic Physicians	http://www.afpweb.org.uk
British Medical Association	http://www.bma.org.uk/ap
British Medical Journal	http://bmj.com/
Canadian Medical Protective Association	http://www.cmpa.org/
Department for Constitutional Affairs	http://www.dca.gov.uk/
US Drug Enforcement Agency	http://www.usdoj.gov/dea/
Drugscope	http://www.drugscope.org.uk
Expert Witness Institute	http://ewi.org.uk/
General Medical Council	http://www.gmc-uk.org/
Home Office (Research Papers)	http://www.homeoffice.gov.ouk/rds/
Journal of Clinical Forensic Medicine	http://intl.elsevierhealth.com/journals/jcfm/
Medical & Dental Defence Union of Scotland	http://www.mddus.com/
Medical Defence Union	http://www.the-mdu.com/
Medical Protection Society	http://www.mps-group.org/
National Criminal Justice Reference Service	http://www.ncjrs.org/
National Institute for Clinical Excellence	http://www.nice.org.uk
OfCom	http://www.ofcom.org.uk/
Royal Society of Medicine	http://www.rsm.ac.uk
World Medical Association	http://www.wma.net

From: *Clinical Forensic Medicine: A Physician's Guide, 2nd Edition*
Edited by: M. M. Stark © Humana Press Inc., Totowa, NJ

Index

A

Abrasions,
  anal intercourse, 109
  features, 138, 139
ADAM, *see* Arrestee Drug Abuse
    Monitoring Program
Alcohol intoxication, *see also* Substance abuse,
  alcohol content in drinks, 306
  assessment questionnaires,
    AUDIT, 411
    brief MAST, 409
    CAGE, 410
  crime association, 305, 306
  deaths in custody, 337, 338
  dependence, 313, 314
  diagnostic criteria, 312, 313
  driving under the influence,
    discouragement of drunk driving,
      breath test expansion, 360
      high-risk offender scheme, 361
      ignition interlocks for repeat
        offenders, 360, 361
      legal limit lowering, 360
    performance effects, 355, 356
    Road Traffic Act legal defenses,
      blood samples, 365–369
      breath testing, 363, 366, 367
      definitions, 361, 362
      failure to provide samples, 366–369
      hospital procedure, 363, 364
      police station procedure, 364, 365
      urine samples, 369
    testing and legislation,
      blood alcohol, 357–359
      breath testing, 358
      postmortem testing, 359, 369–371
      urine testing, 358, 359

      vitreous testing, 359, 370
  effects,
    cardiovascular effects, 312
    central nervous system depression,
      309, 310
    metabolic effects, 312
    nystagmus, 310, 311
    pupillary changes, 311
    slurred speech, 311, 312
  fit for interview considerations, 222, 223
  metabolism,
    absorption, 306, 307, 355
    elimination, 306, 307, 355
    factors affecting,
      drink type, 308
      drug interactions, 308, 309
      duration of drinking, 308
      elimination rate, 309
      food in stomach, 308
      physiological factors and genetics, 308
      sex and weight, 307, 308
  poisoning and death, 312
  simulating pathological states, 313
  withdrawal,
    complications,
      cardiac arrhythmias, 316
      hallucinations, 316
      metabolic disorders, 316
      seizures, 315, 316
    delirium, 315
    uncomplicated, 314, 315
Alkyl nitrites, abuse, 305
Amphetamine,
  dependence, 300
  effects, 300
  tolerance, 300